Obesity

Robin P. Blackstone

Obesity

The Medical Practitioner's Essential Guide

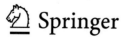

Robin P. Blackstone
Banner University Medical Center
University of Arizona School
 of Medicine – Phoenix
Phoenix, AZ
USA

ISBN 978-3-319-39407-7   ISBN 978-3-319-39409-1 (eBook)
DOI 10.1007/978-3-319-39409-1

Library of Congress Control Number: 2016942485

© Springer International Publishing Switzerland 2016

This work is subject to copyright. All rights are reserved by the Publisher, whether the whole or part of the material is concerned, specifically the rights of translation, reprinting, reuse of illustrations, recitation, broadcasting, reproduction on microfilms or in any other physical way, and transmission or information storage and retrieval, electronic adaptation, computer software, or by similar or dissimilar methodology now known or hereafter developed.

The use of general descriptive names, registered names, trademarks, service marks, etc. in this publication does not imply, even in the absence of a specific statement, that such names are exempt from the relevant protective laws and regulations and therefore free for general use.

The publisher, the authors and the editors are safe to assume that the advice and information in this book are believed to be true and accurate at the date of publication. Neither the publisher nor the authors or the editors give a warranty, express or implied, with respect to the material contained herein or for any errors or omissions that may have been made.

This Springer imprint is published by Springer Nature
The registered company is Springer International Publishing AG Switzerland

Robert N. Pavlich, my father, who should have lived longer.

Foreword

The world of obesity is still a relatively young world. While some of the treatments for the disease of obesity have been around for decades, overall, obesity is still a young disease. Dr. Robin Blackstone phenomenally discusses the current state of obesity in this book in a very insightful and thoughtful manner. Too often in today's literary world, obesity is reduced to statistics, facts, and figures. While these numbers play an integral role in the discussion of obesity, we often forget that each number represents a population that on a daily basis faces obstacles such as weight bias, limited access to care (obesity management and treatment services), oversaturation of harmful and misguided information and more. Dr. Blackstone takes an in-depth look at these issues and provides readers with a glimpse into the world of obesity that is often overlooked and ignored.

Weight bias is one of the last acceptable forms of discrimination in today's society. Individuals affected by obesity face weight bias in almost all areas of life, such as employment, education, health care, pop culture, and more. Study after study shows that weight bias can greatly impact someone's life and has damaging effects on their social, mental, and physical well-being. Yet weight bias is still very prevalent in the world of obesity. We, as a society, need to stand up to weight bias and put an end to it.

Receiving a diagnosis of obesity can often be a difficult moment for most individuals. In fact, it is usually not until an individual develops an obesity-related condition, such as type 2 diabetes, hypertension, or sleep apnea that they would have had the conversation of weight with their healthcare provider. Even more troublesome is the extreme limitations on access to care for obesity treatment. Those battling this disease are often told to "eat less and move more." And for those who may be interested in treatment such as behavioral counseling, pharmacotherapy, or bariatric surgery, they will most likely face very limited coverage of obesity services. Again, this is a clear example of how the world of obesity is so very different from any other disease state, and Dr. Blackstone clearly recognizes these differences.

The one place where the world of obesity is most certainly not lacking would be information. A simple Boolean search for "Obesity and Book" returns more than 51 million hits in a split second. Among the results you will see words like "truth," "myth," "lose," "guaranteed," and others. When it comes to searching for information on obesity, information overload is almost a certain fate for any person. In Dr. Blackstone's book, she has taken great pride in ensuring that the information she shares is evidence-based and has stood the test of time. To me, one of the things that make her book so refreshing is that she knows the world of obesity is an ever-changing landscape. In fact, she embraces this in a remarkable manner. As I stated early on, each one of the 93 million Americans affected by obesity is unique. They are not just simply another number in a statistical fact sheet, and Dr. Blackstone knows this very important point. While obesity is often reduced to a scientific level, she recognizes that every person is unique with different struggles in life.

As President and CEO of the Obesity Action Coalition (OAC), a more than 50,000 member national, nonprofit organization dedicated to helping individuals affected by obesity, I find Dr. Blackstone's take on the obesity epidemic refreshing, enlightening and most of all—human. She has been a pioneer in the field of obesity treatment and has always advocated for the most important variable in the obesity epidemic—the patient. I applaud Dr. Blackstone's efforts and know that she will continue to pave the way in caring for all individuals affected by the disease of obesity.

Joseph Nadglowski, Jr.
OAC President and CEO

Preface

As a provider of medical care, regardless of specialty or level of training, 33 % of your patients are obese and over 60 % are overweight or obese. Within 15 years, it is projected that 50 % of your patients will be clinically obese. Socially we have been taught to ignore this fact and try and reach beyond it to interact with the "real person." While that is an acceptable, even desirable, approach in a social setting, in medicine it is devastating. Obesity is the central paradigm of modern disease. It is the prelude to insulin resistance, high cholesterol, high blood pressure, type 2 diabetes, sleep apnea, and heart disease. If you fail to "see" overweight and obesity in your patients or to take it into account when treating them, you may stem the tide of these obesity-related medical problems for a while, but the patient will lose the battle.

Systematically and with sensitivity, you and your staff must acknowledge the role overweight and obesity plays in your patients' health. Helping them to achieve better health through weight loss and body fat loss will enable you to make all the other therapies you employ for related disease more effective. It will also strengthen your relationships with your patients.

This book will educate you about the current state of the science of obesity as a disease and help you establish a systematic process for recognizing and working with patients who are overweight or obese. Knowing the facts about the nature of obesity based upon scientific, peer-reviewed data may require you to suspend your personal beliefs about obesity. Set aside your preconceived notions, open your mind, and let us get down to the essential medicine every practitioner should know for helping this group of patients win this battle.

Robin P. Blackstone

Acknowledgments

With special thanks

Carrie P. Withey, J.D.
Judge Withey helped make the science approachable by providing clarity in the writing and assistance in copyediting. Her dedication to help people with obesity and their practitioners understand the material presented was matched by her superb craftsmanship in creating a professional text. It would have been impossible to complete this project without her help.

Joy C. Bunt, M.D., Ph.D.
Dr. Joy Bunt filtered the content of the rough draft of the book through the lens of her doctorate in exercise physiology and many years of work with the NIH/NIDDK section in Phoenix, Arizona working with native peoples affected by obesity.

Wendy H. Lyons, RN, BSN, MSL
Wendy worked within the healthcare system for many years, starting as a unit clerk and becoming an RN and the senior Vice President for Community Affairs for a very large hospital system. She knew first hand the affect and cost of obesity and provided insight into the writing from this perspective.

Contents

1 Epidemiology, Measurement, and Cost of Obesity 1
   Obesity in Populations 4
      Child and Adolescent Obesity 4
      Adult Obesity 5
      Obesity Rates Within Minority Groups and Subpopulations...... 7
   Measurement of Obesity 9
      Weight Related Health Indicators (WRHI)................. 9
      Surveys of Health Status in the United States 15
   Healthcare Costs: The Impact of Obesity
   and Obesity-Related Disease 16
      Social, Future, and Personal Cost of Obesity 17
   Implementing Specific Process for Chapter 1 Recommendations..... 19
   Conclusion 20
   References.. 20

**2 Prejudice, Discrimination, and the Preferred Approach
to the Patient with Obesity** 23
   The Patient's Perspective................................. 24
   Discrimination, Prejudice, and Weight Stigma 24
      Creating a Culture of Safety for the Patient with Obesity 25
   The Current Healthcare Environment Is Prejudiced
   Against People with Obesity 25
   Changing the Current Healthcare Environment from Biased
   to Blameless 26
   The Blame Game: Why Blame the Patient for Their Obesity
   When We Do not Blame Them for Their Allergies,
   High Cholesterol, Hypertension, or Cancer?................... 27
   Inability or Unwillingness to Overcome Bias Against Obesity
   and Its Effects 28
   How Obesity Bias Negatively Affects Medical Care
   and Outcomes 29

The Importance of Communicating the Measurement and Identification of Obesity of All Patients Within a Healthcare System.	30
How to Talk with Your Patient About Obesity—The Preferred Approach	32
The Expression of Empathy.	33
The Development of Discrepancy.	34
Implementing Specific Process for Chapter Two Recommendations	35
For Staff and Colleagues.	35
For Patients.	36
Physical Environment of the Workplace	37
Conclusion	37
References.	38

3 The Biology of Weight Regulation and Genetic Resetting™ 41

The Canary in the Coal Mine	41
The Pima Story	42
Research Results: The NIH/NIDDK and the PIMA.	43
Fetal Programming.	45
Application of Research Results to Other Populations.	45
Calories in Do Not Equal Calories Out.	46
The Brain: The Control Center.	47
Neuroanatomy.	48
Genetic Resetting™: Setting the Stage for Obesity.	49
The Double Helix—The Human Genome	50
Epigenetics and Epigenetic Modification (Genetic Resetting™)	51
Imprinting.	51
Intergenerational Metabolic Programming	51
Interactome Networks in Human Disease: Obesity	54
The Gut Brain Axis (GBA): Signals from the Gut to the Brain	55
The Microbiome and Microbiota	55
Why Eat?	57
Hormone Signals to the Brain	57
Taste—Not All in Your Mouth	58
Ghrelin: The "I'm Hungry" Hormone.	58
Glucagon-Like Peptide-1 (GLP-1)	59
Insulin	59
Cognitive Function and Glucose-Related Signaling.	60
Signaling Through the Nervous System.	60
The Sympathetic Nervous System (SNS).	62
Parasympathetic Nervous System: The Vagus Nerve.	63
The Second Brain: The Enteric Nervous System (ENS).	63
Conclusion	63
References.	63

Contents

4 The Biology of Adipose Tissue 67
    Adipose Tissue: Energy Storage and Endocrine Signaling 68
    The Development of Adipose Tissue 68
    The Structure of Adipose Tissue 69
        The Adipocyte.. 69
        Brown Adipose Tissue (BAT) 69
        White Adipose Tissue (WAT) 69
        Macrophages... 71
        Extracellular Matrix (ECM)............................ 71
        Adipose Tissue Blood Flow and Innervation 71
    Lipogenesis and Lipolysis: How Fat Is Stored
    and How It Is Used For Energy............................ 72
    The Tipping Point: Inflammation and Adipose Tissue Dysfunction... 73
    Hypoxia and Inflammation in White Adipose Tissue.............. 74
    Adipokines: Leptin and Adiponectin........................ 76
        Leptin... 76
        Leptin Resistance..................................... 78
        Adiponectin.. 78
    Conclusion 79
    References... 80

5 Obesity-Related Diseases and Syndromes: Insulin Resistance, Type 2 Diabetes Mellitus, Non-alcoholic Fatty Liver Disease, Cardiovascular Disease, and Metabolic Syndrome 83
    Insulin Resistance....................................... 84
        How to Assess a Patient for Insulin Resistance 86
        Mechanisms of Insulin Resistance 87
        Inflammation and Insulin Resistance...................... 90
    Impaired Fasting Glucose (IFG), Impaired Glucose Tolerance (IGT),
    and Prediabetes 90
    Type 2 Diabetes Mellitus (T2DM) 92
    Metabolic Syndrome.................................... 93
    Non-Alcoholic Fatty Liver Disease (NAFLD), Steatohepatitis (NASH)
    and Cirrhosis... 95
        The Role of Microbiota, Intestinal Dysbiosis,
        and Metabolic Endotoxemia in NAFLD 95
    Obesity-Related Cardiovascular Disease 97
        The Obesity Paradox 97
        Dyslipidemia... 98
        Hypertension... 99
        Atherosclerosis, Coronary Heart Disease (CHD),
        and Heart Failure...................................... 101

	Atrial Fibrillation and Stroke	101
	Heart Failure	102
	Conclusion	103
	References	103
6	**Obesity-Related Diseases and Syndromes: Cancer, Endocrine Disease, Pulmonary Disease, Pseudotumor Cerebri, and Disordered Sleep**	109
	Obesity and Cancer	110
	Mechanisms of Cancer Growth and Promotion in Patients with Obesity	111
	Obesity and Breast Cancer	114
	The Challenge of Diagnosing and Treating Cancer in the Patient with Obesity	116
	Obesity and Endocrine Disease	116
	Obesity and Thyroid Hormones	116
	Obesity and Polycystic Ovarian Syndrome	117
	Obesity and Infertility	118
	Obesity and Pulmonary Disease	119
	Abnormalities of Pulmonary Function	119
	Asthma	119
	Obesity Hyperventilation Syndrome	119
	Venous Thromboembolic Disease	120
	Obesity and Pseudotumor Cerebrii	121
	Disordered Sleep	121
	Circadian Rhythm	122
	Sleep	123
	Owl or Lark?	123
	Insomnia and Stress	125
	Obstructive Sleep Apnea	126
	Conclusion	127
	References	127
7	**Pediatric Obesity**	133
	Scope of the Epidemic	134
	Genetic Influence on Childhood Obesity	135
	Types of Childhood Obesity	137
	Common Obesity	138
	Syndromic Obesity	138
	Non-syndromic Obesity	139
	Clinical Consequences of Childhood Obesity	139
	Disordered Sleep	141

Contents   xvii

      Respiratory Problems in Children with Obesity 142
      Gastrointestinal Problems in Children with Obesity 142
      Endocrine Disorders in Children with Obesity 143
   Clinical Assessment of Children with Overweight/Obesity......... 148
   Biobehavioral Susceptibility Model of Child Obesity 152
   Treatment Recommendations for Children with Obesity 153
      Stage 1: Prevention Plus................................. 154
      Stage 2: Structured Weight Management................... 156
      Stage 3: Comprehensive Multidisciplinary Program 156
      Stage 4: Tertiary Care................................... 157
   Conclusion 162
   References... 162

8 Fundamentals of Diet, Exercise, and Behavior Modification 167
   Food and Digestion 168
      Digestion 168
      Recommended Mechanics of Eating....................... 169
      Calories and Kilocalories................................. 170
      Macronutrients.. 170
   Reading a Food Label... 179
   Energy Expenditure 180
      Energy Expenditure: Basal Metabolic Rate (BMR)............ 180
      Energy Expenditure: Thermal Effect of Food (TEF) 180
      Energy Expenditure: Thermogenesis
      (Exercise and Physical Activity)........................... 181
   Mental Health in the Bariatric Population 183
      Specific Psychiatric Disorders Related to Obesity:
      Depression and Anxiety 184
      Food Addiction: Science or Silly? 185
   Conclusion 190
   References... 190

**9 The Assessment of the Adult Patient with Overweight
   and Obesity** 193
   The Health History... 195
      Historical Survey of Weight Gain and Loss.................. 196
      Family History of Obesity and Related Disease 196
      Medications... 196
      Dietary History 199
      Stress Factors 199
      Circadian Patterns 202
      Disordered Sleep Analysis................................ 202
      Lifestyle, Cultural, and Occupational Factors................ 203
      Physical Activity 204
      Obesity-Related Disease 205

	Psychosocial and Psychiatric History	216
	Surgical History	216
	Allergies	216
	Review of Systems	218
	Physical Assessment of Patients with Obesity and Related Diseases	219
	Anthropometrics	219
	Pattern of Body Fat Distribution	219
	Vital Signs	220
	General Observation	220
	Head, Eyes, Ears, Nose and Throat	220
	Chest and Breast Exam	221
	Abdomen	221
	Extremities	222
	Neurologic	223
	Pelvic and Anorectal Exam	223
	Skin, Trunk, and Extremities	223
	Determination of Metabolic Factors	224
	Resting Metabolic Rate	224
	Body Composition Analysis	224
	Diagnostic Tests for Obesity-Related Disease	225
	Conclusion: The Summary Assessment Based on History, Physical Exam and Diagnostic Testing	227
	References	228
10	**Beyond Traditional Management: The Use of Medications in the Treatment of Obesity**	**231**
	The Use of Medications for the Treatment of *Other* Medical Problems in Patients with Obesity	232
	Medications that Cause Weight Gain	236
	Medications for Use as Weight Loss Medications	239
	Historical Perspective of Weight Loss Medications	239
	Indications for the Use of Prescription Medications in a Patient with Obesity	241
	Medications Currently Approved for the Treatment of Obesity	244
	Phentermine	245
	Lorcaserin (Belviq)	246
	Liraglutide (Saxenda)	249
	Orlistat (Xenical, Alli)	252
	Phentermine/Topiramate (Qnexa, Qsymia)	252
	Naltrexone SR/Bupropion SR (NB) (CONTRAVE)	254
	Nutraceuticals	257
	Medications as Related to Bariatric Surgery	257
	Conclusion	258
	References	258

11 Bariatric Surgery 261
National Accreditation in Metabolic and Bariatric Surgery......... 263
Indications/Contraindications for Surgery..................... 264
Mechanism of Action of MBS............................. 266
    Epigenetic Changes 267
    Enteroplasticity 267
    Changes in Reward Pathways 269
    Changes in Energy Expenditure 270
Metabolic and Bariatric Surgery: Procedures and Devices 271
    Laparoscopic Roux-en Y Gastric Bypass (LRYGB) 272
    Laparoscopic Sleeve Gastrectomy (LSG)................. 277
    Laparoscopic Adjustable Gastric Band (LAGB) 279
    Duodenal Switch/Biliopancreatic Diversion (DS/BPD) 282
    Gastric Balloon (GB) and the Vagal Blocking
    Device (VBLOC)................................. 284
Variability in Response to Metabolic and Bariatric Surgery:
Weight Regain...................................... 286
Cholecystectomy After Metabolic and Bariatric Surgery 287
Prehabilitation: Preoperative Assessment and Preparation 288
    Education and Informed Consent 289
    Physical Assessment for Surgery 290
    Social and Psychological Health Assessment Prior to Surgery 292
Enhanced Recovery After Metabolic and Bariatric Surgery 294
    Preoperative Prehabilitation 295
    Perioperative 295
    Postoperative.................................... 295
Health Maintenance After Metabolic and Bariatric Surgery 296
Conclusion 297
References... 297

12 Population Health Management of Obesity 307
Barriers... 309
    Accurate Measurement of Obesity Is Essential............... 309
    Politicizing Obesity Prevents Action..................... 309
    Prevention Versus Recognition and Treatment
    of Existing Disease................................ 310
The Epidemic of Obesity Is a Social Disease................... 311
A New Paradigm: Management of Obesity, not Acceptance
of Obesity... 311
Recognition.. 313
    Measure Every Patient, Every Time 313
    Communicate Level of Risk to Each Patient 314
Education 315

Engagement. 317
    Keys to Personal Engagement 317
Risk Groups in the New Paradigm 318
Measuring Value 320
Population Health and Public Policy 322
Conclusion 324
References 324

Index 327

Chapter 1
Epidemiology, Measurement, and Cost of Obesity

Key Message

Obesity currently affects 78.6 million people (33 %) in the United States and is expected to increase to over 50 % of the population by 2030. The epidemic is fueled by the growing rate of obesity in adolescents of 17 %. Healthcare systems have the responsibility to provide care to this burgeoning group of people.

Accurate measurement and tracking of a patient's BMI is critical. As a screening tool it may identify patients with a BMI of 25 kg/m^2 and above who are classified as overweight and are at risk for progression of weight and obesity-related disease. Identification of this group of people presents a tremendous opportunity to reverse the progression of obesity with traditional and less expensive methods of weight loss and control such as diet and exercise. Patients in the overweight BMI group (25.0–29.9 kg/m^2) have generally not yet experienced amplification of their obesity through genetic resetting™. Current research proves that keeping a patient in the overweight range or bringing a patient to a lower BMI from the obese range will stave off obesity-related disease and save billions of dollars in direct and indirect cost.

This chapter will describe the preferred clinical method of accurately measuring obesity using Weight Related Health Indicators (WRHI), which should include BMI, waist circumference, and body fat percentage. The WRHI should be measured and recorded for every patient at every visit and become part of the patient's ongoing educational and monitoring process. Currently there is no scalable system in place to cope with the demand for treatment or the cost. The stakes are high. The annual cost is $305 billion with $190 billion going to the direct cost of treatment of related disease. A universal platform that employs regular, ongoing measurements of WRHI for every patient at every health care visit will allow a scalable system to be put in place to recognize the development of overweight and obesity and to provide timely opportunities to treat the burgeoning epidemic at its earliest stages.

Learning Objectives

1. Summarize the impact of the prevalence rates of obesity in the adult, childhood, adolescent, and minority populations
2. Describe ways to measure obesity accurately and their relationship to predicting incidence of disease
3. Implement the Weight Related Health Indicators (WRHI): height, weight, BMI, BMI for age with Z Score for children/adolescents, waist circumference, and body fat percentage for all patients seen in the practice
4. Develop an understanding of direct and indirect costs related to obesity

Currently, 30 % of the world's population is overweight or obese. By 2020, it is estimated that over 60 % of the world's population will be overweight or obese. Estimates suggest that the prevalence of severe obesity in 2030 will be 11 %, roughly twice the current prevalence [1].

Obesity disproportionately affects minorities, single mothers, and lower socioeconomic groups. In addition, the rate of obesity within the adolescent age group is escalating [2].

Obesity occurs on a continuum from "overweight" to "clinically severe obesity." The higher a patient's BMI rises, the higher the risk becomes that the patient will develop obesity-related diseases. Similarly, the severity of the obesity-related diseases increases as BMI rises. BMI values are clinically related to risk (Table 1.1).

Accurate measurement and tracking of a patient's BMI is critical as it provides a screening tool to identify patients with a BMI of 25 kg/m^2 and above, who are classified as overweight and are at risk for progression of weight and obesity-related disease. Identification of this group of people presents a tremendous opportunity to reverse the progression of obesity with traditional methods of weight loss and control such as diet and exercise. This is because patients in the overweight BMI

Table 1.1 Classification of overweight and obesity by body mass index (BMI), waist circumference, and associated disease risks

	BMI (kg/m^2)	Obesity class	Disease risk* relative to normal weight and waist circumference	
			Men ≤ 102 cm (≤ 40 in.) women ≤ 88 cm (≤ 35 in.)	Men >102 cm (>40 in.) women >88 cm (>35 in.)
Underweight	<18.5		–	–
Normal**	18.5–24.9		–	–
Overweight	25.0–29.9		Increased	High
Obesity	30.0–34.9	I	High	Very high
	35.0–39.9	II	Very high	Very high
Extreme obesity	≥ 40.0	III	Extremely high	Extremely high

From CDC/NHS Health, United States 2014, Fig. 11, Table 64
*Disease risk for type 2 diabetes, hypertension, and coronary heart disease
**Increased waist circumference can also be a marker for increased risk even in persons of normal weight. Reprinted from National Institutes of Health and National Heart, Lung, and Blood Institute, 1998

group (25.0–29.9 kg/m^2) have generally not yet experienced amplification of the "*genetic reset*™." Current research proves that keeping a patient in the overweight range or bringing a patient to a lower BMI from the obese range will stave off obesity-related disease and save billions of dollars in direct and indirect cost [1].

Once a patient gains weight, the environment begins to impact their genes and changes the way the genes work to control their weight. As the BMI exceeds 30, their "genetic reset™" generally starts to become apparent as a resistance to weight loss, and as the patient continues to gain weight they reach a point of no return. The concept of "*genetic reset*™" is explained in detail in Chap. 3 *The Biology of Weight Regulation and Genetic Resetting*™. **Amplification of the *genetic reset*™ is a critical tipping point for the patient, because the genetic reset™ greatly reduces the patient's ability to reverse or control clinically severe obesity and its related diseases by traditional methods.** In fact, almost the opposite is true: once the amplification of the *genetic reset*™ has occurred, the clinically severely obese patient tends to maintain his or her weight or add additional weight, despite "normal" eating patterns and concerted attempts at traditional methods of weight loss. Research shows that the group of patients with a BMI of 40+ has shown the most rapid growth, and this group has the highest risk for and highest severity of obesity-related disease [3].

As we examine the epidemiology, the method of measurement and cost of obesity in this chapter, four statistical terms are necessary to understand the data presented: incidence, prevalence, QALY, and DALY. Incidence and prevalence are often used interchangeably, however, they have important distinguishing characteristics in regard to the groups of people included.

INCIDENCE is the number of newly diagnosed cases of a disease divided by the population at risk. The population-at-risk is all the persons in the population who do not have the disease at the beginning of the observation period but who are capable of developing the disease. Incidence answers the question: How many people per year newly acquire this disease [4]?

PREVALENCE is the number of people in the population with the disease at a given point in time divided by the total population. Prevalence answers the question: How many people have this disease right now [4]?

QALY (Quality-Adjusted Life Year) measures the value of a specific intervention in economic terms. Health is assigned a value from 1.0 (fully healthy) to 0 (death) multiplied by the time an individual spends in that status (Fig. 1.1). In general an effective intervention benchmark is $50,000 per QALY [5].

DALY (Disability-Adjusted Life Years) is a health gap measure. The DALY measures the gap between the current health status caused by a disease in terms of premature death and disability and the ideal situation that exists when a person lives to life expectancy free of disease and disability. It is the sum of years of life lost (YLL) to premature mortality plus years lived with disability (YLD) [6].

These four statistical terms are important to a medical practitioner's understanding of obesity and obesity-related disease.

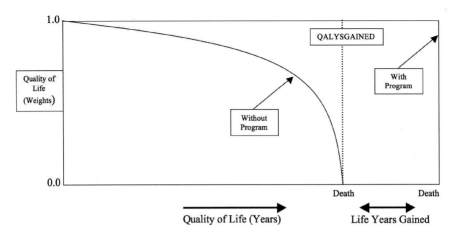

Fig. 1.1 Quality-adjusted life years (QALY) (from http://www.cdc.gov/media/transcripts/t050602.pdf)

Obesity in Populations

Child and Adolescent Obesity

Forty years ago if a child was considered to be a little "pudgy," the prevailing wisdom among doctors and parents was that the child would "grow out of it," and they often did. Times have changed. Experts believe that 110 million children and adolescents are now affected by obesity [7]. **The prevalence of obesity in children and adolescents is 17 %.** Even in early childhood the incidence of obesity is high. Studies show that for children entering kindergarten 14.9 % are overweight and another 12.4 % are obese. By eighth grade 17 % are overweight and 20.8 % are obese. Overweight 5-year olds are more likely to become obese adolescents. Minority children and children from lower socioeconomic families are disproportionately affected. However, ALL groups between kindergarten and eighth grade show significant increases in their prevalence of obesity: 65 % in Caucasian children, 50 % in Hispanic children, 120 % in Black children, and 40 % among children of other races (Asian, Pacific Islander, Native American, and multiracial). The wealthiest 20 % of families have the lowest prevalence of obesity (7.8 %) than any other quintiles of socioeconomic status. The two poorest quintiles have a prevalence of 13.8 and 16.5 % [8].

Despite these sobering statistics, many pediatricians are reluctant to measure and share BMI information with parents and/or the affected children. The reluctance to measure and share this clinically relevant data as part of all routine pediatric examinations is a failure as medical providers to help the family understand and address any overweight issues that may exist. This reluctance can have devastating long-term effects because we fail to identify, educate, and help children who have not yet been genetically reset to favor obesity. They still present as prime candidates to reverse their trend to obesity, particularly when the parents still have the ability to control their children's diet and activities. Teaching children the value of weight maintenance as a part of normal healthy living is essential even if it is a tough conversation to have with parents and kids. The failure to measure and monitor every child's BMI and to encourage and assist the child and the child's parents in addressing any overweight issues sets the child up for an uninformed and defenseless progression to obesity and disease.

The effects of childhood and adolescent obesity are having a negative impact in many ways. Based on 2013 data, current average life expectancy is 78.8 years in the United States: 76.4 for men and 81.2 for women [9]. Life expectancy, however, for future generations is expected to decrease due to the prevalence of childhood obesity and related disease [10]. In addition, the incidence of obesity rates in adolescents (17 %) will have a profound impact on the development of talent for future businesses of all types. Obesity stigma often prevents young people from realizing their full potential. For example, 50 % of applicants to the United States Military fail to qualify for admission due to high BMI. Indeed, many young people will be disabled by obesity-related disease at an early age, thereby reducing their productive years of work. It is estimated that 10 % of children with type 2 diabetes will develop renal failure by young adulthood [11]. Every study of obesity-related mortality makes clear that children who are obese have the most years of life to lose.

In subsequent chapters, we will explore in detail the effects of fetal programming and effects of *genetic resetting*™ with weight gain on childhood and adolescent obesity. The epigenetics of obesity are becoming clear: parents who are obese pass down inheritable physiology to their children. That inheritable physiology is part of what "resets" the child's own genetic expression, which in turn predisposes the child to obesity and type 2 diabetes. Through inheritable epigenetics the incidence of obesity becomes cyclical and increasingly prevalent with each generation.

Adult Obesity

Although the prevalence of obesity appears to be roughly stable in adults, population growth is not. This means the overall number of people with overweight, obesity and related disease is increasing dramatically. The population is estimated to grow from 310 million in 2010 to 439 million in 2030 with a prevalence rate of 42 % for obesity. It is projected that by 2050, over 157 million people will be obese and almost as many will be overweight [12]. In addition, the population is becoming increasingly urbanized with the global urban population growing by 65 million a year. Urbanization reduces daily energy expenditure by 300–400 calories, which in turn increases the population's risk of becoming overweight and obese [13].

Over the past 30 years, the population of overweight and obese adults (BMI of 25 or greater) has increased (Fig. 1.2). In 1980, 28.8 % of men were overweight and/or obese. By 2013 it was 36.9 %. Similarly, in 1980 29.8 % of women in the U.S. were overweight and/or obese. By 2013 it was 38 % of women. The World Health

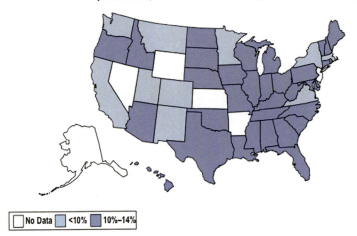

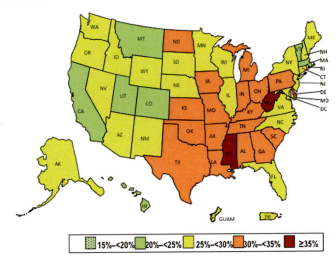

Fig. 1.2 a Obesity trends among U.S. adults, BRFSS, 1990 (from http://www.cdc.gov/media/transcripts/t050602.pdf) **b** Prevalence of self-reported obesity among U.S. adults by state and territory, BRFSS, 2013 (from http://www.cdc.gov/obesity/downloads/dnpao-2013-state-obesity-prevalence-map-508tagged.pdf)

Organization (WHO) estimates that, in the year 2010, overweight and obesity caused 3.4 million deaths (5 %), and resulted in 3.9 % of YLL and 3.8 % of disability adjusted life years (DALY) worldwide. **No country in the world reduced the prevalence of obesity-related disease between 2000 and 2013.** Obesity ranks third in social burdens created by human beings after smoking and armed violence [14].

Obesity Rates Within Minority Groups and Subpopulations

Statistics bear similarly alarming news for specific subgroups of populations. For example, groups of young adults age 20–44 years, Black and Hispanic subpopulations and subpopulations with secondary education or less all showed an increase in their prevalence of obesity and type 2 diabetes [15] (Fig. 1.3).

Native Americans

Native Americans are another such subpopulation. Similar to the increase in the population at large, the overall population of Native Americans is expected to experience large growth relative to their current numbers. It is estimated their populations will increase from 235,000 in 2010 to 918,000 in 2050, with a correlating increase in their rates of obesity and type 2 diabetes [12].

Baby Boomers

The United States has experienced dramatic growth in the number of older people during this century. As a result, the aging population presents major implications for national health care needs. By 2030, 25 % of United States residents will be age 65 or older (1 in 5) due to the aging of the "baby boomers" i.e., people born between 1946 and 1964 [12]. Women represent a significant subgroup within the baby boomer population. In 2003–2004, the obesity rate among women aged 60 years and older was 31.5 %. Six years later, in 2010–2012 that rate increased to 38.1 % [2].

Gender

When it comes to obesity and type 2 diabetes in general, a gender gap appears to exist between men and women. Women are more affected by obesity than men in most countries, but in some countries that gap is more pronounced. In Egypt, for example, the prevalence of obesity in men is 21 % as compared to Egyptian women at 45 %. In the United States black women (57.5 %) are far more affected by obesity than black men (38.1 %) [14].

(a)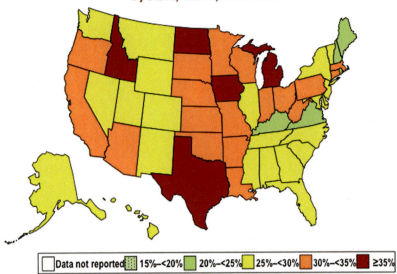

(b)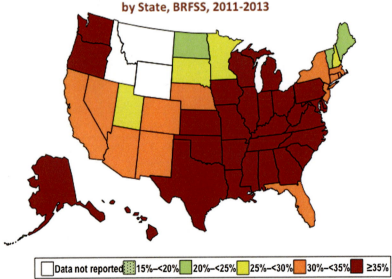

Fig. 1.3 a Prevalence of self-reported obesity among hispanic adults, by state, BRFSS, 2011–2013 (from http://www.cdc.gov/obesity/data/table-hispanics.html) **b** Prevalence of self-reported obesity among non-hispanic black adults, by State, BRFSS, 2011–2013 (from http://www.cdc.gov/obesity/data/table-non-hispanic-black.html)

Socioeconomic Status

The incidence of obesity and type 2 diabetes is affected not only by race, but also by socioeconomic status. In the United States, we describe the impact of economic status as a function of the total yearly income of a family compared to the poverty level established by the federal government. Quartiles of poverty status are defined as follows:

1. Poor: families with income less than 125 % of the poverty line, including people with negative income;
2. Low: families with income equal to or greater than 125 % but less than 200 % of the poverty line;
3. Middle: families with income equal to or greater than 200 % but less than 400 % of the poverty line; and
4. High: families with income equal to or greater than 400 % of the poverty line.

People in the poor income quartile have higher levels of obesity (26.4 %) and extreme obesity (6.8 %) compared to those in the high-income quartile (23.6 % and 3.3 %, respectively) [16]. In studies unadjusted for socioeconomic differences in income, Black adults are more affected by obesity than Caucasian adults. However, when the studies are adjusted for socioeconomic differences, the two groups are close to the same: Black adults and Caucasian adults living in the same social context with similar incomes have relatively similar levels of obesity [17, 18]. These studies indicate that racial disparity in obesity rates disappears if socioeconomic conditions are the same, thus suggesting that social context is a contributor to obesity prevalence. This is important to consider when searching for public policies that will be effective in fighting obesity and obesity-related disease.

Measurement of Obesity

Weight Related Health Indicators (WRHI)

Imagine a healthcare provider trying to quantify a patient's blood pressure without using a sphygmomanometer. Similarly, overweight and obesity are difficult for the healthcare provider to quantify without any clinically accurate measurement upon which to rely. Weight Related Health Indicators (WRHI) allows a healthcare provider to quantify obesity through easily obtained physical measurements at a routine office visit. Like all clinical measurements, WRHI measurements should be obtained in a standardized fashion. The act of clinically measuring the patient for WRHI and then sharing that information with the patient should become part of the patient's ongoing educational and monitoring process. The WRHI criteria that should be measured for every patient at every visit includes the following:

- Body Mass Index (in Children/Adolescents BMI for Age/Z Score) using *measured* height and weight
- Waist Circumference
- Body Fat Percent

A recent study of primary care physicians working in the United States military system showed that using clinical measurements such as the WRHI listed above allowed physicians to more accurately recognize and quantify obesity and the related risk of metabolic disease [19]. Implementing a consistent process in every healthcare office to measure the WRHI will give providers the information they need to medically evaluate and, if necessary, treat the patient. *It is critical that measurement of WRHI be completed in every patient, every time they come into the healthcare setting for any reason.* It is equally critical that the WRHI information is shared with the patient and its significance from a health care impact explained. If a relatively healthy person comes in for allergies and the opportunity to measure his/her WRHI and communicate those measurements to him/her is not seized, a golden opportunity to impact that patient's overall health is lost.

Height and Weight

The measurement of height and weight is usually straightforward and ubiquitous. However, the importance of accuracy in measuring height and weight is crucial for purposes of determining BMI and correlating this information to an individual's level of obesity and associated risks. Implementing standardized procedures for doing these measurements, using correctly calibrated scales and equipment, and providing proper training for staff that will perform these measurements are all essential steps to getting accurate results. Allowing patients to self-report their height and weight is not reliable. Many men under-report their height and many women under-report their weight. In measuring height and weight of severely obese patients, it may be necessary to use special equipment specifically designed to handle the extra weight and for staff to be trained in how to provide the patient with easy, safe access to the equipment.

Body Fat

Obesity is defined as an excess of total body fat: generally 20–25 % in men and 30–35 % in women. The classic way of measuring body fat is water displacement, however, that method is difficult to implement in most clinical settings. Another field method of measuring body fat involves skinfold thickness but this method is variable and unreliable. A reasonable alternative is to use an impedance-type scale that calculates body fat. If there are a number of severely obese patients in your practice, an impedance scale that is designed to handle the extra weight is needed. Impedance scales may not be accurate unless shoes and socks are taken off, therefore it should be cleaned carefully between patients. One note of caution:

impedance scales should NOT be used in people with pacemakers. Although impedance tends to vary with the amount of water (hydration) present in the body, measuring body fat by impedance nonetheless helps in educating both the medical provider and the patient about body fat percentage and over time will help establish trends. There is quite a bit of new data about the relationship of muscle and lean tissue to the energy balance signaling of the body. The amount of fat versus lean tissue has a role to play in overall risk of disease.

The distribution of body fat has an impact on whether the person has obesity-related disease and the distribution of body fat is a heritable trait. Fat depots also have unique characteristics and biological consequences. In general, people that carry their weight in the abdominal cavity primarily have a higher incidence of obesity-related disease.

Waist Circumference

Waist circumference has been shown to be an independent predictor of risk to health as it relates to overall BMI. Waist circumference measurements take into account the location of fat distribution in the body. High-risk central obesity is generally defined as a waist circumference of more than 102 cm (40 in.) for men and 88 cm (35 in.) for women. Waist circumference is measured at the top of the hips and with the tape measure going around the belly button. Waist circumference is NOT measured at the skinny part of the waist; for accuracy it must be measured at the top of the hips and anteriorly at the level of the navel. In addition to waist circumference, some practitioners obtain a measurement of the patient's waist-to-hip ratio. Waist-to-hip ratio is measured around the buttocks.

Correctly measured waist circumference requires very little other than fundamental education and training of the people who do the baseline measurements in the office.

Waist circumference measurement and waist-to-hip ratio are both considered effective in quantifying levels of obesity and relationship to disease. The question is whether the waist-to-hip ratio offers any additional information over and above what waist circumference supplies to either the provider or the patient about their risk of disease. Studies seem to support the idea that the two measurements are similar in terms of conveying risk [20–23]. Therefore, it is recommended that waist circumference be measured as one of the critical WRHI, leaving the waist-to-hip measurement optional.

Body Mass Index and Body Adiposity Index

Body mass index (BMI) is a measure of weight adjusted for height. BMI is an imperfect tool because BMI is unable to distinguish overweight due to excess fat from overweight due to excess lean mass. It is an "anthropometric" or physical measurement of an individual person. Despite its limitations, BMI is currently the most commonly used measure for assessing obesity in adults.

The idea of measuring BMI started in the early 1800s. Adolphe Quetelet (1796–1874), a Belgium mathematician, astronomer and statistician, proposed the Quetelet Index in a paper published in 1832 entitled "The Average Man and Indices of Obesity" (Fig. 1.4). Quetelet recognized the necessity of adjusting weight for differences in body size when comparing levels of obesity in people. This idea of adjustment was later renamed the BMI in 1972 by Ancel Keys, PhD (1904–2004) (Fig. 1.5). Thanks to the scientists who did the groundwork in BMI, we now have a formula for measuring BMI.

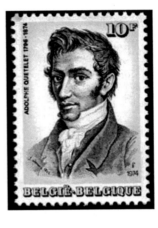

Fig. 1.4 Adolphe Quetelet (from Eknoyan [49], with permission)

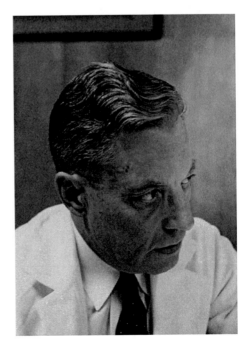

Fig. 1.5 Ancel Keys (from University of Minnesota, http://www.epi.umn.edu/cvdepi/multimedia/photographs/, with permission)

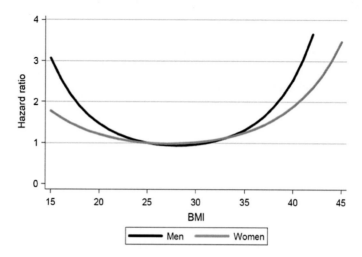

Fig. 1.6 Body mass index and mortality (data from Zajacova 2008, Brookings Institute)

The coding for obesity has received a major upgrade in the new ICD-10 system. In the ICD-10 codes obesity falls under the classification E: Endocrine, nutritional and metabolic diseases. E66.01 is the code for clinically severe obesity due to excess calories. "Z" code 68 indicates BMI in adult's age 21 and older. Z codes range from 68.1 BMI 19 or less, adult to 68.45 BMI 70 or greater, adult. Z codes should not be confused with the "Z score" that is used to correct BMI for age. In the ICD-10 codes the Z codes for children age 2–20 are Z68.51–Z68.54.

BMI is correlated with mortality (Fig. 1.6). BMI as an indicator of obesity and survival risk is not without its complexities. BMI cannot be measured without accurate scales. Calculations in children and adolescents must be adjusted for age. BMI may lack correlation with body fat in people with a high proportion of lean muscle tissue to fat so that athletes with a high BMI may still have a low body fat percentage and waist circumference may be within normal range. BMI may be inaccurate based on inconsistency of height measurements. Finally, BMI may be insensitive to the increased prevalence of disease at lower BMI in certain special populations.

Alternative methods of measuring BMI exist. One of those alternative methods is the use of the Body Adiposity Index (BAI) [24]. The BAI correlates directly with body fat percentage and is applicable across populations.

$$\text{Body Mass Index(BMI)} = \text{weight(lb)} \times 702/\text{height(inches)}^2$$

$$\text{Body Adiposity Index(BAI)} = \text{Hip circumference(inches)}/\text{height in inches}^2 \times 1.5) - 18$$

Measuring hip circumference, however, is often difficult in more obese patients due to both the large size of the abdomen especially if an abdominal pannus exists and the difficulty in defining an accurate hip circumference. At this time the BAI has not been widely adopted in part because of the difficulty with measuring hip circumference and the lack of historical perspective. For this reason, the continued use of BMI augmented with waist circumference and body fat percentage to correlate with fat distribution location is recommended to determine the amount and clinical relevance of these indicators.

Measurements in Special Adult Populations—Asian Americans

Not all populations are affected with clinical severity of disease at the same level of BMI. Asian Americans, due to the marked difference in body habitus, primarily accumulate weight in their abdominal cavity. Abdominal fat is metabolically very active and causes severe obesity-related disease; specifically type 2 diabetes, at a lower BMI. The World Health Organization recommends that "overweight" in Asian populations should begin at a BMI of 23 and "obesity" should begin at a BMI of 25. In Japan a BMI of 25 is defined as obese, and in China a BMI of 28 is defined as obese. The group of Asian Americans is very heterogeneous, consisting of multiple subgroups. A comprehensive review of the pertinent data for Asian Americans suggests that screening for type 2 diabetes in Asian Americans should actually begin at a BMI of 22 [25].

The Edmonton Obesity Staging System

One of the ways to make the BMI and waist circumference (anthropometric measures) more relevant to individuals is to use a clinical staging system. This adds the clinically relevant data that allows you to distinguish an individual's risk for mortality by including an assessment of their burden of obesity-related disease. Why is that needed? Individuals who have the same BMI could have differences in body fat, presence of obesity-related disease and severity of that disease. Conversely, people who have the same amount of body fat or waist circumference can present with a range of BMI [26, 27].

The most widely validated system is the Edmonton Obesity Staging System (EOSS). Proposed in 2009, it uses established and familiar paradigms of clinical staging similar to the New York Heart Association Functional Classification and staging systems for cancer and renal failure [28].

The Edmonton classification system has been shown to predict increased mortality independent of BMI or waist circumference using the National Health and Nutrition Examination Survey (NHANES) from 1988–1994 and 1999–2004 [29]. A lower EOSS stage is associated with more weight loss. Higher EOSS stages required more concentrated intervention time to achieve an equal result [30].

The importance of using the Edmonton system for those patients with a BMI of 30 kg/m^2 or greater (obese) is that it will help identify those individuals who need more intense medical intervention, pharmaceutical treatment or surgery.

Practioners can download the EEOS pocket card staging tool at: http://www.drsharma.ca/wp-content/uploads/edmonton-obesity-staging-system-pocket-card.pdf.

The clinical system for measuring obesity should now involve two specific steps. First, the WRHI (BMI, waist circumference, and body fat percentage) should be used to identify those patients who should then be further staged with the Edmonton Staging System.

Measurements in Children and Adolescents

BMI is used in both adults and children, however, in growing children it must be adjusted for age and gender using the CDC's BMI-For-Age chart (www.cdc.gov/growthcharts).

For example, a 5-year-old boy with a BMI of 20 is likely to be obese, but a 15-year-old boy with a BMI of 20 is likely to be lean. For BMI to be meaningful in children it must be compared to a reference standard that accounts for the age and gender. National reference standards now exist in the United States and the United Kingdom and are being developed in other countries. The International Obesity Task Force (IOTF) has also produced an international BMI reference. There is controversy about whether a national or international reference standard is best. In 2004, the data was standardized to an external reference and a standardized "Z score" can now be assigned for children and adolescents. "Z scores" correspond to growth chart percentiles. "Z scores" range from −3 to +3, with zero being normal weight [31].

Another significant BMI measuring issue when dealing with children is the transition from adolescent measurements (BMI adjusted for age) to adult BMI measurements. Of the reference standards currently available, the IOTF reference provides the best transition formula from the child/adolescent definition of overweight/obesity to the adult definition for overweight/obesity. For example, an 18-year-old girl with a BMI of 25.5 would be considered overweight under the adult definition and considered normal weight under the child/adolescent definition [32]. In the UK, between 1987 and 1997 waist circumference of children increased more than BMI, so surveillance alone by BMI For Age may not be adequate [33]. Using both BMI For Age/Z scores and waist circumference may give the clinician more confidence in identifying those children whose high BMI poses the greatest health risk. A comparison of different anthropometric measurements to predict metabolic syndrome in children shows that using waist circumference in combination with BMI provides a measure of success in identifying children at risk [34].

Surveys of Health Status in the United States

The United States has the highest mean BMI among all high-income countries. We know this thanks to important ongoing studies done by the National Center For

Health Statistics and ongoing surveys done by the NHANES (National Health and Nutrition Examination Survey). The NHANES is a program of studies designed to assess the health and nutrition status of adults and children in the United States. As a survey tool it is unique in that every participant included in the survey visits the physician and undergoes interviews and physical examinations. The NHANES examines a nationally represented sample of 5000 people each year. The findings from the NHANES are used to determine the prevalence of major diseases and risk factors for disease. The NHANES shows that 1 in 3 adults have a BMI over 30, meaning that 1 in 3 adults in that survey are in the category of obese with moderate health and survival risk.

A second U.S. survey, The Behavioral Risk Factor Surveillance System (BRFSS), is the nation's largest telephone survey. This survey collects data from U.S. residents regarding their health. The BRFSS annually interviews 400,000 adults 18 years or older by telephone, using participant's self-reported weight and height data and other health information, as opposed to clinically measured data. The BRFSS shows 1 in 4 adults have obesity. The discrepancy in statistics between the NHANES and the BRFSS might be due to the fact that obesity is underestimated when the data is self-reported. Under-reporting by individuals has been statistically correlated: a cut point of BMI 40 would actually be a BMI 37.3 in self-reporting men and BMI of 37 in self-reporting women [35].

When working with and considering an individual patient's overall health and healthcare needs, practitioners need to take into account the patient's heritage; background, and physique in order to better assess risk. Patients face an increasing burden of disease with increased BMI. This should be recognized by the provider and addressed with the patient in any encounter within the healthcare system. Despite its limitations, BMI is currently the most widely used approach to clinically identify individuals who are overweight or obese and to calculate their risk for related disease.

Standardized measurements of the WRHI and discussion of the results with the patient are crucial steps in establishing communication with the patient around their health without introducing discrimination. The WRHI will send a strong message to both the health care team and the patient about the status of the patient's health and, when necessary, the medical issues presented by overweight and obesity will have been introduced for discussion in subsequent visits.

Healthcare Costs: The Impact of Obesity and Obesity-Related Disease

Obesity and obesity-related disease, left unchecked, will continue to drive healthcare costs to record highs. Healthcare professionals are usually more focused on treating individual people than on the overall cost of care. To the extent the focus is on cost, awareness of the individual's private cost as opposed to the societal cost of care is given the attention. Obese patients with related disease will be part of panels of patients that medical providers and healthcare systems will be called upon to manage exceptionally well in order to reduce overall societal costs, keep patients healthy, and maintain a satisfactory level of personal reimbursement for medical services. Bundled insurance payments to healthcare systems may not be able to take into account the high acuity in these panels because many do not include accurate WRHI. If measurement of obesity and related disease is not taken into account then value-based health care will be not be obtained. In this sense, obesity is a hidden challenge to current risk stratification. The cost of treating obesity in an ever-aging population is spiraling out of control. The goal of stemming the tide and reversing the trend is compelling.

Social, Future, and Personal Cost of Obesity

Social cost is the expense to an entire society resulting from some articulable event —in this case obesity. Private cost is the cost to the individual patient. Future cost is calculated based on assumptions made about the prevalence of disease in the future.

Healthcare cost breaks down into two areas: direct costs and indirect costs. Direct costs include inpatient services, outpatient services, laboratory evaluations, diagnostic tests, drugs, and insurance. Direct costs are relatively easy to measure. Indirect costs relate to the loss of productivity caused by absenteeism, disability pension costs, and premature disability and death. The impact of indirect cost is also expressed in terms of QALY's and DALY's, as defined earlier. A QALY measures the extent of health gain that results from healthcare interventions while a DALY measures the YLL to disability. Indirect costs are obviously more difficult to quantify than direct costs.

Social Cost

The global economic cost of obesity is about $2 trillion annually, or 2.8 % of global gross domestic product (GDP). The health burden of obesity includes several other related high-cost diseases: cardiovascular disease, hypertension, diabetes, cancer, sleep apnea, osteoarthritis, and depression. In the United States the number of obese individuals with coronary heart disease (CHD) is estimated to increase to 5.6 % to 540,000 by 2050. Similarly there is estimated to be a 7 % increase in diabetes (separate from CHD) and mortality [36]. In 2014, the American Society of Clinical Oncology (ASCO) issued a report warning that obesity will soon overtake tobacco as the No. 1 risk factor for cancer. That report confirms that obesity is associated with increased risk of the following types of cancer: breast (post-menopausal), colon, rectal, esophageal, endometrial, pancreatic, kidney, thyroid, and gallbladder [37]. The relationship between obesity and depression has also been well documented: 43 % of adults suffering from depression are obese, and 55 % of people taking antidepressant medications for depression are obese [38].

Diabetes contributes significantly to rising heath care costs. Over 40 % of U.S. citizens 20 years or older are diabetic or prediabetic [39]. The American Diabetes Association estimates that in 2012 the total cost of diabetes care was $245 billion, an increase of 41 % since 2007. In addition, patients with diabetes spend an additional $13,700 per year out of pocket on medical care. The lifetime risk of diabetes has increased from 30 to 40 %, with a life-shortening effect of 13 years. Significantly, a 7 % weight loss accompanied by moderate exercise has been shown to decrease the incidence of type 2 diabetes by 58 % [40]. Thus, weight loss in obese individuals, if it can be achieved and sustained, would significantly reduce the cost of diabetes-related heath care.

Lost productivity accounts for about 70 % of the total global cost of obesity. As measured in DALY's (disability-adjusted life years), the loss due to obesity was 71 % due to premature death and 29 % due to disability. The U.S. economic loss in productivity is estimated to be $390–580 billion annually.

The cost of obesity in the United States is estimated to be from $147 billion to $190 billion per year. This represents approximately 7 % of total annual health care spending [1]. If the cost of treatment of obesity-related disease is included, the total cost of care may be as high as $663 billion a year, or 4.1 % of GDP [36].

Future Cost

The projected future cost of treating obesity and obesity-related disease is staggering. It is estimated that 3 out of 4 Americans and 7 out of 10 citizens of the United Kingdom will be overweight or obese by 2020 [41]. Given our rapidly aging population, there could be as many as 65 million more adults in the U.S. who are obese in 2030 than in 2010. Approximately 24 million of those 65 million (37 %) will be over age 65. Arthritis, CHD, and type 2 diabetes are the highest contributors to healthcare costs and people will incur half of those costs over age 65. The primary source of funding for treatment of these patients will be nationally funded payment mechanisms such as Medicare [42]. Based on the known progression to obesity when adolescents become adults, it is estimated that adult obesity will increase from 330,000 in 2010 to more than 9,700,000 in 2050. Overweight adolescents who become obese adults may increase future obesity rates from 5 to 15 % in 2035, producing more than 100,000 more cases of CHD [36]. Finally, with respect to future costs, obesity and related diseases are estimated to represent a loss of 24.5–48.2 million quality-adjusted life-years (QALYs) in the U.S. in the interval between 2010 and 2030.

Personal Cost

In addition to societal and future costs associated with obesity, there are private patient costs as well. These may include: (1) out-of-pocket costs for medical care, treatments, and procedures not covered by insurance; (2) lost or lower wages due to obesity discrimination or disease and disabilities caused by obesity; (3) higher insurance premiums correlating with increasing degrees of overweight; and (4) the cost of assistance or adaptations necessary to function in daily life due to obesity-related disabilities. Individuals with obesity have 30 % higher medical costs than a normal weight person. Compared to normal weight patients, obese patients incur 46 % more inpatient costs, spend 80 % more on prescription drugs, and have 27 % more costs in outpatient and physician visits [43]. In addition, it is estimated that individual consumers spend over $50 billion annually on over-the-counter and/or non-reimbursed weight loss treatment products. Over a lifetime the cost for a person with obesity is $92,235 [44].

Private insurance pays for roughly one half of the cost of health care in the United States. In fact, the higher insurance premiums that cover the cost of employees with obesity are estimated to be $7.7 billion of the $18.9 billion overall cost [45]. Similarly, the Center for Medicare and Medicaid spends over 20 % of its budget for obesity-related healthcare costs (8.55 % for Medicare and 11.8 % for Medicaid), which accounts for 12.9 % of overall private payer spending [46]. The percent of private payer spending may increase sharply in the future under the Affordable Care Act because under the Act insurers are now covering people within exchanges who are minorities and/or those at or near the poverty level who have a statistically higher prevalence and severity of obesity and obesity-related diseases.

For individual U.S. employers, absenteeism due to obesity represents a $8.65 billion per year expense. Overall the cost of absenteeism due to obesity was 9.3 % [47]. The annual cost from presenteeism (the practice of coming to work despite illness, injury, anxiety) resulting in reduced productivity accounts for 44 % and 38 % of total costs, respectively, for men and women with obesity. Men having a BMI of 40 or more is equivalent to one month of lost productivity which costs employers approximately $3792 per year [48].

Clearly, a strategic nationwide effort to decrease obesity by even 1 % of 2010 prevalence would have a major cost savings effect. The more aggressive the decline in the rate of obesity, the greater the savings to all stakeholders.

Implementing Specific Process for Chapter 1 Recommendations

A. Implement **measured** WRHI for all patients every time they are seen in the healthcare environment:

   1. BMI (Adults) or BMI for Age/Z Score (Children and Adolescents)
   2. Waist Circumference
   3. Body Fat Percent

B. Standardize a process within the local healthcare environment for collecting the WRHI on each patient and educate staff on the correct process for collecting, recording, and updating the WRHI information within the electronic health record with particular attention to the correct coding of obesity in ICD-10.

Conclusion

Our global population is increasingly becoming overweight, obese, and suffering from obesity-related diseases. This is the healthcare epidemic of the present and the healthcare crisis of the future. While the subjects of overweight and obesity are common topics that receive a lot of written analysis, we are doing nothing significant in our individual day-to-day operations as healthcare providers to stem or turn the tide. At many levels of healthcare and public policy obesity remains a disease that is largely unseen, untreated, or ignored. To date there has been no compelling or strategic proposal made for a scalable population management process that would effectively measure and manage all patients who are clinically overweight and/or obese. Chapter 12 will propose just such a process—a process based on the new science of obesity that will provide a scalable, systematic, clinical approach for the universal measurement, recognition, treatment, and prevention of obesity.

References

1. Finkelstein EA, Khavjou OA, Thompson H, Trogdon JG, Pan L, Sherry B, Dietz W. Obesity and severe obesity forecasts through 2030. Am J Prev Med. 2012;42(6):563–70.
2. Ogden CL, Carroll MD, Kit BK, Flegal KM. Prevalence of childhood and adult obesity in the United States, 2011–2012. JAMA. 2014;311(8):806–14.
3. Andreyeva T, Sturm R, Ringel JS. Moderate and severe obesity have large differences in health care costs. Obes Res. 2004;12(12):1936–43.
4. World Health Organization Expert Committee on Health Statistics. 1959;164:783–4.
5. Neumann PJ, Cohen JT, Weinstein MC. Updating cost-effectiveness—the curious resilience of the $50,000-per-QALY threshold. N Engl J Med. 2014;371(9):796–7.
6. World Development Report 1993. Investing in Health. Oxford: The World Bank, Oxford University Press; 1993.
7. Call AM, Caprio S. Obesity in children and adolescents. J Clin Endocrinol Metab. 2008;93 (11) Suppl 1:S31–6.
8. Cunningham SA, Kramer MR, Narayan KMV. Incidence of childhood obesity in the United States. N Engl J Med. 2014;370(5):403–11.
9. Kochanek KD, Murphy SL, Su J, Arias E. Mortality in the United States; 2013. www.cdc.gov.
10. Olshansky SJ, Passaro DJ, Hershow RC, Layden J, Carnes BA, Brody J, Hayflick L, Butler RN, Allison DB, Ludwig DS. A potential decline in life expectancy in the United States in the 21st Century. N Engl J Med. 2005;352(11):1138–45.
11. Dean H, Flett B. Natural history of type 2 diabetes diagnosed in childhood: long term follow up in young adult years. Diabetes. 2002;51(2):A24.
12. Vincent GK, Velkoff VA. US Census Bureau The Next Four Decades The Older Population in the United States: 2010 to 2050. www.census.gov/population/www/projections/2008projections.html.
13. James WP. The fundamental drivers of the obesity epidemic. Obes Rev. 2008;9(1):6–13.
14. Ng M, Fleming T, et al. Global, regional and national prevalence of overweight and obesity in children and adults during 1980–2013: a systematic analysis for the global burden of disease study. Lancet. 2014;384(9945):766–81.

15. Geiss LS, Wang J, Cheng YJ, Thompson TJ, Barker L, Li Y, Albright AL, Gregg EW. Prevalence and incidence trends for diagnosed diabetes among adults aged 20–79 years, United States, 1980–2012. JAMA. 2014;312(12):1218–26.
16. Agency for Healthcare Research and Quality Medical Expenditure Panel Survey (MEPS) Statistical Brief #364: obesity in American: Estimates for the U.S. Civilian Noninstitutionalized Population Age 20 and older, 2009.
17. Thorpe RJ, Kelley E, Bowie JV, Griffith DM, Bruce M, LaVeist T. Explaining racial disparities in obesity among men: does place matter? Am J Mens Health. 2014;PMID: 25249452.
18. Bleich SN, Thorpe RJ, Sharif-Harris H, Fesahazion R, Laveist TA. Social context explains race disparities in obesity among women. J Epidemiol Community Health. 2010;64(5):465–9.
19. Warner CH, Warner CM, Morganstein J, Appenzeller GN, Rachal J, Greiger T. Military family physician attitudes toward treating obesity. Mil Med. 2008;173(10):978–84.
20. DeKoning L, Merchant AT, Pogue J, Anand SS. Waist circumference and waist-to-hip ratio as predicators of cardiovascular events: meta-regression analysis of perspective studies. Eur Heart J. 2007;28:850–6.
21. Zhang X, Rexrode KM, van Dam RM, Li TY, Hu FB. Abdominal obesity and the risk of all-cause, cardiovascular, and cancer mortality: sixteen years of follow-up in US women. Circulation. 2008;117:1658–67.
22. Vazquez G, Duval S, Jacobs DR, Silventoinen K. Comparison of body mass index, waist circumference and waist/hip ratio in predicting incident diabetes: a meta-analysis. Epidemiol Rev. 2007;29:115–28.
23. Borne y, Nilsson PM, Melander O, Hedblad B, Engstrom G. Multiple anthropometric measures in relation to incidence of diabetes: a Swedish population-based cohort study. Eur J Public Health. 2015;PMID: 25817208.
24. Bergman RN, Stefanovski D, Buchanan TA, Sumner AE, Reynolds JC, Sebring NG, Xiang AH, Watanabe RM. A better index of body adiposity. Obesity. 2011;19(5):1083–9.
25. Hsu WC, Araneta MRG, Kanaya AM, Chian JL, Fujimoto W. BMI cut points to identify at-risk Asian Americans for type 2 diabetes screening. Diabetes Care. 2015;38:150–8.
26. Wellens RI, Roche AF, Shamis HJ, Jackson AS, Pollock ML, Siervogel RM. Relationships between body mass index and body composition. Obes Res. 1996;4:35–44.
27. Gallagher D, Heymsfield SB, Heo M, Jebb SA, Murgatroyd PR, Sakamoto Y. Healthy percentage body fat ranges: an approach for developing guidelines based on body mass index. Am J Clin Nutr. 2000;72:694–701.
28. Sharma AM, Kushner RF. A proposed clinical staging system for obesity. Int J Obes. 2009;38:289–95.
29. Padwal RS, Pajewski NM, Allison DB, Arya M, Sharma MD. Using the Edmonton obesity staging system to predict mortality in a population-representative cohort of people with overweight and obesity. CMAJ. 2011;183(14):F1059–66.
30. Canning KL, Brown RE, Wharton S, Sharma AM, Kuk JL. Edmonton obesity staging system prevalence and association with weight loss in a publicly funded referral-based obesity clinic. J Obes. 2015;619–734.
31. World Health Organization. Training Course on Child Growth Assessment. Geneva: WHO; 2008.
32. Must A, Anderson SE. Body mass index in children and adolescents: considerations for population-based applications. Int J Obes. 2006;30:590–4.
33. McCarthy HD, Jarrett KV, Crawley HF. The development of waist circumference percentiles in British children aged 5.0–16.9 year. Eur J Clin Nutr. 2001;55:902–7.
34. Wicklow VA, Becker A, Chateau D, Palmer K, Kozyrskij A, Sellers EA. Comparison of anthropometric measurements in children to predict metabolic syndrome in adolescence: analysis of prospective cohort data. Int J Obes. 2015;PMID: 25869598.
35. Sturm R, Hattori A. Morbid obesity rates continue to rise rapidly in the US. Int J Obes. 2013;37(6):889–91.

36. Lightwood J, Bibbins-Domingo K, Coxson P, Wang C, Williams L, Goldman L. Forecasting the future economic burden of current adolescent overweight: an estimate of the coronary heart policy model. Am J Public Health. 2009;99:2230–7.
37. Ligibel JA, Alfano Catherine M, Courneya KS, et al. American society of clinical oncology position statement on obesity and cancer. J Clin Oncol. 2014;32(31):3568–74.
38. Zipf G, Chiappa M, Porter KS, et al. National health and nutrition examination survey: plan and operations, 1999–2010. National Center for Health Statistics. Vital Health Stat. 2013;1(56).
39. Cowie CC, Rust KF, Ford ES, Eberhardt MS, Byrd-Holt DD, Li C, Williams DE, Gregg EW, Bainbridge KE, Sayday SH, Geiss LS. Full accounting of diabetes and pre-diabetes in the U.S. population in 1988–1994 and 2005–2006. Diabetes Care. 2009;32:287–94.
40. Diabetes Prevention Program Research Group. The diabetes prevention program (DPP): description of lifestyle intervention. Diabetes Care. 2002;25(12):2165–71.
41. Sassie F. Obesity and the economics of prevention: fit or fat. Paris: OECD Publishing; 2010.
42. Wang YC, McPherson K, Marsh T, Gortmaker SL, Brown M. Health and economic burden of the projected obesity trends in the USA and the UK. Lancet. 2011;378:815–25.
43. Finkelstein EA, Trogdon JG, Cohen JW, Dietz W. Annual medical spending attributable to obesity: payer-and service-specific estimates. Health Aff. 2009;28:822–31.
44. Kasman M, Hammond RA, Werman A, Mack-Crane A, McKinnon RA. An in-depth look at the lifetime economic cost of obesity. Brookings Institute. 12 May 2015.
45. Hammond RA, Levine R. The economic impact of obesity in the United States. Economic Studies Program, Brookings Institution. Aug 2010.
46. Withrow D, Alter DA. The economic burden of obesity worldwide: a systematic review of the direct costs of obesity. Obes Rev. 2011;12:131–41.
47. Andreyeva T, Luedicke J, Wang YC. State-level estimates of obesity-attributable costs of absenteeism. JOEM. 2014;56(11):1120–7.
48. Finkelstein EA, DaCostaDiBonaventura M, Burgess SM, Hale BC. The costs of obesity in the workplace. JOEM. 2010;52(10):971–6.
49. Eknoyan G. Adolphe Quetelet (1796–1874)—the average man and indices of obesity. Nephol Dial Transplant. 2008;23(1):47–51.

Chapter 2
Prejudice, Discrimination, and the Preferred Approach to the Patient with Obesity

Key Message

Discrimination and prejudice against people who suffer from obesity is an unacceptable treatment environment within healthcare. In the last 10 years, prejudice against obesity has increased by 66 %. Obesity bias and discrimination is widespread both in society and among healthcare workers. In the healthcare environment, bias leads to inconsistent evaluation and management of obesity, discourages the patient from seeking care, and increases the cost of care. To eliminate bias, practitioners and staff must first identify their personal attitudes and misinformed beliefs about obesity. This can be done through the use of specific survey tools. Physicians and health care staff should adopt nonjudgmental ways of talking effectively with patients using motivational interviewing techniques (MIT) and self-determination theory. After that, a framework can be developed that provides consistent, blameless, sensitive and effective care for those patients who suffer from obesity. An important part of that unbiased framework of care is routine clinical measurements of each person's level of obesity through the universal use of Weight Related Health Indicators (WRHI) (i.e. measurements of BMI, Waist Circumference and Body Fat Percentage). Many overweight patients are in denial or simply unaware of their level of obesity and their potential health risks. Thus, measuring and recording the patient's WRHI and then sharing that information with the patient every time they encounter the healthcare system is of paramount importance if we want the patient to be fully informed and engaged in their own care.

Learning Objectives

1. Understand key principles regarding obesity-related prejudice and discrimination.
2. Identify personal attitudes and misinformed beliefs that may contribute to obesity bias in the practice for all staff and providers.
3. Learn and incorporate Motivational Interviewing Techniques (MIT) in all patient interviews with a focus on the patient with obesity.

4. Develop a framework to provide a blameless, sensitive, and engaging environment for staff and providers to identify, understand, and optimally treat those patients who suffer from obesity.
5. Communicate the Weight Related Health Indicators (WRHI) to patients in each visit using the Weight Related Report Card (WRC).

The Patient's Perspective

The feelings expressed below are a compilation of many patients' perspectives, and are very common among patients who are obese. It is essential for health care providers to recognize and understand the magnitude of these feelings.

> I was big even as a young boy. Looking back at photographs from my elementary school, I immediately see that I was so much larger than the rest of the kids. These photographs always show me in the middle, with thin people on either side. It was humiliating when I was the only one left standing as teams were being picked. A teacher would eventually assign me to a team, but the other team members clearly resented the burden of having me on their team, and I rarely actually played the game. As a teen-ager I took comfort in food. Food never criticized you. I wasn't really athletic, but "found myself" in my schoolwork. Using my brain gave me some positive feedback. As I got older my weight became a more substantial problem. I was treating my anxiety and my boredom with food but I felt helpless to stop it. Food gave me comfort.
>
> I started to try and do something, anything, about my weight, realizing how much it was affecting my opportunities and my social interactions. My attempts to lose weight have led me to trying different diets, reading a handful of books, and surfing the Internet for new information or clues, but honestly I have no idea what is true about obesity and what is not. I guess the reason for my obesity is obvious: I eat too much, I don't exercise regularly, and I'm emotionally screwed up. The answer from professionals and healthcare providers is simply to reverse those factors. But it feels impossible for me to achieve and sustain weight loss. Repeated cycles of failure to overcome my weight problem have devastated my self-image. I have become progressively defensive, angry, depressed and withdrawn. The media and the Internet constantly reinforce my poor self-image.
>
> I can't remember at what point in time I realized that the looks I get from people around me are looks of disgust and loathing. No matter how good a person I try to be, or how much I try to please others, my good characteristics can't seem to break through. I feel there is literally no help for me. Even when I go to the doctor I am not sure they really see "me". The fact that I am 100 lb overweight doesn't seem to matter anymore – I don't think they really understand, or know how to help me.

As a medical practitioner, it is essential that you put yourself in the shoes of the person with obesity. The pain of obesity is profound and life changing. It must be met with empathy and direct, specific clinical care; not with bias, avoidance, or confrontation.

Discrimination, Prejudice, and Weight Stigma

Patients suffering from obesity experience widespread discrimination and prejudice everywhere they turn. The "big" person sitting in your front office is the residual personality forged from years of assumptions and negative reactions from society in general. A "big" person is unique in our environment. They may find it difficult to fit in, socially or physically. People avoid making eye contact with them when they are trying to find a seat on the plane. They cannot fit in many of the seats or booths in a restaurant. People watch what they order, and how and what they eat. The person with obesity often encounters open scrutiny from strangers, and can suffer verbal abuse and negative judgment from society as a whole. All of which, in turn, fosters depression and despair, adding to insecurity about their ability and self-image that may already be felt by a person with obesity. In adolescents who are obese, this discrimination often results in bullying and physical abuse [1].

Some of the most painful discrimination is suffered at the hands of family members, romantic partners, and friends. Women are more often victimized than men in these settings. In the workplace, up to a third of people with obesity are paid less and experience discrimination that includes wrongful termination, not being promoted or not even being hired [1].

The media is another source of discrimination, portraying people with obesity as bumbling, stupid, or negligent, and depicting obesity as a personality flaw, a lack of personal control, or as the object of humor [2]. The media often will focus on the cost of obesity to society for example in the increased cost of health care. The expense of obesity may also drive prejudice.

August 12, 2009, David Leonhardt of the NYT wrote about Delos "Toby" Cosgrove, MD CEO of the Cleveland Clinic, "Cosgrove says that if it were up to him, if there weren't legal issues, he would not only stop hiring smokers. He would also stop hiring obese people."

Creating a Culture of Safety for the Patient with Obesity

Before engaging in the specific treatment of obesity and related disease, I was no more "aware" of the patient with obesity than the average practitioner. I recall the day that we brought new chairs into the gastric bypass clinic that were "roomier" for bigger people. The first patient who came in sat down and then burst into tears, saying she had never been in a doctor's office where she had been able to sit comfortably and without embarrassment in a chair. What may seem like an obvious office necessity to you may be a symbol of acceptance and care to your bigger patients, signaling a supportive, empathetic environment.

– Robin Blackstone, MD

The Current Healthcare Environment Is Prejudiced Against People with Obesity

Americans persist in their prejudice against the person who is overweight and obese. In the last 10 years, prejudice against obesity increased 66 %, while prejudice against age and race remained relatively constant [3].

Physicians have the same level of prejudice as the general public and this bias prevents patients from seeking timely and effective medical care [4, 5]. Over 50 % of primary care physicians view patients with obesity as unattractive, awkward, ugly, and noncompliant. Moreover, 44 % of physicians feel they are unqualified to treat obesity and 31 % of physicians feel that treating obesity is futile. These same physicians rate the treatment for obesity as being less effective than 9 out of 10 treatments for other chronic diseases [6]. Research further shows that physicians believe that only 2.5–3.15 % of their patients are motivated to lose weight. However this view that patients with obesity are not motivated for change is incorrect. In fact, 30 % of female patients and 21 % of male patients with obesity are very motivated to change [7].

Physicians are not the only health care providers who are biased against the obese. Medical students report that the patient with obesity is most often the target of humor during training [8]. The same bias exists in nurses, dieticians, and exercise physiologists. The very group of people being counted on to care for the obese are so influenced by their own bias that, wittingly or unwittingly, they cannot help but negatively affect the quality of care.

What is your own personal reaction when you see a person who is obese? Do the feelings that come to mind invoke incredulity, curiosity, disgust, or revulsion? Do you immediately assume that person is ignorant? Lazy? Self-indulgent? These negative reactions are rarely hidden successfully from patients and they compromise a provider's ability to connect with their patient and engage them in their own health. On a broader and more far-reaching scale these negative assumptions and reactions provide the wrong leadership model for the clinical setting.

Changing the Current Healthcare Environment from Biased to Blameless

Changing the current healthcare environment from one of bias and prejudice to one of understanding and blameless support requires the identification and quantification of obesity bias in the staff, colleagues, and oneself. To this end, both **explicit** (deliberate/verbal behavior) and **implicit attitudes** (spontaneous/nonverbal behavior) are areas where physicians and staff need (1) sensitivity training, and (2) Motivational Interviewing Technique (MIT) training [5]. Explicit attitudes are easier to monitor and regulate if a no-tolerance policy against deliberate/verbal obesity bias is implemented; this in turn creates a blameless and safe clinical environment.

Tackling the implicit cues that patients receive, however, is more difficult. It may be best to start by doing an in-house survey. Consider administering the Implicit Association Test and the Fat Phobia Scale to yourself, your staff, and your colleagues in your particular healthcare setting. This will identify the level of obesity bias that exists, and will identify specific areas of improvement that can be discussed as a group.

Controlling and ultimately conquering obesity bias in the healthcare setting is not accomplished simply by providing staff with sensitivity and MIT training. A second, even more critical step is necessary: making staff and colleagues aware of the **biological bases** that causes obesity. Understanding the most current science surrounding the biological bases for obesity may be the single most effective catalyst that transforms the current healthcare environment from one of bias and blame to one of engaged understanding and optimal treatment.

The Blame Game: Why Blame the Patient for Their Obesity When We Do not Blame Them for Their Allergies, High Cholesterol, Hypertension, or Cancer?

Blame is assigned to the patient with obesity primarily due to one fact: the person with obesity is widely believed to be personally responsible for the lack of control over his/her weight.

Physician bias in believing that the patient is personally responsible, as surveyed in the Fat Phobia Scale, correlates with negative attitudes toward the obese [9]. Large-scale surveys of physicians cite lack of physical activity as the main cause of obesity, with consumption of high-fat and high-sugar foods as the second highest cause. Both of these perceived "causes" of obesity are directly attributed to the personal choices of the patient. In addition, 50 % of physicians feel there is an additional psychological or emotional component that contributes to the patient's lack of self-control, and may prevent patients from achieving weight loss [6]. Indeed, physicians often cite the patient's emotional "addiction to food". Addiction is a medical term attributed to a *physiologically* and *biologically* driven impulse, not an emotional or psychological impulse.

Based upon these widespread but outdated beliefs, physicians may feel it is acceptable not to bother "treating" obesity at all. Alternatively, the physician may become inconsistent in their efforts to address and treat obesity, leaving most patients with obesity to cope with their disease on their own.

The view that the patient with obesity is personally responsible for his/her excessive weight is, at best, medically incomplete. Obesity is primarily a physiologically/biologically driven disease; *not* primarily a psychologically/emotionally driven one. Psychological issues complicate obesity not unlike obesity-related disease complicates obesity. The current, widespread beliefs and discrimination surrounding obesity is based on an outdated and incorrect understanding of science.

The history of medicine contains a multitude of examples where prevailing, widespread beliefs were simply wrong. For instance, for many years physicians were taught and believed that stress, and the subsequent increase in acid production in the stomach, was responsible for peptic ulcer disease. Treatments were proposed and enacted upon thousands of patients based on this understanding. Then one day, a scientist demonstrated that the causative agent of peptic ulcer disease was a simple bacterium, *Helicobacter pylori*. The disease was treatable with antibiotics. Ulcer disease disappeared virtually overnight. Once the underlying medicine and science was correctly understood, effective treatment was established.

The science of obesity is in a similar state of misunderstanding. The limited education we give patients and the methods recommended to manage obesity are based largely upon societal preconceptions and one's own personal beliefs, not on the most current, informed science. It is no wonder the outcomes of one's "treatment" are poor and the disease recurrence (weight regain) rate is so high.

Inability or Unwillingness to Overcome Bias Against Obesity and Its Effects

If the bias against obesity in a particular healthcare environment is so strong it cannot be overcome that particular healthcare environment should limit the inclusion of obese patients. Initiation of the doctor–patient relationship in the clinical setting is voluntary. The American Medical Association (AMA) provides guidance to physicians in Rule 10.5, permitting the refusal of services to a patient if the required treatment is: (1) beyond a physician's level of competence, (2) not medically indicated, or (3) incompatible with the physician's personal, religious, or moral beliefs [10].

Although physicians are not allowed to refuse care based on race, gender, sexual orientation, gender identity, or any other criteria that constitutes treating a protected class of persons unequally in a manner that is malicious or damaging (i.e., invidious discrimination), this prohibition does NOT extend to overweight or obese persons, who account for nearly 66 % of the general population. More significantly, that 66 % of the population routinely seeks health care primarily because they have become sick with obesity-related diseases. Obviously, excluding 66 % of the population from your practice would be impractical and perhaps unethical. To remain relevant and have a successful practice, each provider needs to understand, educate, and overcome personal bias. These changes will better serve the majority of patients. Key questions to ask oneself are:

1. Are personal beliefs biased?
2. Is that bias promoting a subtle discrimination against the patient with obesity, thereby making your recommendations less effective or so off-putting that the patient with obesity does not seek timely care?
3. Are personal beliefs influencing the cost of care because patients who experience bias avoid care? Has the team considered how bias affects care and outcomes [11]?

How Obesity Bias Negatively Affects Medical Care and Outcomes

Discrimination and obesity stigma create a perfect storm. It starts with the fact that even patients with BMI in the overweight range of 25–39.9 kg/m² can have increased levels of obesity-related disease. As BMI increases, so does the prevalence of related disease (Fig. 2.1).

Large research trials have shown that patients with obesity-related disease (including type 2 diabetes, hypertension, high cholesterol/lipids, obstructive sleep apnea, degenerative joint disease, and/or gastroesophageal reflux) who also experience discrimination and stigma are more likely to avoid seeking medical care until the disease manifests in a higher acuity [12].

For example, breast and colorectal cancer are both associated with increased frequency and acuity at the time of diagnosis in patients with obesity. Yet regular cancer screening is less frequently accomplished in patients with obesity, despite the fact that preventive screening for both breast and colorectal cancer significantly increases detection rates [13]. This is just one example of how obesity bias negatively affects medical outcomes.

Discrimination and obesity stigma also affect the physiology of patients. In one carefully controlled study, the stress response of women exposed to video clips featuring jokes and vignettes about overweight and obesity was measured by their rising cortisol levels. The initial hypothesis was that women who were obese would have an increase in their level of stress and cortisol. Surprisingly, the results demonstrated that ALL women, including normal weight women, had an increased level of stress and free cortisol after viewing the material featuring abuse of the patient with obesity. This physiological connection between the patients' exposure

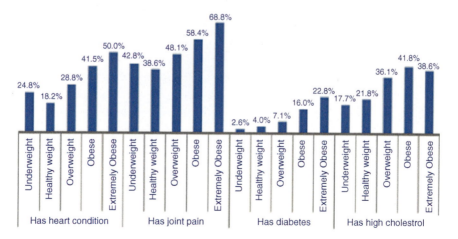

Fig. 2.1 Percentage with selected comorbidities by BMI categories, adults age 20 and older, 2009 MEPS (from Carroll and Rhoades [18])

to discrimination and increased stress may trigger additional adverse effects such as hypertension, high heart rate, increased blood glucose, and other physiological health risks that are caused or exacerbated by higher cortisol levels [14].

The Importance of Communicating the Measurement and Identification of Obesity of All Patients Within a Healthcare System

Many overweight patients are in denial or simply unaware of their level of obesity and their potential health risks. Thus, measuring and recording the patient's personal Weight Related Health Indicators (WRHI) (BMI, Waist Circumference and Body Fat Percentage) and sharing that information with the patient every time they encounter the healthcare system is of paramount importance if we want the patient to be informed of his/her current health status, and potential health risks [15].

Some physicians and psychologists have advocated NOT measuring or sharing BMI factors with the patient, as they are concerned the patient may get angry and defensive, or view it as discriminatory. Their main objection to measuring the level of obesity appears to be that it will increase stigma [16]. This view may be true when measurement and communication of BMI is haphazard and inconsistently applied from patient to patient. But rather than abandon measurement and effective education around the result, the goal can still be achieved in a way that avoids discrimination and bias. Making the measurement and communication of WRHI part of the standard process for all patients for every visit will accomplish this goal. Measuring and sharing a patient's Weight Related Health Indicators should be no different than measuring and sharing a patient's blood pressure, pulse, or temperature. In addition, this feedback should be provided to patients in a timely way so that it provokes a consultation/discussion of BMI and obesity-related disease, when warranted, at the earliest opportunity.

One way to facilitate that essential communication step with the patient to promote education and understanding of weight-related health is for patients to receive a color-coded "Weight Related Report Card" containing their vital statistics of BMI, Waist Circumference and Body Fat Percentage. The color assigned would reflect the individual's level of risk and reflect a composite risk score that accounts for how the waist circumference and body fat percentage affect risk (Table 2.1). This allows you to accurately and succinctly capture and communicate the weight-related health indicator (WRHI) data in a way that makes sense to patients. The electronic health record will allow validation of the risk scoring system by correlating the personal clinical history of the patient over time with the development of their personal history with obesity and related disease in a real-world setting.

For example, the patient with a normal BMI (less than 25 mg/kg^2) would receive a green card, unless his/her weight circumference or body fat percentage were above healthy levels, than they would be in the yellow zone. This allows for special

Table 2.1 Adult weight related report card based on weight related health indicators

		Range	Points	Score
BMI		18.5–24.9	0	
		25.0–29.9	1	
		30.0–39.9	2	
		>40	3	
Waist circumference	Male	≤40 in	0	
		≥40 in	1	
	Female	≤35 in	0	
		≥5 in	1	
Body fat %	Male	≤25	0	
		≥5	1	
	Female	≤35	0	
		≥35	1	
Health report card			Total Points	

Total Points	Health Report Card
0	Green
1	Green
2	Yellow
3	Orange
4	Red
5	Red +

populations, which carry weight centrally, to be more accurately evaluated in regards to risk. The patient with a BMI of 25–29.9 kg/m^2 might also receive a green card if his/her waist circumference and body fat are within a healthy range. On the other hand, they may get a yellow or orange card urging caution if either waist circumference or body fat percentage are outside healthy guidelines. The patient with a BMI of 30–39.9 kg/m^2 most often will receive an orange or red card, indicating a more advanced level of risk; however the system also accounts for the athlete who maintains a higher BMI but healthy weight circumference and body fat percentage (green/yellow). A patient with a BMI of 40 kg/m^2 or greater receives a red card, indicating that they are in the danger zone and need to take steps to immediately address the health risks they face regardless of any other factors. Risk is a concept often difficult for patients to grasp. The use of color-coded cards would provide a familiar paradigm of risk that people are used to seeing: yellow means caution, proceed with care and knowledge. Red means that continuing unchecked may result in a fatal accident at worst and a ticket at best. The patient may get away with running a red light now and then, but eventually the risk of negative consequences increases. This system of using the Weight Related Report Card (WRC) would open the door to an ongoing conversation between doctor and patient about obesity and its corresponding health risks. The WRC system might also provide an immediate, visible signal to the healthcare provider and team that there may be more going on medically with the patient in regards to a standard physical complaint. It allows for the rapid assessment of weight gain between visits and may suggest an association with a particular intervention, like prescribing an antidepressant or other drug that causes weight gain. A patient may say, "Last time I was here with an ear infection I was in the yellow zone, now I am orange. What should I do?" The Health Report Card for WRHI is a communication tool.

If **ALL** patients were to receive information about their BMI, there would be no "singling out" and no discrimination. Some patients may feel a measure of discomfort initially in being given their WRHI statistics and WRC, having themselves been in denial of the level of their obesity for some time. However, as they voluntarily seek help by coming to see a medical practitioner in the first place, where better to find it than with a trusted healthcare provider who approaches the problem with quantitative data, empathy, and a clear understanding of the new science of obesity.

Measuring patients' BMI and discussing the results with them may also avoid the "black hole" of obesity management. Consider this common scenario: The healthcare provider mentions, almost in passing, that the patient needs to "push away from the table" and get some exercise, or similar words to that effect. In a follow-up visit, it becomes clear that the patient has failed to lose weight, and the patient may feel the despair of failure. Likewise, the provider may feel frustration at what he/she perceives as a lack of compliance. This scenario is repeated over and over until both sides simply stop talking about obesity. Avoiding this "black hole" of treatment requires a deeper understanding of the actual biology and pathophysiology of obesity that, in turn, will translate into a treatment paradigm that actually works [17].

In sum, changing the biased culture in our healthcare environment is the crucial first step to effectively treating obesity and obesity-related disease. Discrimination and obesity stigma must be recognized and overcome. Personal beliefs and those of the staff should be objectively examined. Sensitivity to the patients' perception of stigma should be discussed, and specific training should be implemented to diminish and eliminate discrimination and bias in the workplace. Creating a blameless and supportive environment will allow you to approach this sensitive and difficult topic with empathy.

The second step in effectively recognizing and treating obesity and obesity-related disease is to implement a mandatory, universal, non-discriminatory protocol of measuring every patient's WRHI as outlined in Chap. 1. Those objective, clinical measurements can be used, where appropriate, to open a dialogue about obesity, obesity-related disease, and treatment.

How to Talk with Your Patient About Obesity—The Preferred Approach

Human beings have a tendency to judge others. Therefore, medical providers are trained to avoid the countertransference of negative judgment to patients while simultaneously remaining aloof from personal responses that might endanger the therapeutic relationship. This aloofness and distance is not the best way to engage patients in their own care. Patients want and need a personal response to them as people. In the latest Medical Expenditure Panel Survey (MEPS), overweight and obese patients received a doctor's advice about exercise or about the dangers of eating high-fat foods less than 50 % of the time [18]. Effective treatment requires an authentic interest in the patient's health. The traditional method in obesity treatment involves encouraging a patient to personally change his/her behavior through food intake and exercise. This foundation of behavior change will be a part of every treatment strategy currently available. To achieve that goal, the best tool is Motivational Interviewing Techniques (MIT). When these interviewing techniques are used consistently they are effective with patients who suffer from obesity [19].

MIT is defined as "a client-centered, **directive** method for enhancing intrinsic motivation to change by exploring and resolving ambivalence [20]." There are four tenets of MIT:

1. The expression of empathy
2. The development of discrepancy
3. Rolling with resistance
4. Support for self-efficacy

The Expression of Empathy

The first foundational tenet and best predictor of behavior change in the patient is the expression of empathy by the provider. In order to maximize this approach, it is critical that the provider/staff members first acknowledge and resolve any personal bias about overweight and obesity within themselves in order to achieve empathy in an authentic way.

There is a scale that is used to measure empathy to determine if the correct MI techniques are being used. It is called the Motivational Interview Treatment Integrity Scale. It measures "global empathy" as well as MIT "spirit," and includes an "assessment of evocation" (i.e., eliciting a patient's own reasons for change), "collaboration" (actively partnering with the patient), and "autonomy" (helping the patient understand that change only comes from within themselves). There are six recognized physician/provider behaviors that positively or negatively affect the provider's MIT "spirit" score

- Closed Questions (negative effect; avoid using)
- Open Questions (positive effect)
- Simple Reflection—a signal of understanding (positive effect)
- Complex Reflection—a signal of understanding that adds meaning to their reflection (positive effect)
- MIT Consistent Behaviors—asking permission, affirming their intention, emphasizing their control (positive effect)
- MIT Inconsistent Behaviors—advising without permission, confronting, directing (negative effect; avoid using)

The patient with obesity is in a classic decisional conflict: they are aware at some level that their obesity is having a profound effect on their health and life [21]. They will have tried many commercial methods of addressing it (buying books, dieting, joining a gym, going to a commercial weight loss program, etc.) but they really do not know much about why they are obese or what will really work.

The Development of Discrepancy

The discrepancy conundrum is that the patient with obesity does not fully understand the risks of obesity or the benefits of treatment. Once the motivational interviewing techniques are used to initially engage the patient, you need to go further and develop discrepancy within the patient using the same interviewing techniques to organize their thoughts. The development of discrepancy involves engaging the patient in exploring the pros and cons of his/her current level of obesity and discussing what action can be taken to affect change. In short, discrepancy involves developing awareness in the patient of the difference between their current state of health and their broader goals and values. This is the "active ingredient" of transformation [22].

After years of doctors appointments, many patients experience confrontation from their healthcare providers as an approach to coaxing behavior change. The confrontation approach is ineffective and is often born of the frustration a healthcare provider feels about a patient's perceived lack of compliance and lack of results. Many providers feel a sense of accomplishment when they diagnose hypertension or diabetes and prescribe a medication. On subsequent visits, the patient often has normal blood pressure or blood sugar as a result of the treatment protocol. The management of obesity is less gratifying in the short run and frustration can lead to confrontation rather than the empathy required to facilitate long-term behavior change. Consistency of effort, the essence of successful obesity management, is necessary.

Instead of confronting the patient, developing a sense of discrepancy will, in turn, develop self-determination in the patient. Self-determination theory begins with external regulation (like being on a two week "induction" diet) where external controls (the prescribed menu and "rules") are present and the process only works when those external controls are in place. The next step is introjected regulation, where a person puts pressure on himself/herself to exhibit certain behavior. This is very similar to what takes place when a patient adopts a set of rules (i.e., for the next few weeks I will be on a "maintenance" diet plan) and the patient then constantly deals with their compliance or noncompliance with rules they have set up for themselves. This creates an energy sink for the patient, causing constant conflict within them.

Most patients with obesity are either in external or introjected regulation. Ideally, the best place for a patient to be is in "integrated regulation," when they become intrinsically motivated to achieve certain goals that are part of their core values. "Intrinsic motivation" is most often discussed in the context of psychological behavior change [23]. Under the traditional model of treating obesity, the focus is on a psychological or emotional construct, not a physiological one. We should, however, be open to the idea that this model is incomplete. Intrinsic motivation can be viewed as incorporating an understanding of how the biology of obesity interacts with psychological/emotional motivation. MIT can help the patient manipulate their biology to achieve better health using consistent behavior to change physiology through epigenetic manipulation.

In regards to the current treatment of obesity, certain maxims are clear. First, in order to break through the decisional conflict of a patient struggling to overcome obesity, the patient must know their own burden of disease by getting consistent, reliable, objective feedback on their specific measurements of Weight Related Health Indicators for BMI, waist circumference, and body fat percent. Second, that information must be communicated to them on a consistent, unbiased, and sequential basis using a tool such as the WRC. Third, they need education about obesity as a biologic and physiologic response to the environment and they must be taught what treatment will work and what will not work. Fourth, the patient's expectations should be aligned with the realities of current therapeutic options. Fifth, successful treatment requires consistent follow-up and motivational/nonconfrontational support delivered with empathy. Simply asking about weight or talking generally about losing weight is not sufficient to engage patients in behavior change. It is necessary to know and use MIT in each encounter.

Implementing Specific Process for Chapter Two Recommendations

Implementing a philosophy of unbiased and effective empathy will require putting in place a specific process. The first step is a commitment on behalf of the leadership of the healthcare environment to establish a clinical philosophy of unbias and a therapeutic environment of empathy and effective treatment for the patient with obesity.

For Staff and Colleagues

- Survey staff, colleagues and self using the Implicit Association Test and Fat Phobia Scale to reveal bias.
- Require sensitivity training for all staff that includes education on the biology of obesity.
- Train staff on the accurate assessment of the WRHI and provide the WRC to each patient in each visit. Decide on a process for implementation within your healthcare setting.
- Invest in teaching staff and colleagues MIT and Self-Determination Theory.

- Include questions in patient experience surveys regarding obesity bias and stigma.
- Create a culture of "no tolerance" for jokes or comments that stigmatize obesity.
- Walk the talk: require that office snack foods brought into the practice be healthy, and do not accept "food" donations from patients unless they are healthy.

For Patients

- Communicate to patients in each visit using the WRC based on their WRHI. It is critical to accurately verify the **measured** height and weight of a patient, not just take their word for it. Most patients think they are taller than they are (Table 2.2)—Example of use of the WRC).
- WRCs are color-coded to communicate risk based on BMI, Waist Circumference (≤ 40 in for men and ≤ 35 in for women), and Body Fat Percent (≤ 25 for men and ≤ 35 for women).
- Measuring all patients across the board will reduce bias by not singling anyone out, and will provide essential clinical information to the patient, the provider and the healthcare system. It will make the level of obesity "real" and create an opportunity for engagement and support.
- Invite and encourage patients with a higher risk (yellow, orange or red WRC) to make an appointment with a trained weight specialist to enable the patient and healthcare team to gain a deeper understanding of the patient's personal clinical context (biology) of obesity, to assess related disease, and to develop a plan to

Table 2.2 Adult Weight Related Report Card based on Weight Related Health Indicators

		Range	Points	Score
BMI		18.5–24.9	0	
		25.0–29.9	1	1
		30.0–39.9	2	
		>40	3	
Waist circumference	Male	≤ 40 in	0	
		≤ 40 in	1	1
	Female	≤ 35 in	0	
		≥ 35 in	1	
Body fat %	Male	≤ 25	0	
		≥ 25	1	1
	Female	≤ 35	0	
		≥ 35	1	
Health report card		Total Points		3

Total Points	Health Report Card
0	Green
1	Green
2	Yellow
3	Orange
4	Red
5	Red +

lower risk. This kind of comprehensive visit will be outlined in the therapeutic chapters of this book.
- Establish a unique section in the electronic health record (EHR) that includes the WRHI data and WRC in dashboard format for easy recovery and sequential monitoring by the team.

Physical Environment of the Workplace

Provide a physical environment that is complementary to the culture you have established. Ensure that the equipment in your office can accommodate the level of obesity you are seeing:

- Chairs in the waiting room (make them all big to avoid stigma)
- Calibrated scale that measures body weight and body fat percent to at least 600 lb
- Extra large gowns (patients who are healthy body weight will feel good in larger gowns as well)
- Blood pressure cuffs appropriately sized

Conclusion

Discrimination and obesity bias are widespread both in society and among healthcare workers. Stigma in the healthcare environment leads to inconsistent evaluation and management of obesity, discourages the patient from seeking timely care, and increases the cost of care. The value proposition is not met adequately in this type of treatment environment and diminishes the patient experience.

The myth that obesity is a personal choice and not a matter of biology is the single biggest fallacy driving physician attitudes and behavior. Chapters 3 and 4 demonstrate the misconceptions of this paradigm and lay to rest the foundation of blame that has been the cornerstone of poor and inconsistent treatment of obesity by the medical community. Consistency in the management of obesity is a requirement of the healthcare provider. Every patient should be objectively measured at every appointment. Their WRHI should be clinically reported as a part of their medical history and should be directly communicated via the WRC to the patient.

To engage patients in their own health care, MIT and Self-Determination Theory should be implemented in a ubiquitous way throughout the healthcare environment. In order to establish an unbiased culture and to ensure effective treatment of obesity, educating all health practitioners about the biology of obesity is also of paramount importance. In addition, sensitivity testing and training must be ongoing to eliminate the explicit and implicit bias against obesity that may persist. Physically, the healthcare environment should reflect the enlightened culture of the practice in order to provide safe and optimally effective understanding and treatment.

References

1. Puhl RM, King KM. Weight discrimination and bullying. Best Pract Res Clin Endocrinol Metab. 2013;27:117–27.
2. Heuer CA, McClure KJ, Puhl RM. Obesity stigma in online news: a visual content analysis. J Health Commun. 2011;16:976–87.
3. Andreyeva T, Puhl RM, Brownell KD. Changes in perceived weight discrimination among Americans, 1995–1996 through 2004–2006. Obesity. 2008;16(5):1129–34.
4. Jay M, Kalet A, Ark R, McMCacken M, Messito MJ, Richter R, Schlair S, Sherman, Zabar A, Gillespie C. Physicians' attitudes about obesity and their associations with competency and specialty: a cross-sectional Study. BMC Health Serv Res. 2009;9:106–17.
5. Sabin JA, Marini M, Nosek BA. Implicit and explicit anti-fat bias among a large sample of medical doctors by BMI, race/ethnicity and gender. PLoS ONE. 2012;7(11):e48448.
6. Foster GD, Wadden TA, Makris AP, Davidson D, Sanderson RS, Allison DB, Kessler A. Primary care Physician's attitudes about obesity and its treatment. Obes Res. 2003;11(10):1168–77.
7. Befort CA, Greiner KA, Hall S, Pulvers KM, Nollen NL, Charbonneau A, Kaur H, Ahluwalia JS. Weight-related perceptions among patients and physicians: how well do physicians judge patients' motivation to lose weight? J Gen Intern Med. 2006;21:1086–90.
8. Puhl RM, Heuer CA. The stigma of obesity: a review and update. Obesity. 2009;17:941–64.
9. Pantenburg B, Siorski C, Luppa M, Schomerus G, Konig H, Werner P, Riedel-Heller SG. Medical students attitudes towards overweight and obesity. PLoS ONE. 2012;7(11):e48113–8.
10. American Medical Association Rule 10.5.
11. Lynch HF. Discrimination at the doctor's office. NEJM. 2013;368(18):1668–70.
12. Schwartz MG, Chambliss HO, Brownell KD, et al. Weight bias among health professionals specializing in obesity. Obes Res. 2003;11:1033–77.
13. Wolfe BA. Presidential address-obesity discrimination: what can we do? Surg Obes Relat Dis. 2012;8:495–500.
14. Schvey NA, Puhl RM, Brownell KD. The stress of stigma: exploring the effect of weight stigma on cortisol reactivity. Psychosom Med. 2014;76:156–62.
15. Warner CH, Warner CM, Morganstein J, Appenzeller GN, Rachal J, Greiger T. Military family Physician attitudes toward treating obesity. Mil Med. 2008;173(10):978–84.
16. Must A, Anderson SE. Body mass index in children and adolescents: considerations for population = based applications. Int J Obes. 2006;30:590–4.
17. Ahmad NN, Kaplan LM. It is time for obesity medicine. Virtual Mentor. 2010;12(4):272–7.
18. Carroll W, Rhoades J. Agency for healthcare research and quality medical expenditure panel survey (MEPS) Statistical Brief #364: obesity in American: Estimates for the U.S. Civilian Noninstitutionalized Population Age 20 and older, 2009.
19. Barnes RD, Ivezaj V. A systematic review of motivational interviewing for weight loss among adults in primary care. Obes Rev. 2015;16:304–18.
20. Miller WR, Rollnick S. Motivational interviewing helping people change september. 3rd ed. New York: Guilford Press; 2012.
21. Markland D, Ryan RM, Tobin VJ, Rollnick S. Motivational interviewing and self-determination theory. J Soc Clin Psychol. 2005;24(6):811–31.

References

22. Miller WR. Motivational interviewing. III. On the ethics of motivational intervention. Behav Cognit Psychother. 1994;22:111–23.
23. Pollak KI, Alexander SC, Coffman CJ, Tulsky JA, Lyna P, Dolor RJ, James IE, Brouwer JN, Manusov JRE, Ostbye T. Physician communication techniques and weight loss in adults. Am J Prev Med. 2010;39(4):321–8.

Chapter 3
The Biology of Weight Regulation and Genetic Resetting™

Key Message

The biggest myth in healthcare is that obesity is a self-induced, self-controlled problem cured by eating less and getting more exercise. Despite decades of treating obesity with traditional methods of dieting and exercise, progress has not been made. While these traditional methods are successful and repeatable in people who are merely overweight (BMI of less than 30), patients with obesity (BMI of 30 kg/m² or greater) have generally progressed beyond the "tipping point" after which traditional methods of weight loss become less effective. The new science of obesity indicates that this "tipping point" at which genetic resetting™ occurs is reached when adipose tissue dysfunction occurs. It is becoming clear that obesity is less an ongoing personal choice than a fact of biology: once obesity is established at a certain level of adiposity dysfunction, the person with obesity rarely escapes its grip or consequences.

Learning Objectives

1. Understand the difference between coding and non-coding genes and how the environment affects them.
2. Understand the genetic resetting™ that occurs when a person reaches the tipping point indicating adipose tissue dysfunction or "sick" obesity.
3. Understand how genetics, genetic resetting™, and the environment all impact an individual's propensity to develop sick obesity.
4. Understand how hormones send signals to the brain that impact an individual's feeling of hunger, feeling of satiety, and response to food.

The Canary in the Coal Mine

There is a legendary group of Native Americans who currently live in the Sonoran desert of Arizona: the Gila River Pima Indians. They are genetically related to the Pima Bajo that reside in Maycoba, Mexico. To study the natural history of obesity and its most impactful related disease, type 2 diabetes mellitus (T2DM), the story of these two groups of Native Americans is the place to start. Their story and contribution to medical research give us a new and critical understanding of how people become and remain obese.

The O'Odham Pima and the Pima Bajo have been partners in research with the National Institute of Health (NIH) and the National Institute for Diabetes and Digestive and Kidney Diseases (NIDDK) since 1965 and 1991, respectively. These studies prove that, over time and under certain conditions, the American Pima Indians have developed a genotype that favors obesity and T2DM. In other words, a majority of the American Pima Indians have experienced "genetic resetting™." This genetic resetting™ influences the MC4R receptor in the brain, which in turn is linked to thermogenesis and ultimately fosters a propensity to obesity [1]. The Pima/NIH/NIDDK studies show that this hardwiring of physiology by genetic resetting™ makes it physiologically difficult for an individual to get back to a healthy weight once obesity has been established. The studies further show that the weight loss is made even more difficult if the individual was "programmed" during gestation to favor obesity and T2DM. As a medical community we are extremely grateful to the Pima for their willing collaboration on these studies, as it has allowed us to significantly advance our understanding of obesity and T2DM in an unprecedented way.

The Pima Story

Around 300 BC a group of native Pima Indians migrated from Mexico to the Gila River Valley. There, using the Gila River, they built a sophisticated system of canals that allowed them to flourish economically, growing many crops including corn, beans, cotton, tobacco, and vegetables. They called themselves the O'Odham Pima or River People.

Although the O'Odham Pima migrated to Arizona, other genetically related native Pima Indians, known as the Pima Bajo, remained in a geographically isolated area around Maycoba, Mexico. In fact, up until 1991, the general public's only access to the population of Pima Bajo in Maycoba was over a rope bridge. Thus, the Pima Bajo in Maycoba have largely maintained their natural way of life, living off the land and remaining fairly isolated from the processed foods and more sedentary lifestyle of the modern world. In 1854, amid the territorial expansion of the United States and the Gadsden Purchase, the land that would eventually be known as the state of Arizona became a territory and gradually the two groups of Pima lost contact with each other.

Generations of the O'Odham Pima lived and thrived in the Arizona territory for centuries, growing their own crops and living off the land. In the early 1900s, the water of the Gila River that irrigated the extensive crops of the O'Odham Pima was diverted upstream and over time the river literally ran dry. The lack of water eventually destroyed the O'Odham Pima's ability to farm and caused widespread, chronic famine. The O'Odham Pima's way of life, their economy, and the balance between their food intake and their level of physical activity changed forever. Where once the O'Odham Pima had lived in peace and prosperity, they now had to deal both psychologically and physically with a drastic and devastating change in culture [2].

When the O'Odham Pima lost their connection to the land they became more urbanized; eventually becoming known as the Gila River Pima Indian Tribe. With urbanization and modernization the traditional diet evolved from all-natural organic homegrown food to a diet of modern processed food [3]. In 1929, the building of the Coolidge Dam and gradual water allotments restored the ability of the Gila River Pima to irrigate and grow crops, however, the epigenetic damage of the years of famine and processed food diet influenced the phenotype dramatically. Much of the produce grown by the tribe was not consumed but rather sold at market or fed to livestock [4]. The change in diet and lack of exercise from working the land promoted obesity to develop in the O'Odham Pima, bringing very high rates of T2DM.

Research Results: The NIH/NIDDK and the PIMA

The history of T2DM in the Gila River O'Odham Pima is startling: In 1900, only 1 case of diabetes was recorded in the O'Odham Pima [5]. In 1937, the O'Odham Pima were diagnosed with 21 cases of T2DM [6], a prevalence rate similar to the prevalence rate of the United States general population. By 1965 the O'Odham Pima had the **highest** prevalence of T2DM in the world [7]. A 10-year longitudinal study comparing the O'Odham Pima with a group of predominantly Caucasian people in Rochester, Minnesota indicated that the prevalence of diabetes in the O'Odham Pima was 19 times higher [8]. *The O'Odham Pima appear to have developed a unique predilection to obesity and T2DM* (Fig. 3.1).

In stark contrast to the rates of obesity and T2DM in the O'Odham Pima, the Pima Bajo of Maycoba, Mexico continued to maintain low rates of obesity and low rates of T2DM. The question became: why the significant difference?

A longitudinal study published in 1995 comparing the two groups of Pima resulted in many key observations supporting the current biological model of obesity and pathophysiology of T2DM. That study documented a prevalence of T2DM of 6.9 % in Pima Bajo versus 38.0 % in the Gila River O'Odham Pima, confirming that T2DM in the Pima Bajo was only 1/5 of the incidence of the O'Odham Pima. The prevalence of obesity in Pima Bajo men and women was 6.5 % and 19.8 % as compared to 63.8 % and 74.8 % in O'Odham Pima men and women [9]. In addition, this study included the group of nonnative, non-Pima people living in Maycoba, Mexico, so they could distinguish differences in obesity and type 2 diabetes rates in people who shared a similar environment with the Pima Bajo but who were not genetically related. The incidence for T2DM in this group of Non-Pima Mexicans in the 1995 study was only 2.6 %.

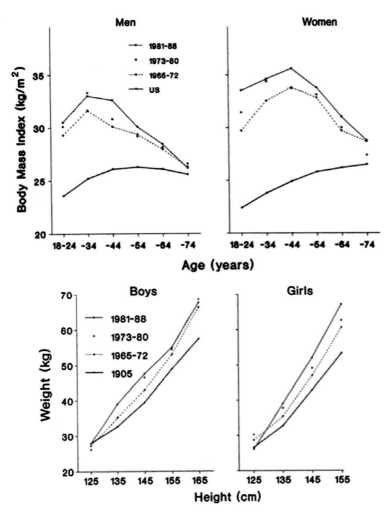

Fig. 3.1 Mean BMI in Pimas for three periods and in the US white population (from Knowler et al. [4], with permission)

A report comparing levels of T2DM and obesity between 1995 and 2010 show the remarkable result of increased exposure of the Maycoba Pima Bajo to the processed food of the modernized world and introduction of technology [10] (Table 3.1).

The difference between the prevalence in men and women is associated with increased work-related physical activity in men.

Table 3.1 Comparison of the prevalence of Mexican Pimas ($n = 359$) and Non-Pima Mexicans ($n = 251$) in Maycoba, Mexico 1995–2010

	T2DM 1995	T2DM 2005	Obesity 1995	Obesity 2005
Mexican Pima (M/F)	5.8 %/9.4 %	6.1 %/13.4 %	6.6 %/18.9 %	15.7 %/36.3 %
Non-Pima Mexicans (M/F)	0.0 %/4.8 %	8.6 %/9.5 %	8.5 %/29.5 %	20.5 %/42.9 %

Data from Esparza-Romero et al. [10]

Fetal Programming

The Pima/NIH/NIDDK research indicates a strong correlation between parents' high BMI and the onset of early adolescent obesity in their offspring and suggests that fetal programming is occurring. Fetal programming occurs when the intrauterine environment programs the developing fetus for future chronic diseases. In the case of the Pima Indian population, it has been shown that fetal programming is exacerbating the genetic predisposition of the Pima to obesity and type 2 diabetes. More specifically, fetal programming is responsible for a marked increase in obesity and type 2 diabetes within the 5–24 year-old age group as a whole, but particularly in children born to mothers with gestational diabetes [11, 12]. As the saturation of epigenetic changes has increased from generation to generation, the prevalence of diabetes has increased.

The Gila River O'Odham Pima in the United States demonstrate the serious consequences of transgenerational epigenetically driven mal-adaption to the environment: Currently 50 % of all O'Odham Pima over the age of 35 have T2DM and 63.8 % of the men and 74.8 % of the women are obese [13].

Application of Research Results to Other Populations

The research results of the Pima/NIH/NIDDK studies have now been replicated in nonnative populations and are generalizable to a number of diverse populations including (1) obese men in Utah, (2) people from France, (3) people from the United Kingdom, (4) the Chinese, (5) the Amish; and (6) people participating in the Framingham Heart Study [14].

Moreover, genetic analysis based upon the Pima/NIH/NIDDK research demonstrates that at least one major gene influences the risk of obesity and type 2 diabetes, and the "resetting" of this gene's expression, in turn, affects the age of onset of diabetes. Similarly, in many populations BMI has been genetically linked to obesity and T2DM on Chromosome 11 (d1154464) and Chromosome 1 (1a21-a24) [15].

The Pima story is critical to our understanding of how people become and remain obese. Their story and the studies run by the NIH and the NIDDK demonstrate that American Indians likely have a genetic variant that influences the MC4R receptor in the brain that is linked to thermogenesis. The studies indicate that the propensity for increased food intake and decreased energy expenditure relates to that gene expression variation and can occur in MC4R over time and under certain circumstances. When this hard wiring of physiology by genetic changes (i.e. genetic resetting™) occurs, it can make it almost impossible for individuals to change back to a healthy weight once obesity has been established. It is even more difficult if the person was fetally programmed during gestation to obesity, T2DM, and related metabolic disease [1].

The relatively small population of 11,000 Gila River O'Odham Pima Indians has contributed deeply to our understanding of obesity and Type 2 Diabetes. This narrative summarizes only a small portion of the important information arising out of the study of these good people. Their story and their willingness to partner with the NIH and the NIDDK for purposes of medical research provide critical and new insight into how people become and remain obese. More importantly, they may also have given us new ideas of how to attack the world's increasing burdens of obesity, T2DM, and other obesity-related diseases.

Calories in Do Not Equal Calories Out

The most often cited piece of advice for people trying to lose weight is to simply eat less and get more exercise. This assumes that the Law of Conservation of Energy is the operative guiding principle: total energy of an *isolated* system is constant. Translated into obesity language: The amount of energy you ingest (food and drink) less the amount of energy you expend through exercise results in weight gain, weight loss, or if they are equal, weight maintenance. The capacity for energy storage in the human body is impressive. A lean person stores 2–3 months of their energy needs in their adipose tissue. An obese person can store almost a year of energy. Humans as biological entities have to obey the law of thermodynamics, so if a person is obese, it means that over an extended period of time that person took in more energy than he or she used. Once an excessive amount of energy is accumulated and stored it becomes very difficult to get back to a lean physiology or to get lean and stay lean. Put another way, if your patient were to ingest 100 calories less every day but keep his activity constant, over 5 years that patient should lose about 50 lb (based on the law of thermodynamics). Instead, he ends up losing only 10 lb. If the same patient were to increase his amount of exercise by 100 calories per day, a similar result would take place, resulting in a loss of only 10 additional pounds. The question is why do certain people tend to become overweight and obese, and once they are obese why are they unable to achieve or maintain weight loss? Studies show this is true regardless of how personally motivated the person is to lose weight. *If an obese individual loses 100 lb and now weighs the same as a lean person of the same weight, that formerly obese person can only eat half as* much as the lean person in order to maintain the same weight, even if they continue the same exercise routine. What is the set of conditions that cause this to be true?

The Brain: The Control Center

The brain is the command center of the human body. The input to the brain does not connect through the frontal lobe where consciousness dwells, but rather through the hypothalamus of the midbrain. This part of our brain predates *Homo sapiens*. The hypothalamus and the impulse to eat is much less under conscious control than people realize. You can think of the brain as a "black box" whose only input is from the five senses, the chemical composition of the foods you eat and the input from body tissues (Fig. 3.2). When the brain senses that you are "losing weight" it makes an adjustment in its signals in an attempt to reestablish the status quo. In other words, the brain attempts to return you to the weight dictated by your physiology by sending signals to your body about hunger and satiety. If a person has been exercising, the brain reads this as an increase in energy consumption and it will send signals that influence intake of more food. If food intake has been mechanically restricted by "dieting," only a certain amount of weight loss can occur before the brain reacts to defend its physiologic set point by changing the body's metabolic rate and decreasing the amount of energy burned. As a health care provider, a recommendation that a patient lose weight to improve their health may be made, and if the patient complies, the result will be variable. If the weight loss is attempted with exercise, they will generally lose little or no weight. Feeling better and looking better is often achieved with exercise but it usually does not result in

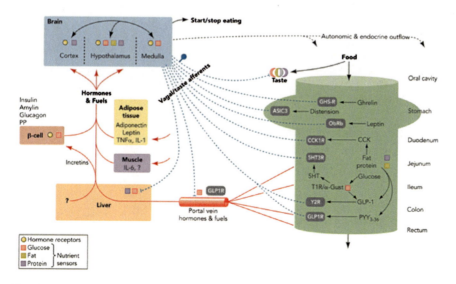

Fig. 3.2 Nutrient sensing by the brain (from Zheng and Berthoud [18], with permission)

significant weight loss. Decreasing portions and consistently curtailing food consumption or changing the content of the food eaten, may achieve initial success with weight loss, but the overall result is usually regain of weight that has been lost. Behavior modification through dieting or increased exercise works through manipulating the biological system of the body that controls weight. That system is constantly trying to achieve equilibrium. When dieting modifies caloric intake, or energy expenditure is increased by exercising, the status quo of the body's system is upset. At a lower level of adiposity, in the "overweight" category as opposed to the "obese" category, the patient has a better chance of being successful and their efforts are repeatable. Once the patient reaches a certain "tipping point" of obesity, the chances of success become increasingly difficult to achieve.

Inability to maintain weight loss is due in part to the fact that a formerly obese person will have to eat fewer calories to stay at the same weight as someone who was never obese [16]. Although this is often interpreted by the provider as noncompliance, it is just physiology. The brain's defense of the physiologic set point in that individual has taken place through this process of "metabolic adaptation" facilitated by genetic resetting™ [17] (Fig. 3.3).

Neuroanatomy

How does this input from outside the brain get processed? Within the hypothalamus (midbrain) is an area called the Arcuate Nucleus that contains two sets of "first order" neurons that give signals that cause either thermogenesis or storage. The first order neurons (POMC and AGRP/NPY) act on the second order neurons in the paraventricular nucleus and lateral hypothalamus to affect food intake and energy expenditure through action on the MC4R receptor pathway.

Activation of the parasympathetic system (AGRP/NPY) by the hormone ghrelin causes an *increase* in food intake and *decrease* in energy expenditure. Activation of

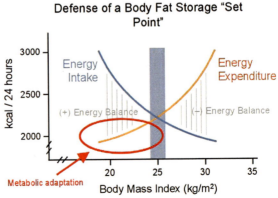

Fig. 3.3 Defense of the body set point (from Weigle [17], with permission)

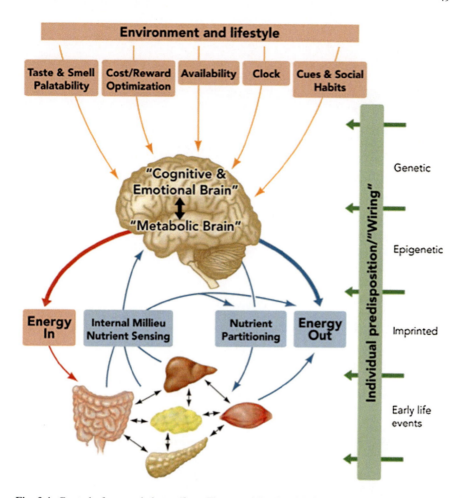

Fig. 3.4 Control of energy balance (from Zheng and Berthoud [18], with permission)

the sympathetic system (POMC) by leptin and insulin cause a *decrease* in food intake and an *increase* in energy expenditure. In short, the brain receives specific input from these neurons that activate or deactivate MC4R pathways.

Body weight is the result of a complex and highly regulated system in which the brain is the command center controlling numerous inputs [18, 19] (Fig. 3.4).

Genetic Resetting™: Setting the Stage for Obesity

Understanding genetics and how a genetic propensity to obesity occurs is the starting point. There are a number of mechanisms through which inherited genes and epigenetic modifications of genes during fetal development impact the onset of chronic disease in childhood and adulthood. Obesity is a heritable disease. If one parent is obese there is a 25–50 % chance the child will be obese. If both parents are obese the chance of obesity rises to 75 % [5]. Up to 67 % of human obesity is inherited as a polygenetic trait. Multiple studies of monozygous twins (twins thought to have 100 % identical genes) and dizygous twins (twins that share about 50 % of the same genes) have been cited to verify that about two thirds of obesity is heritable [20, 21].

The Double Helix—The Human Genome

It is a myth that environment is more important than genetics in the evolution of obesity. This myth was based upon the belief that inherited traits, while open to modification by the environment, were not heritable. It turns out that while modifications to the double helix of DNA (genotype) rarely occur, the "epi" genetic non-coding genes (RNA) do respond to the environment and allow for change to occur in the genetic expression of those genes.

The story of the discovery of genes specifically in the form of a double helix began in 1860 when a Swiss chemist, Friedrich Miescher, first identified a substance inside the nucleus of white blood cells that was different than other proteins. Eventually this came to be called deoxyribonucleic acid or DNA. Eventually, James Watson and Francis Crick proposed the double helix configuration of DNA [22].

DNA is essentially a blueprint of biological guidelines. DNA also contains highly complex RNA (ribonucleic acid) that instructs and directs the development and functioning of all living organisms and some viruses. There are about 20,000 genes distributed on 23 pairs of chromosomes. These 23 chromosomes and the genes they contain make up the human genome [23].

Due to the "double helix" nature of DNA, there are two genes (one from each parent) that are inherited. Genotype and DNA remain constant from one environment to another and from one generation to another. It changes or evolves extremely slowly, if at all. When scientists first presented the paradigm of the human genome, they believed that only 3 % of the billion bases in DNA made up the actual protein encoding genes. They further believed that 97 % was just random pieces of DNA embedded like bits of refuse in the sea of the double helix. It was not until 2012 that ENCODE scientists recharacterized that random 97 % of "junk" DNA as the essential regulatory switches, signals and directions that govern the interactions of genes and their likely response to the environment. It should be noted that the rules for how the 3 % coding genes evolve are not the same as the rules for how the 97 % non-coding regulatory genes evolve. In fact, although the coding genes are similar between mice and humans, the regulatory genes are different. The copying of DNA to RNA is a frequent process and that is the purpose of non-coding regulatory genes.

With the discovery of the regulatory genes there appears to be a convergence of the genes linked to disease with the appearance and location of these new regulatory genes. Studying both the coding genes and the regulatory genes and how the environment may impact them is leading to a better understanding of the disease of obesity.

Epigenetics and Epigenetic Modification (Genetic Resetting™)

While the genome itself (double helix) is not open to modification by the environment except over thousands of years, the **expressions** of the genes are exquisitely sensitive to the environment. Research and science have produced a new definition of "epigenetics": "the study of phenomena and mechanisms that cause chromosome-bound heritable changes to gene expression that are not dependent on changes to DNA sequence" [24].

The impact that environment can have on the genome with respect to obesity and the propensity to develop obesity is based upon the epigenetic modification or "resetting" of the regulation of genes. Epigenetic modification or genetic resetting™ can occur in utero as a result of the metabolic environment of the mother. This is called metabolic programming. It can be triggered by gestational diabetes in the mother or by imprinting, where one allele inherited from either the mother or the father is "silenced," allowing the other to be expressed. Epigenetic modification or genetic resetting™ takes place in both germ line and somatic cells, and these changes are inheritable. Epigenetic inheritance explains how populations like the Pima Indians of Arizona have achieved such high rates of prevalence of obesity and T2DM within just a few generations.

Imprinting

Imprinting is a type of epigenetic inheritance that occurs when a single copy of the gene from either the mother or father is silenced, allowing the other allele to be expressed. This is commonly found in genes that affect fetal growth. Prader-Willi, a syndromic type of childhood obesity, occurs from this mechanism. Imprinting is a relatively rare cause of obesity.

Intergenerational Metabolic Programming

While imprinting is a fairly rare cause of obesity; another type of metabolic programming transmitted through the fetal/embryonic environment has been demonstrated to occur frequently. If a woman develops gestational diabetes, the fetus is exposed to a high glucose environment that causes an increase in the risk of obesity and T2DM at an earlier age in the offspring. The prevalence of T2DM in Pima Indian children age 5–19 years who were exposed to an intrauterine environment associated with diabetes has increased over the last 30 years from 18 % (1967–1976) to 35 % (1987–1996). The propensity for early obesity and type 2 diabetes that develops when genetic resetting™ has occurred means that the propensity is inherited over and over again in a repeating cycle. There has been a remarkable rise in gestational diabetes in non-Native American populations, indicating there may be an increased propensity for obesity in general populations of children in utero. In other words, it is likely the same cycle has begun to manifest itself in non-Indian populations [25].

Further evidence that gestational malnutrition in general affects our adult offspring's health comes from studies conducted with people who suffered through the Dutch Hunger Winter of 1944. When the Germans cut off the food supply to a region of the Netherlands. Calories were rationed and during one five month period at the height of the famine the population was allocated only 400–800 calories per day. Women during this period still became pregnant and had children. The children were for the most part born at normal weight despite gestational malnutrition in the mother. Children born to these mothers, however, grew up to have higher BMI, increased blood glucose and higher lipids and incidence of heart disease [26]. Thus, both high birth weight and low birth weight have been shown to affect health in adulthood.

Convincing data on epigenetic modification or genetic resetting™ comes from a study by Anita Ost and colleagues on fruit flies (Drosophila). The study showed that feeding **male** Drosophila a high sugar diet before mating resulted in high triglyceride levels and modifications in the F1 generation. If a Drosophila in the F1 generation was fed a water, the Drosophila did not gain weight. If, however, that F1 generation Drosophila was fed sugar water, it gained weight quickly. After identifying the mechanism through which this modification occurred, the study then focused on the effects on chromatin and gene expression and mapped it to a specific area of the X chromosome. The deregulation, or modification, of two encoding proteins, one of which is SuVar, was shown to be involved in shaping the chromatin. It is this SuVar pathway that is impacted when the genetic resetting™ occurs, thereby authorizing a propensity for obesity.

The study went on to explore other species of mammals, including mice and humans, and similar genetic resetting™ was found. Obesity epigenetic modifications are passed on through both the father and the mother's genetic contribution to their children. Importantly the human studies included sets of monozygotic twins, one of whom was normal weight and the other obese. The obese twin had a genetic depletion in the SuVar pathway. Thus, even in twins with identical inherited DNA, the concept of fetal metabolic programming and genetic resetting™ explained why one twin was obese and one was not [27, 28] (Fig. 3.5).

Genetic Resetting™ explains the variability in response to treatment of obesity and related disease. Physicians can no longer assume that patients have not complied with recommendations when they fail to lose a substantial amount of weight

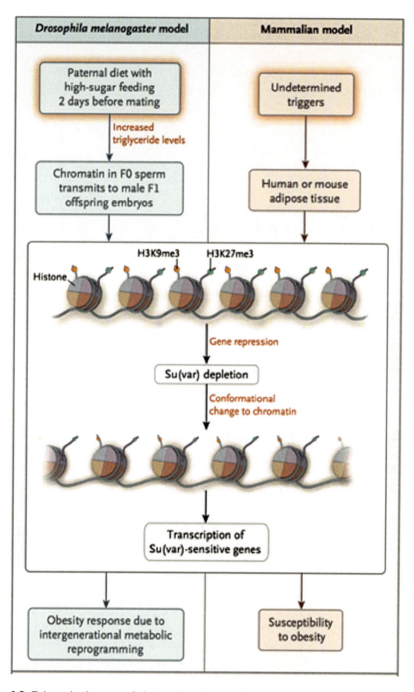

Fig. 3.5 Epigenetic signature of obesity (from Ozanne [28], with permission)

or regain weight. Each individual will respond somewhat differently to the same stimulus (diet, exercise, or pharmaceuticals) based on their genetic makeup and epigenetic changes in response to the environment.

Interactome Networks in Human Disease: Obesity

Perhaps the most important health-related discovery in the twenty-first century was the sequence and mapping of all genes of our species, Homo Sapiens. The Human Genome Project (HGP) was completed in April of 2003 by an international team of scientists. Since that time a group of scientists working in the ENCODE project have mapped that 97 % "junk DNA" that provides the non-coding "regulatory" signals and signposts that allow the body system to work. The totality of the resulting interactions is called the human interactome. It is increasingly clear that the impact of a specific gene product is not restricted to that one gene but spreads along and impacts gene products that are unrelated. An example of how this becomes important in medicine is demonstrated by pharmaceuticals: a prescription drug has site-specific interactions as its primary purpose, but also has "side effects." Side effects are the "other" signs or symptoms we see that develop in the patient who takes the drug. The drug may be serving its site-specific purpose, but may also cause diarrhea, vomiting, or itching. In a micro molecular sense, the side effects are the result of the drug interacting with the genetic "network" outside the primary target. Similarly, a disease phenotype (i.e., how a disease is expressed) is a result of pathobiological processes resulting from the interaction within these genetic coding and non-coding networks.

The complexity of the genetic network is challenging and the field of network medicine is evolving. There are many types of networks that can be mapped that reflect various ways of looking at how the body works on the molecular level and how it works in the disease state. These networks can then be cross-mapped in order to identify areas where similar molecules, processes, and epigenetic phenotypes are clustered. These clusters are then examined for genes and non-coding elements that are critical to a particular disease process. While the testing for these "candidates" to identify the genes of interest is often carried out in other species, once a gene of interest has been identified the testing can then be completed in humans that have and do not have the disease in order to determine relevance in human disease. The field of network medicine is quickly evolving and one major area of focus is the area of endocrine disorders: specifically obesity and T2DM [29].

Once a human baby is born, a complex set of interactions between the body's organisms and the brain begin to govern the health of that individual, including the governance of body weight and metabolism. Examining this set of interactions will yield more insight for the future as it relates to a person's body weight, propensity for obesity, and related disease. In the next section we will review the major signal drivers from the internal environment (i.e. the intestines, pancreas, muscle, and fat tissues) and the outside environment (i.e., stress, anxiety, sleep, and reward).

The Gut Brain Axis (GBA): Signals from the Gut to the Brain

The initiation of signaling takes place even before any food actually enters your mouth. It is the result of stimulation through olfactory senses, visualization of food, and even sounds that may stimulate the body's anticipation of eating. It has been shown that all of these mechanisms of stimulation prepare the body for food intake.

Of all the inputs the brain receives that impact body weight, the information the brain gets from the food we eat is the most consistent and necessary input. Eating is essential to sustain life. Taking in adequate calories and nutrients is essential. Food boils down to a set of chemicals. Different foods have different chemical signatures. Fat, carbohydrates and proteins are all significantly different chemical signals. The sensing of these chemical signals causes the brain to generate certain responses.

The Microbiome and Microbiota

Often called the "second genome," the human microbiome is a population of more than 100 trillion microorganisms that live somewhere within or on our bodies. It includes all the bacteria and archaea that support life and digest our food, synthesize essential components of nutrients, and protect us from disease.

Archaea constitute a group of single cell microorganisms. Initially classified as bacteria, they differ in that they do not have a cell nucleus or any other membrane-bound organelles. They do have genes and metabolic pathways that are related to the functions of gene transcription and translation. These organisms use a wide range of energy sources to fuel their work. They reproduce asexually. Initially the thought was that archaea only lived in extreme environments like hot springs. They have now been found to be present in many habitats, including the human colon and navel. Archaea in plankton are probably one of the most numerous organisms on the planet. In human beings they are involved in the digestion of food.

The Human Microbiome Project (HMP) is dedicated to characterizing these microbial communities and is looking for interactions that influence health and disease. Scientists increasingly regard the microbiome as a new "organ system" that, while established at birth, changes as we grow in response to internal and external signals. The microflora or microbiota in the gut is estimated to consist of 10^{14} bacteria and archaea, with 1100 prevalent species and about 160 species per individual [30]. Eating not only nourishes the individual but nourishes all the microflora that live within the gut. Depending on what food is eaten, different species live and grow and other species become less prominent. Some species of gut microbes are important to the story of obesity.

Most of the data that has been generated thus far in regards to obesity has been done using a mouse model. The data show that obese mice have different microbes in their intestine than lean mice. The type of bacteria that populate the intestines of obese mice is very efficient at extracting calories from food and in causing those calories to be stored as fat [31]. Initial work in this field demonstrated that the type of foods a mouse was fed influenced the type of microbes in their intestine. Diets high in fat and sugar and simple carbohydrates encourage the growth of the population of microbes that is good at extracting calories out of food and promoting fat storage. If these bacteria (microbes) from an obese mouse are transplanted to a thin mouse, the thin mouse becomes obese [32].

More recently, three different clusters of microbial compositions called "enterotypes" have been identified that are not nation or continent specific. While studies show there was no correlation with Bacteroides and Firmicutes, the studies identified genomic biomarkers that correlated strongly with BMI [33].

Most intestinal (gut) bacteria are established at birth. Children who are born by vaginal delivery acquire many of the bacteria of the mother. When a child is born by caesarian section, the bacteria established are different. Also, breast milk has some critical ingredients that feed the good bacteria in the intestine. During the period of time when many children began to be bottle fed with synthetic milk products, a polysaccharide was left out of commercially manufactured milk. That polysaccharide provided an essential nutrient to bacteria believed to be favorable to weight maintenance. The combination of increased caesarian sections and bottle feeding contributed to some health problems in the baby boomer generation, by promoting an environment of less favorable types of microbes in their intestines [34].

Ongoing research and ongoing reporting of results in humans are necessary to enhance the understanding of the microbiome and its role in obesity and health. The scientific community is working hard to understand how microbes in the gut can be manipulated by eating specific supplements. In the meantime, avoiding fat and sugar is a good place to start.

It is clear that changing our food "environment" affects both epigenetics and the microbiome. The Developmental Origins of Health and Disease hypothesis has proposed that early life from conception into early childhood, when the body is developing, is a time when stressors result in epigenetic changes in the individual that persist to cause disease throughout their lives. Classic Mendelian genetics does not account for these phenomena so attention has turned to epigenetic modifications and the most significant ones may be due to changes in the food we eat. Over the last 40 years, preserving food has become commonplace and is accomplished by adding chemicals that stabilize food in jars and cans. These preservatives contain endocrine disrupting chemicals that act as "obesogens" during the developmental period to cause the type of epigenetic modifications that can result in long term susceptibility of individuals to disease through disruption of steroid hormone pathways [35]. The term "obesogen" has been expanded to "Metabolic Disruptors" to better describe the effect of these chemicals on health and disease [36].

Why Eat?

It may seem evident that without food our bodies could not function. There are groups of people who eat very little compared to others and seem in many ways to be healthier. The function of eating is to use food to get the energy the body's cells need to do their own work. Food goes through three stages to become energy. First, digestion takes place in the gut where food is broken down into "monomer" units: proteins into amino acids, carbohydrates into sugar and fat into free fatty acids and glycerol. Second, these monomer units are then further processed in the cytosol through a process called glycolysis. Each molecule of sugar becomes two molecules of pyruvate and generates 4 units of energy (ATP) without the benefit of oxygen, so this happens even in anaerobic animals. For most animals (like humans) who require oxygen to live, the pyruvate ends up in the energy-producing powerhouse of the body: the mitochondria. Third, the mitochondria turn glucose from sugar and fat into energy through a process called oxidative phosphorylation. This energy producing process is very efficient as about 50 % of the food you eat turns into usable energy [37]. Like all manufacturing processes, there is a "cost" in energy. The usual aerobic process of glycolysis (oxidative phosphorylation) produces a net total of 38 ATP.

When the body switches from aerobic to anaerobic metabolism, only 2 ATP are generated. This difference becomes important when the stored energy in the body (adipose tissue) is used for fuel. In conditions of chronic over nutrition, the flow of fatty acids from adipose tissue overwhelms the machinery that manufactures energy. The body begins to function in an "anaerobic" mode where less energy is produced on a chronic basis [38].

Hormone Signals to the Brain

Much of the input that is received by the brain in regards to how the human body is functioning comes from the tissues in the body. This includes adipose tissue (adipokines), stomach and intestines tissue (incretins), pancreas tissue (insulin), and muscle tissue (myokines). The hormones in these tissues are the key hormones involved with hunger, satiety and energy homeostasis. The most active area of drug development for the treatment of obesity and related disease is in the creation of drugs that can interact with the receptors for these hormones.

Taste—Not All in Your Mouth

Even before food actually gets into the mouth the body is "prepared" for eating through visualization, sound and particularly the smell of food. This is called the "cephalic" phase of eating. The physiology of smell is particularly complex and sophisticated. Multiple inputs signal the brain that eating is about to start. Once food actually is placed in the mouth a whole host of hormones modulate what the response of the brain is to that food. *This is accomplished in part by the "chemical sensors" or taste buds that exist not only on the tongue, but also all along the gastrointestinal track.* The taste cells in the mouth detect sweet, bitter, sour and salt. Recently, receptors for fat and umami (protein) have also been documented [39]. As food passes along the digestive track it changes into its component parts (amino acids, peptides, sugars, and bitter compounds) that cause the local release of the hormone GLP-1 [40]. The small intestine also has chemosensors that result in specific signals being sent to the brain. Some of the key early information from the mouth is mediated through the sensory system of taste, adding information on texture and temperature of food.

Ghrelin: The "I'm Hungry" Hormone

Scientists have identified ghrelin as the only hormone in the body that stimulates appetite. Kojima and Kangawa identified Ghrelin, a 28 amino acid peptide, in 1999. The largest group of ghrelin producing cells is located in the stomach but it is also produced in small quantities in the small intestine, pancreas and brain. Ghrelin transmits a signal of starvation to the hypothalamus portion of the brain via the vagus afferent nerve. This activates the AGRP/NPY parasympathetic pathway and stimulates hunger (orexigenic). When a person is fasting the level of ghrelin starts to rise, peaking just before eating. Ghrelin production correlates to the times of day when one usually eats. Ghrelin levels decline rapidly after eating in response to the release of insulin and the increases in intestinal osmolality. Ghrelin is generally lower in persons with obesity than in those who are lean, with the exception of the obese child who has Prader–Willi syndrome, a monogenic form of obesity. Ghrelin is uniquely activated in the body in a way that is different than any other known hormones. This unique activation is present in all animals including fish from the depths of the Antarctic Ocean.

When a high fat diet is consumed, ghrelin resistance is induced by dysregulation of the signal to the vagus nerve. The resistance to ghrelin develops when the brain develops localized micro-inflammatory changes that inhibit the reception of the correct signaling, thus affecting ghrelin levels [41].

Ghrelin has a number of other functions in the body. It controls the secretion of insulin and is involved with promoting adiposity through storage of fatty acids. In addition, it crosses the blood brain barrier affecting the amygdala and eases anxiety as a type of endogenous stress coping agent. It causes the release of corticosteroid hormones as well [42].

Glucagon-Like Peptide-1 (GLP-1)

Glucagon-like Peptide-1 (GLP-1) is one of the incretins, meaning its primary function involves the release of insulin. In the process of eating, insulin release is first stimulated by ghrelin. As food progresses down the gastrointestinal (GI) tract, insulin release is stimulated by GLP-1. GLP-1 is primarily secreted in the small intestine in proportion to the amount of calories ingested, but it is also secreted to a small extent in the pancreas and the brain.

It takes about 10 min for GLP-1 to appear after ingestion. GLP-1 is the most potent cause of feeling "full," primarily through the action of insulin on the POMC receptors in the brain. People who eat very fast may not be able to generate this signal of satiety in a way that helps them control overeating. In addition to stimulating insulin release, GLP-1 generates a feeling of fullness by delaying gastric emptying after a meal, as well as acting on the pancreas to increase the number of beta cells that produce insulin.

Synthetic GLP-1 has been developed and is being used to decrease weight and improve T2DM. Part of the challenge in using synthetic GLP-1 is that there is a strong variability in response. One patient may lose weight and have improvement and another may not, or no reaction occurs. This unpredictable response may be due to genetic variability in the GLP-1 receptor [43].

Insulin

Insulin was discovered in part because scientists were searching for a cure for diabetes. The clinical features of diabetes were described over 3000 years ago in Egypt: excessive thirst, continuous urination and severe weight loss. These signs are commonly seen in type 1 diabetes. Physicians in India were the first to note that the urine of affected people attracted flies and ants. They called the urine "madhumeha" or "honey" urine. Apollonius of Memphis was the first person in 230 BC to use the term "diabetes" which means in Greek "to pass through". It was treated with bloodletting and dehydration.

Insulin was first injected into 14-year-old Leonard Thompson on January 11, 1922, and it resulted in a buttock abscess and systemic illness. A refinement of the fluid was made and he was injected again on January 23, 1922. His blood glucose fell from 520 to 120 mg/dl and urinary ketones disappeared. He lived another 13 years before dying of pneumonia. The discovery of insulin to treat diabetes became the flagship that convinced the public of the value of medical research [44].

The pancreas secretes insulin. The primary action of insulin is to get glucose out of the blood and into the cell by increasing the number of "glucose transporters" in the cell membrane. The most common insulin transporter molecule is called GLUT 4 and has been identified in adipose, cardiac, and muscle tissue. The translocation of GLUT 4 to the membrane of a cell occurs within 30 min of insulin stimulation.

Insulin resistance occurs when the ability of insulin to maintain enough transporters is impaired along with its ability to translocate GLUT 4 to the cell membrane. When we have sufficient energy for our needs, then insulin promotes the storage of glucose in the liver as glycogen, and it promotes the storage of free fatty acids in adipose tissue [45].

Cognitive Function and Glucose-Related Signaling

The three hormones we have reviewed, ghrelin, GLP-1, and insulin, all play a role in cognitive function. We often see an accelerated cognitive decline in patients with obesity. Type 2 diabetes also accelerates the decline that comes with aging [46, 47]. The physiology of these key hormones is different in an obese and diabetic patient than it is for patients with normal weight. Thus, it makes sense that some of the cognitive clinical differences we see in our obese patients are being driven at the molecular level by these same hormones [48].

A number of other gut peptides involved in the metabolism and signaling between the gut and the brain are also important in metabolism: CCK (Cholecystokinin), GIP (Glucose-dependent insulinotropic peptide), Oxyntomodulin and Peptide YY [49].

Signaling Through the Nervous System

The signaling system consists of the central nervous system (CNS), the autonomic nervous system (ANS), the enteric nervous system (ENS), and the hypothalamus, pituitary and adrenal glands (HPA).

The CNS includes the brain and spinal cord and often includes the retina and optic nerve (cranial nerve 2), the olfactory nerve (cranial nerve 1) and the olfactory epithelium. The olfactory nerves are the only direct communication between the CNS and the outside world.

The ANS consists of the sympathetic and parasympathetic nervous systems and is responsible for much of the process of living that we do not think about: body temperature, heart and breathing rates, blood pressure, **digestion and metabolism**.

The CNS and ANS cannot develop without the microbiome (the colonization of the intestinal bacteria) [50]. Without the signaling pathways provided by these neural networks to the brain, the body systems would not be able to communicate with the brain, nor would the brain be able to respond [18]. At one point the hypothalamus was thought to be central to the signaling pathways, but it is now believed that information input comes into many different parts of the brain: the forebrain, midbrain, and hindbrain. The areas that are receiving and sending input are all connected to each other and the signaling is coordinated (Fig. 3.6).

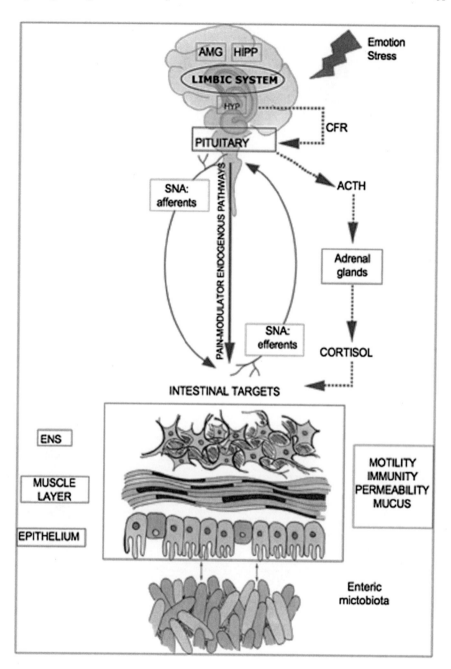

Fig. 3.6 Microbiome (from Carabotti et al. [50], with permission)

The Sympathetic Nervous System (SNS)

The sympathetic nervous system is part of the ANS and easily recognized as part of the system that exerts cardiovascular control. It also plays a key role in the regulation of energy homeostasis. The sympathetic system is activated by peripheral reflexes (arterial baroreflexes, chemoreceptors, and hormonal input) as well as circulating molecules generated throughout the body that cross the blood brain barrier to exert a direct affect on the medulla. For example, the SNS exerts control over peripheral process like blood pressure through input from and to the heart and kidney. The SNS modulates resting metabolic rate and thermogenesis based on changes in energy state, food intake, and exposure to cold and carbohydrate consumption. The effects of sympathetic tone depend on whether an individual is fasting or postprandial. Organs integral to metabolism like liver, pancreas, and skeletal muscle are also innervated by the parasympathetic system. Adipose tissue on the other hand, is only innervated by the sympathetic system. The sympathetic system is an important regulator of lipid mobilization, directly stimulating lipolysis. Leptin, an adipokine that crosses the blood brain barrier, is a direct modulator of adipose function [51] (Fig. 3.7).

In people with obesity, insulin resistance in the sympathetic system shows overactivation with higher levels of noradrenaline. Direct measurement of sympathetic activity shows a decrease in muscle sympathetic nerve activity in people with obesity. Insulin resistant individuals with central obesity display blunted responses after a meal compared to normal weight individuals [52].

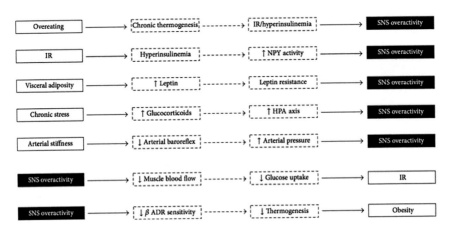

Fig. 3.7 Central nervous system and metabolic disease (from Thorp and Schlaich [51], with permission)

Parasympathetic Nervous System: The Vagus Nerve

All cranial nerves are part of the Parasympathetic Nervous System, a key-signaling highway in the ANS. The vagus nerve runs from the brainstem, along the esophagus, to the liver, stomach and small intestine. The vagus nerve communicates the presence and volume of food through mechanical distension and stretch as well as by signals generated by paracrine action (a hormone released locally that acts on the nerves). For example, afferent vagal fibers detect ghrelin and leptin made in the mucosal lining cells of the stomach. The vagus nerve has the ability to provide input to the brain throughout the gut in this way (90 % of its function) and also to communicate a response from the brain to the gut.

The Second Brain: The Enteric Nervous System (ENS)

The muscular walls of the gastrointestinal system, esophagus, stomach and intestines contain over 100 million neurons. This ENS network works together to control much of gut behavior in an automatic way, without specific input from the brain. The ENS also provides the electrical signals that move food through the intestines [53].

Conclusion

Obesity is much more complicated than an individual eating too much, exercising too little, or having a general lack of self-discipline. The chronic disease of obesity is the result of metabolic change and genetic resetting™. The environment surrounding a baby in the uterus and both internal and external environments after birth influence an individual's propensity to be obese. In fact, if obesity rates continue to climb and genetic resetting™ continues to occur, human beings may become increasingly affected from one generation to the next.

References

1. Muller YL, Thearle MS, Piaggi P, Hanson RL, Hoffman D, Gene B, Mahkee D, Huang K, Kobes S, Votrubs S, Knowler W, Bogardus C, Baier LJ. Common genetic variation in and near the Melanocortin 4 receptor gene (MC4R) is associated with body mass index in American Indian adults and children. Hum Genet. 2013;133:1431–41.
2. Russell F. The Pima Indians. The 26th annual report of the Bureau of American Ethnology. Washington, DC, 1904-05. Tucson, AZ: University of Arizona Press; 1975.

3. Ravussin E, Valencia ME, Esparza J, Bennett PH, Schulz LO. Effects of a traditional lifestyle on obesity in Pima Indians. Diabetes Care. 1994;17:1067–74.
4. Knowler WC, Pettitt DJ, Saad MF, Charles MA, Nelson RG, Howard BV, Bogardus C, Bennett PH. Obesity in the Pima Indians: its magnitude and relationship with diabetes. Am J Clin Nutr. 1991; 53:1543S–1551S.
5. Hrdlick A. Physiological and medical observations among the Indians of Southwestern United States and Northern Mexico. Bulletin. 1908;34:1–347.
6. Joslin EP. The universality of diabetes: A survey of diabetic morbidity in Arizona the frank billings lecture. J Am Med Assoc. 1940;115(24):2033–8.
7. Bennett PH, Burch T, Miller M. Diabetes mellitus in American (Pima) Indian. Lancet. 1971;298(7716):125–8.
8. Knowler WC, Bennett PH, Hamman RF, Miller M. Diabetes incidence and prevalence in Pima Indians: a 19-fold greater incidence than in Rochester, Minnesota. Am J Epidemiol. 1978;108:497–505.
9. Schulz LO, Bennett PH, Ravussin E, Kidd JR, Kidd KK, Esparza J, Valencia ME. Effects of traditional and western environments on prevalence of type 2 diabetes in Pima Indians in Mexico and the U.S. Diabetes Care. 2006;29:1866–71.
10. Esparza-Romero J, Valencia ME, Urquidez-Romero R, Chaudhari LS, Hanson RL, Knowler WC, Ravussin E, Bennett PH, Schulz LO. Environmentally driven increases in type 2 diabetes and obesity in Pima Indians and Non-Pimas in Mexico over a 15-year period. The Maycoba Project. Diabetes Care, PMID: 26246457; 2015.
11. Pettitt DJ, Baird HR, Aleck KA, Bennett PH, Knowler WC. Excessive obesity in offspring of Pima Indian women with diabetes during pregnancy. E Engl J Med. 1983;308:242–5.
12. Dabelea D. The predisposition to obesity and diabetes in offspring of diabetic mothers. Diabetes Care. 2007;30(2):S169–74.
13. Schulz LO, Chaudhari LS. High-risk populations: the Pimas of Arizona and Mexico. Curr Obes Rep. 2015;4:92–8.
14. Pakov ME, Hanson RL, Knowler WC, Bennett PH, Krakoff J, Nelson RG. Changing patterns of type 2 diabetes incidence among Pima Indians. Diabetes Care. 2007;30(7):1758–63.
15. Baier LJ, Hanson RL. Genetic studies of the etiology of type 2 diabetes in Pima Indians. Diabetes. 2004;53:1181–6.
16. Jou C. The biology and genetics of obesity—a century of inquiries. NEJM. 2014;370(20):1874–8.
17. Weigle DS. Appetite and the regulation of body composition. FASEB J. 1994;8:302–10.
18. Zheng H, Berthoud HR. Neural systems controlling the drive to eat: mind versus metabolism. Physiology. 2008;23:75–83.
19. Lenard NR, Berthoud HR. Central and peripheral regulation of food intake and physical activity: pathways and genes. Obesity. 2008;16(3):S11–22.
20. Sorensen TIA, Price RA, Stunkard AJ, Schulsinger F. Genetics of obesity in adult adoptees and their biological siblings. Br Med J. 1989;298:87–90.
21. Garver WS, Newman SB, Gonzales-Pacheco DM, Castillo JJ, Jelinek D, Heidenreich RA, Orlando RA. The genetics of childhood obesity and interaction with dietary macronutrients. Genes Nutr. 2013;8:271–87.
22. Pray L. Discovery of DNA structure and function: Watson and Crick. Nat Educ. 2008;1(1):100.
23. Griffin DK. Is the Y chromosome disappearing? Both sides of the argument. Chromosome Res. 2012;20(1):35045.
24. Deans C, Maggert KA. What do you mean, "epigenetic"? Genetics. 2015;199:887–96.
25. Dabelea D. The predisposition of obesity and diabetes in offspring of diabetic mothers. Diabetes Care. 2007;30(2):S169–74.
26. Roseboom TJ, van de Meulen JHP, Ravelli ACJ, Osmond C, Barker DJP, Bleker OP. Effects of prenatal exposure to the Dutch famine on adult disease in later life: an overview. Mol Cell Endocrinol. 2001;185:93–8.

References

27. Ost A, Lempradl A, Casas E, Weigert M, Tiko T, Deniz M, et al. Paternal diet defines offspring chromatin state and intergenerational obesity. Cell. 2014;159:1352–64.
28. Ozanne SE. Epigenetic signature of obesity. NEJM. 2015;372(10):973–4.
29. Stevens A, De Leonibus C, Hanson D, Dowsey AW, Whatmore A, Meyer S, Donn RP, Chatelain P, Banerjee I, Cosgrove KE, Clayton PE, Dunne MJ. Network analysis: a new approach to study endocrine disorders. J Mol Endocrinol. 2014;52:R79–93.
30. Tilg H, Kaser A. Gut microbiome, obesity, and metabolic dysfunction. J Clin Invest. 2011;121 (6):2126–32.
31. Turnbaugh PJ, Ley RE, Mahowald MA, Magrini V, Mardis ER, Gordon JI. An obesity-associated gut microbiome with increased capacity for energy harvest. Nature. 2006;444(7122):1027–31.
32. Ley RE, Backhed F, Gordon J, et al. Obesity alters gut microbial ecology. Proc Natl Acad Sci USA. 2005;102(31):11070–5.
33. Arumugam M, Raes J, Pelletier E, Le Pasiler D, Yamada T, Mende DR, et al. Enterotypes of the human gut microbiome. Nature. 2011;473(7346):174–80.
34. Stevens EE, Patrick TE, Pickler R. A History of Infant Feeding. J Perinat Educ. 2009;18 (2):32–9.
35. Newbold RR. Impact of environmental endocrine disrupting chemicals on the development of obesity. Hormones. 2010;9(3):206–17.
36. Heindel JJ, vomSall FS, Blumberg B, Bovolin P, Calamandrei G, Ceresini G, et al. Environ Health. 2015. doi:10.1186/s12940-015-0042-7.
37. Alberts B, Johnson A, Lewis J, et al. How Cells Obtain Energy from Food. In: Molecular biology of the cell. 4th ed. New York: Garland Science; 2002.
38. Lodish H, Berk A, Zipursky SL, et al. Oxidation of glucose and fatty acids to CO_2. In: Molecular cell biology. 4th ed. New YOrk: W. H. Freeman; 2000.
39. Laugerette F, Passilly-Degrace P, Patris B, Nieot I, Febbraio M, Montmayeau JP, Besnard P. CD36 involvement in orosensory detection of dietary lipids, spontaneous fat preference and digestive secretions. J Clin Invest. 2005;90:4521–4.
40. Chaudhari N, Roper SD. The cell biology of taste. JCB. 2010;190(3):285–96.
41. Naznin F, Toshinai K, Waise TM, Namkoong C, Moin AS, Sakoda H, Nakazato M. Diet-induced obesity causes peripheral and central ghrelin resistance by promoting inflammation. J Endocinol. 2015;. doi:10.1530/JOE-15-0139.
42. Bali A, Jaggi AS. An integrative review on role and mechanisms of ghrelin in stress, anxiety and depression. Curr Drug Targets. 2015. PMID: 25981609.
43. Jensterle M, Pirs B, Goricar K, Dolzan V, Janez A. Genetic variability in GLP-1 receptor is associated with inter-individual differences in weight lowering potential of Liraglutide in obese women with PCOS: a pilot study. Eur J Clin Pharmacol. 2015. PMID: 25991051.
44. Zajac J, et al. The main events in the history of diabetes mellitus. Principles of diabetes mellitus. New York: Springer; 2010. p. 3–16.
45. Steiner DF, Phillipson LH. Insulin Biosynthesis, Secretion, Structure and Structure-Activity Relationships. In: De Groot LJ, Beck-Peccoz P, Chrousos G, Dungan K, Grossman A, Hershman JM, Koch C, McLachlan R, New M, Rebar R, Singer F, Vinik A, Weickert MO, editors. Endotext [Internet]. South Dartmouth (MA): MDText.com, Inc. 2000.
46. Sellbom KS, Gunstad J. Cognitive function and decline in obesity. J Alzheimers Dis. 2012;30 (2):S89–95.
47. Messier C. Impact of impaired glucose tolerance and type 2 diabetes on cognitive aging. Neurobiol Aging. 2005;265:S26–30.
48. Chan JSY, Yan JH, Payne VG. The impact of obesity and exercise on cognitive aging. Front Aging Neurosci. 2013;5(97):1–8.
49. Perry B, Wang Y. Appetite regulation and weight control: the role of gut hormones. Nutr Diabetes. 2012;2(1):E26.
50. Carabotti M, Scirocco A, Maselli MA, Severi C. The gut-brain axis: interactions between enteric microbiota, center and enteric nervous systems. Ann Gastroenterol. 2015;28:203–9.

51. Thorp AA, Schlaich MP. Relevance of sympathetic nervous system activation in obesity and metabolic syndrome. J Diabetes Res. 2015;. doi:10.1155/2015/341583.
52. Straznicky NE, Lambert EA, Nestel PJ, McGrane MT, Dawood T, Schlaich MP, et al. Sympathetic neural adaptation to hypocaloric diet with or without exercise training in obese metabolic syndrome subjects. Diabetes. 2010;59(1):71–9.
53. Avetisyan M, Schill EM, Heuckeroth RO. Building a second brain in the bowel. J Clin Invest. 2015;125(3):899–907.

Chapter 4
The Biology of Adipose Tissue

Key Message

Body fat (white adipose tissue) stores energy and produces multiple chemical signals that communicate a state of health throughout the body. At a certain point in the development of obesity, fat becomes sick, causing adipose tissue to dysfunction. Adipose tissue dysfunction is the key tipping point in metabolic disease. Adipose tissue dysfunction is the final common pathway of inflammation and it induces insulin resistance locally (adipose) and distally (muscle, liver). A simple increase in fat storage is not sufficient to cause metabolic disease. Inflammation is the triggering event that causes adipose tissue to become sick and dysfunctional, leading to metabolic disease. This chapter will discuss the components of adipose tissue and the characteristics of different fat cells. It will also explain the role of hypoxia on inflammation and discuss the key metabolic steps that lead to adipose tissue dysfunction.

Learning Objectives

1. Describe the different types of fat cells (adipocytes) and other components of adipose tissue and the unique characteristics of each.
2. Discuss the role of hypoxia in the development of inflammation of adipose tissue.
3. Outline the key metabolic steps that lead to adipose tissue dysfunction.

Shakespeare acknowledged our perception of obesity in the character of Falstaff in Henry the IV. Falstaff gains weight because of the irresponsibility with which he carries out his duties as a nobleman. He hides his self-loathing in cleverness and humor, while also hiding the flaws in his soul. His weight fluctuates during the course of the play similar to the weight fluctuations experienced by many patients with obesity that try to diet. When he is given an office and has to walk, Falstaff slims down. Falstaff has a grand strategy: to earn his place in the court and get back his soul by dieting. Shakespeare's use of obesity is strangely prescient of current popular misconceptions. The stigma of obesity that was memorialized in Falstaff echoes throughout time [1].

Scientific knowledge about "fat" or adipose tissue has come a long way since Shakespeare. Since then, the science and physiology of adipose tissue has been advancing. The more we study it, the more it becomes clear that adipose tissue dysfunction is at the heart of most modern disease.

Adipose Tissue: Energy Storage and Endocrine Signaling

Adipose tissue (fat) is the most variable organ in the body. In a malnourished human, adipose tissue may account for only a few percent of body mass whereas in severely obese patients it can be over 50 % of the total mass of the body [2]. The primary role of adipose tissue is the storage of excess energy. Obesity is defined as an excessive accumulation of adipose tissue. Adipose tissue is also increasingly recognized as an "endocrine organ". In 1994, Douglas Coleman and Jeffery Friedman discovered the adipokine (cell signaling protein produced by adipose tissue) called leptin. Their studies of leptin demonstrated that adipose tissue plays a critical role in the signaling and regulation of metabolism. Since that time, over 600 adipokines have been discovered [3]. These protein and chemical signals exert a major influence over the complex system of metabolism, hunger, and satiety. Adipose tissue has multiple components and contributes to both health and disease.

The Development of Adipose Tissue

Adipose tissue first appears in the fetus during the second trimester. Subcutaneous adipose tissue develops before intra-abdominal adipose tissue and brown adipose tissue (BAT) develops before white adipose tissue (WAT). The primary location of fat storage is in adipocytes located in a specific location called a "depot." The primary fat depot is in the subcutaneous tissue of the body. The ability of subcutaneous fat cells to take up a large amount of lipid acts as a "buffer" to prevent fat from accumulating in places where the metabolic consequences are more impactful. In particular, intra-abdominal storage of fat is associated with a higher incidence of insulin resistance and "metabolic" diseases like diabetes.

Adipose depots are heterogeneous, with different locations expressing different compositions of cell types and different responsiveness to postnatal environmental factors.

Adipose tissue is highly structured and contains a number of different cell types, including stem cell-like precursors called preadipocytes, adipose cells (White, BRITE/Beige, and Brown), macrophages (resident in fat tissue as well as recruited by hypoxia and other stimulation to the fat depot), extracellular matrix and blood vessels, lymph vessels and nerves. The vast majority of the cells in adipose tissue are not mature adipocytes. This complex milieu is dynamic, not static, and intimately related to multiple stimuli.

Adipose tissue is a large reservoir of mesenchymal stem cells that are progenitors of multiple cell lines in the postnatal human [4]. The $CD24^+$ mesenchymal stem cell in adipose tissue matures into preadipocytes and adipocytes under the influence of specific chemical signaling [5, 6]. Preadipocytes occupy a perivascular "niche" prior to differentiating into adipocytes. Adipocytes have markers of shared lineage with other types of cells in the body including muscle (BAT and BRITE cells) and vascular endothelium (WAT) [7].

The Structure of Adipose Tissue

The Adipocyte

There are three types of fat cells (adipocytes): White, BRITE (also called Beige), and Brown. Each has its own unique properties. White adipocytes and BRITE/Beige adipocytes are derived from precursor cells that look like cells in nearby types of tissue, while Brown Adipocytes come from muscle-like precursor cells.

Brown Adipose Tissue (BAT)

Brown (BAT) is made up of brown adipocytes that are highly oxidative. Areas in the body that have a concentration of BAT, once believed to exist only in infants, have been identified in adult humans. Brown adipocytes have an abundance of mitochondria. In most tissue types, mitochondria are the central organelle of a cell that converts fatty acids to energy. Brown adipocytes are unique in having a specific uncoupling protein 1 (UPC1) that allows mitochondria to convert fatty acids to heat. There are hopes that humans can lose weight by increasing the activity or amount of BAT; however, it is unclear whether there is enough BAT to increase thermogenesis to a degree necessary to control weight [8, 9].

White Adipose Tissue (WAT)

White adipocytes are the main components in WAT. The function of the white adipocyte is to store triglycerides that can be mobilized as energy during periods of fasting and to produce protein hormones that influence metabolism (Figs. 4.1 and 4.2).

The overall number of adipocytes is stabilized during childhood and early adolescence. In some fat depots, the number of fat cells can increase (hyperplasia) however, most of the increase in adipose tissue mass comes from the storage of

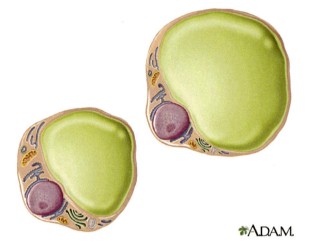

Fig. 4.1 White adipocte (copyright © 2016 A.D.A.M., Inc. All rights reserved)

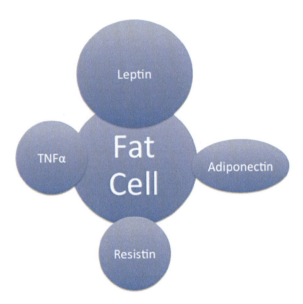

Fig. 4.2 Adipocte as an endocrine cell (data from Kershaw and Flier [48])

increasing amounts of lipid within each cell (hypertrophy). The capability of subcutaneous WAT to hyperplasia and hypertrophy "buffers" other organs against ectopic fat storage [10]. In times of chronic overeating, the buffering capacity of subcutaneous adipose tissue depots is exceeded, causing storage in ectopic locations and continuous lipolysis.

White adipocytes can be remodeled under certain stimuli to transform into a more oxidative phenotype resembling brown fat cells [11]. This "browning" of white adipocytes results in the BRITE (brown and white—also called beige) cell. BRITE cells share lineage with brown adipocytes and generate heat energy. BRITE cells are stimulated in response to cold, exercise, and lactate. The "browning" of WAT to acquire adipocytes with the BRITE phenotype may be a response to the lactate produced by oxidative stress [12]. When the stimulus stops the cell goes back to white [13].

Macrophages

Macrophages exist as resident cells within white fat depots and they are also recruited to white fat in response to injury or hypoxia. Some macrophages (M1) are pro-inflammatory and associated with immune defense and insulin resistance. Macrophages produce a number of hormone proteins that contribute to inflammation, IL-6 being perhaps the most studied. Other macrophages (M2) are involved in tissue repair and may also play a role in preventing excessive free fatty acid during weight loss/lipolysis. M2 macrophages also secrete catecholamine in response to stress, like exposure to cold, and are implicated in the browning of fat cells. As adipose tissue accumulates, neutrophil infiltration precedes macrophage infiltration. Phenotypic switching to pro-inflammatory macrophages causes chronic low-grade inflammation [10].

Extracellular Matrix (ECM)

The extracellular matrix (ECM) provides structural support to adipose tissue and produces biochemical signals that influence mesenchymal stem cell differentiation. Preadipocytes play an important role in the development and maintenance of healthy ECM. The ECM has the capability of undergoing extensive remodeling to accommodate expanding fat mass. When the ECM has to react to chronic injury including hypoxia and adipose cell death, it forms a fibrotic architecture that impairs the function of adipocytes and other types of parenchymal cells. This loss of elasticity may cause ectopic storage of fat in metabolically more active sites.

Adipose Tissue Blood Flow and Innervation

Blood flow is an important conduit of oxygen, lipid transportation, and hormonal signaling. A lean individual in a fasting state has higher blood flow than people with obesity. People with obesity have lower capillary density in abdominal fat and subcutaneous fat, despite having larger blood vessels [14]. The lower blood flow in the patient with obesity is further impaired if they are insulin resistant. During exercise the blood flow to muscle is increased but the blood flow to fat is decreased [15]. The sympathetic nervous system is involved in regulating blood flow and fatty acid mobilization in WAT and BAT and mediated through catecholamines or by "alternatively activated" macrophages that stimulate lipolysis and thermogenic gene expression in brown fat [16].

Lipogenesis and Lipolysis: How Fat Is Stored and How It Is Used For Energy

Dietary fat is a source of energy, second only to glucose. Both glucose and fat are metabolized for energy production concurrently. Relative contributions depend on the state of the body at any given time including genetics, diet, activity level, and environment. Fat is released from fat depots through a process called lipolysis.

Dietary fat has three possible fates: it can be stored as fat in adipocytes, it can be used for energy, or it can be reconstituted as very low-density lipoproteins and recycled.

Dietary fat has to be handled in a special way by the body in order to be absorbed. Think about trying to wash a dinner plate with fat on it: when you try to clean it with just water the fat sticks to the plate because fat is insoluble in water. In order to get the fat off the plate you have to use soap. Similarly, when you ingest fat as part of a meal, it cannot be absorbed through the wall of the intestine without special treatment to make the fat absorbable.

Digestion starts in the mouth. Small amounts of lipase produced in the mouth and stomach begin the process. The liver produces bile that flows through the bile ducts into the duodenum and mixes with fat coming from the stomach. The bile is like soap; it breaks down and emulsifies fat. The bile acids stimulate the production of enzymes from the pancreas, including pancreatic lipase. Pancreatic lipase is the primary enzyme that breaks down dietary fat into monoglycerides and free fatty acids. Pancreatic lipase is so efficient in breaking down fat that only less than 10 % of dietary fat remains unchanged in the intestine. Two key fatty acids are produced in this process: short chain fatty acids and long chain fatty acids.

Short chain fatty acids (12 carbons or less) are absorbed directly through the wall of the intestine. They enter the blood stream, and move directly to the liver where they are processed for energy.

Long chain fatty acids (more than 12 carbons) and cholesterol are not transported to the liver but are processed in the epithelial cells that line the intestine and are then transported through the lymph system for storage in fat cells (adipocytes). The majority of all absorbed fatty acids are processed through the lymphatic system and stored in adipocytes, a process called lipogenesis. In a state of chronic overnutrition, triglycerides are stored as fat in subcutaneous depots. When it is needed, stored fat is liberated and used for energy.

The primary source of energy is glucose. Early during a fasting period, glycogen stored in the liver is broken down into glucose. There is only enough glycogen to last for a few hours. After that, as starvation continues, the body uses glucose made from proteins and fat. Fat is broken down into fatty acids and glycerol. Fatty acids are used by skeletal muscle for energy, conserving glucose for use by the brain. As fasting continues, fatty acids are converted in the liver to ketone bodies that can be utilized by the brain for energy. Most tissues in the body can use fatty acids as an energy source. Exercising muscle uses both glucose and fatty acids with the relative contribution depending on the intensity of the exercise.

When energy is needed, fatty acids are liberated through the process of lipolysis. When lipolysis occurs in a person with obesity, it produces excessive glucose and fatty acids flow into the mitochondria. An increased demand for the processing of these substrates results in apoptosis, DNA damage, and maladaptive signaling within inflammatory pathways [17]. The resulting toxic internal environment is termed lipotoxicity. Clinically, the patient with lipotoxicity experiences increased fatigue and premature aging. Changes in fatty acid synthesis and metabolism occur when a person is in a state of insulin resistance and has type 2 diabetes. Insulin enhances fat storage.

Not all people who have an excess of body fat become metabolically sick. On the other hand, there are lean people who have a relatively small amount of central body fat who develop metabolic disease.

The Tipping Point: Inflammation and Adipose Tissue Dysfunction

The tipping point within human beings that distinguishes those simply having a high BMI from those being sick with a particular amount of fat tissue (adipose tissue dysfunction) is related to the presence of inflammation within the adipocytes (fat cells) (Fig. 4.3). Inflammation is widely considered to be the instigator of metabolic disease. The etiology of inflammation is probably not the result of just one defect, but the resulting state of multiple defects, the sum of which may indicate the level and intensity of metabolic disease [18]. A few strong theories have emerged that cite hypoxia as one critical stimulus of adipose tissue dysfunction.

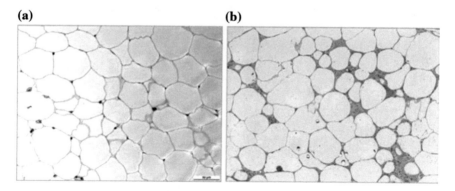

Fig. 4.3 **a** Insulin sensitive obesity. **b** Insulin-resistant obesity

Hypoxia and Inflammation in White Adipose Tissue

Oxygen is a critical nutrient for the body. Ambient oxygen in the air is about 21 % but the level of oxygen in the tissue is lower. Sensing of oxygen occurs first in the carotid body and on a molecular level in tissues that utilize oxygen by hypoxia inducible factor (HIF1). When available oxygen is low, as it is at higher altitudes for example, multiple adaptations take place throughout the body. At the cellular level, this adaptation is controlled by HIF1. This reduces the production of harmful reactive oxygen species (Fig. 4.4). When hypoxia occurs, there is an increase in Cori Cycle activity precipitated by the increase in HIF1. Hepatic lactate uptake and gluconeogenesis are increased. The shift to the Cori Cycle requires less oxygen but the energy production is limited to 2 ATP for each molecule of glucose metabolized and a consumption of 6 ATP for each of 2 ATP formed from lactate (Fig. 4.5). Thus, going to a higher altitude results in an energy wasting state with production of glucose and an increase in basal metabolic rate, as energy is required for the process to take place.

A low oxygen or hypoxic state can also exist within body tissues. A well-known example occurs when a tumor becomes hypoxic. As it grows, the tumor consists of rapidly dividing cells that require an extremely high amount of energy. The blood supply cannot keep pace with the rapid growth and the tumor outgrows its blood supply.

Why is hypoxia important to a discussion about adipose (fat) tissue and obesity? There is evidence that WAT becomes hypoxic as the fat cells increase in number and

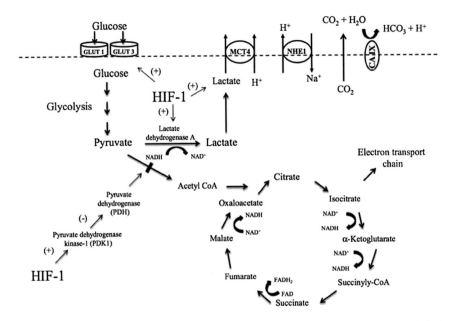

Fig. 4.4 Inflammation of omental adipose tissue (from Palmer and Clegg [20], with permission)

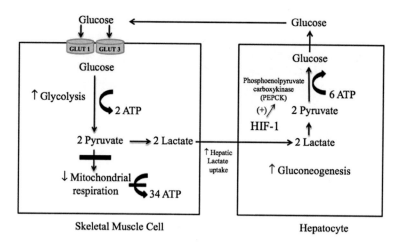

Fig. 4.5 Cori Cycle activity enhanced by hypoxia (from Palmer and Clegg [20], with permission)

overall mass expands in size. This is similar to the growing tumor because the fat cells' need for energy outstrips the supply and hypoxia results. When hypoxia occurs, there is a decrease in the removal of fatty acids from blood circulation and the WAT loses its ability to "buffer" fat stores, thereby encouraging ectopic deposits of WAT. At the cellular level, hypoxia causes a shift from oxidative energy production to lactate production [19]. Lactate is not simply the result of the switch to anaerobic metabolism. Lactate is a complex signaling chemical that sets up a state of insulin resistance in muscle and is, in part, responsible for metabolic disease in people who are obese [20]. Hypoxia also encourages the invasion of macrophages into WAT and the activation of macrophages that are already a part of the WAT. These macrophages make powerful inflammatory proteins, including IF-6. In individuals who are obese, high levels of circulating inflammatory markers are consistently demonstrated.

WAT is poorly vascularized. In a person who is obese, blood flow does not increase in response to feeding [21]. Recent studies of continuously measured levels of interstitial oxygen showed that people with obesity actually had higher oxygen levels (80 mm Hg) versus lean individuals (60 mm Hg) [22]. In addition, the utilization of oxygen in the adipocytes of a person with obesity is lower than that of a lean person. The increased levels of oxygen in the interstitium may be due to lower oxygen utilization within the adipocytes. The adipocytes of persons with obesity have a lower metabolic rate compared to persons who are lean [23]. There is additional evidence for hypoxia in white fat cell depots. This evidence is seen in the increase of macrophages, the increase in the level of lactate, and the amplification of oxygen-sensitive genes that increase the production of leptin. Hypoxia within adipose tissue contributes to dysfunction through multiple pathways in a strongly interconnected network of disease.

A study of moderate hypoxia (15 %) shows an increase in insulin sensitivity in men with obesity, indicating that the response to hypoxia may actually be a type of "protective" mechanism [24]. A short abrupt change in total body oxygenation (sleep apnea) seems unlikely to produce the hypoxia that increases inflammation. Therefore the current belief is that hypoxia in a setting of insulin resistance and the production of inflammatory markers may initially be protective, but eventually becomes detrimental to the environment, further worsening the metabolic situation and enhancing lipolysis.

Currently there is ongoing work to clarify the relationship between hypoxia and metabolic disease. Patterns of fat distribution and the severity and duration of hypoxia may be important factors for determining levels of inflammation. In other words, severity of inflammation due to hypoxia may vary depending on fat depot locations.

Hypoxia plays a role in stimulating inflammation in adipose tissue, but there are also other ways to account for the inflammatory cascade.

Adipocytes die as part of the natural process of revitalization of the tissue. This process is called apoptosis. Cell death calls inflammatory macrophages to the area. The macrophages surround the dead adipocyte and form a crown-like structure that triggers a local inflammatory response. Crown structures are also seen in inflammation associated with cancer, particularly in the breast [25].

Inflammation has a cascade-like effect on other body tissues by interrupting the balance between storage of fatty acids and mobilization of fatty acids. Inflammation also produces chemicals signals that impair the signaling of insulin. It also promotes fibrosis, promoting more insulin resistance in the adipose tissue itself [26].

Inflammation and insulin resistance are part of the internal environment of obesity and are often precipitated by products of the adipocyte itself: adipokines.

Adipokines: Leptin and Adiponectin

Adipokines from adipose tissue regulate a wide variety of physiologic process in the body and affect far more types of tissue than previously realized. These adipokines are highly integrated into the system of metabolic control [27] (Fig. 4.6). In addition, they are increasingly regarded as biomarkers of the relative health or sickness of adipose tissue and even predictors of mortality from metabolic disease [28]. Adipokines have been used on a limited basis to treat specific deficiencies and have wider applications for the treatment of disease in the future despite significant challenges in translational research [29].

Leptin

Leptin is known as the "satiety hormone". It is a hormone that controls hunger and the feeling of satiety. Leptin is secreted by adipose (fat) tissue, so the more overweight a person is, typically the higher the level of leptin.

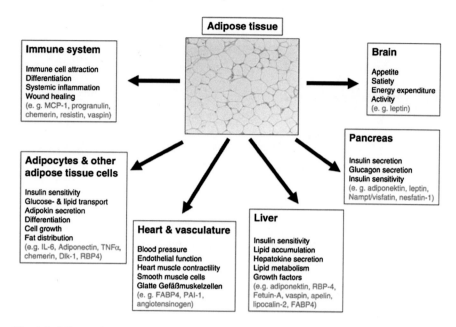

Fig. 4.6 Adipose tissue and adipokine regulation of physiology (from Bluher and Mantzoros [49], with permission)

The discovery of leptin in 1994 changed the science of obesity in a profound way because it helped to demonstrate the connection between adipose tissue and disease. Leptin has a number of properties that are important to our understanding of how metabolism works. In humans, leptin is produced in proportion to BMI (higher burden of adipose tissue = more leptin) and acts as a hormone that mediates a wide range of effects on the brain, heart, liver, and muscle [30].

The release of leptin is pulsatile and is affected by sleep. It follows a circadian rhythm [31]. Therefore, the time of measurement can be important in obtaining accurate information about leptin levels in the body. The levels of leptin are highest between midnight and early morning, and lowest in the afternoon. Both lean people and people with obesity have similar rhythm but there are higher concentrations of leptin in persons with obesity [32]. Women have greater concentrations at the same BMI than men [33]. When a human goes into a fasting state, there is a rapid decline in leptin levels that precedes loss of fat and triggers a compensatory mechanism to conserve energy [34]. When leptin levels fall, changes in thyroid hormone levels and sympathetic tone with subsequent decreased energy expenditure combine to drive the patient to regain weight [35].

Scientific interest in leptin was driven by the idea that it might be able to be used therapeutically to treat obesity. Currently, leptin is used to treat congenital leptin deficiency, a rare autosomal dominant disease caused by mutations in the leptin gene. However, in terms of a wider application, it has not proven to be useful.

Specifically in the setting of hyperleptinemia, administration of additional leptin does not result in weight loss, due to insulin resistance [33].

Leptin Resistance

Although persons with obesity have higher levels of leptin, they tend to be resistant to or develop a tolerance for the hunger-inhibiting action of leptin [30]. In trials of obese patients, even the highest dose of exogenous leptin produced less than 7.1 kg of weight loss with significant variability in the response [36]. Initially, leptin resistance was thought to be due to mutations of the leptin receptor. In humans, however, such a mutation is rare [37]. We now know that obesity in humans impairs the transport of leptin across the blood–brain barrier because the molecules that transport leptin become saturated and sluggish [38]. Different parts of the brain get activated at different thresholds of leptin concentration [39]. Complex feedback mechanisms actually create a conundrum: infertility and insulin resistance can occur both with leptin deficiency and leptin excess [40]. Leptin signaling is almost shut down in persons with obesity who have developed adipose tissue dysfunction and tipped over into disease [41, 42]. Solving the riddle of leptin resistance is an ongoing and important therapeutic goal in finding a way to treat adipose tissue dysfunction and obesity.

Adiponectin

Adiponectin is an anti-inflammatory hormone that was discovered in 1995. Adiponectin is secreted exclusively by adipocytes and it regulates the metabolism of lipids and glucose. It also influences the body's response to insulin. The concentration of adiponectin is low in persons with obesity. Adiponectin is an anti-inflammatory and it promotes insulin sensitivity. It is a good biomarker, and is easily detectable in the blood. It is not pulsatile, so the time of collection is not as important. It acts centrally to increase energy expenditure [43]. It is inversely correlated with metabolic disease and is a marker for heart disease and type 2 diabetes [44]. Female centenarians have higher levels of adiponectin than BMI-matched women of other ages [45]. Efforts are underway to produce an effective agonist for adiponectin that might increase longevity in persons with obesity [46].

Pro-inflammatory Adipokines: *Leptin*, Interleukin-6 (IL-6), Tumor Necrosis Factor Alpha (TNFα), Retinol Binding Protein 4 (RBP4); Resistin, Chemerin [47].

Anti-inflammatory Adipokines: *Adiponectin*, Apelin, Omentin-1, Visceral Adipose Tissue-Derives Serine Protease Inhibitor, Secreted Frizzled-Related Protein 5 [47].

Conclusion

There are hundreds of adipokines—some inflammatory and some anti-inflammatory—that contribute to overall health. In addition to energy storage, adipose tissue has a profound potential to regulate health or disease. The tipping point at which adipose tissue dysfunction causes disease is related to the development of inflammation. Inflammation and dysfunction of adipose tissue are central players in the study of obesity-related disease (Fig. 4.7).

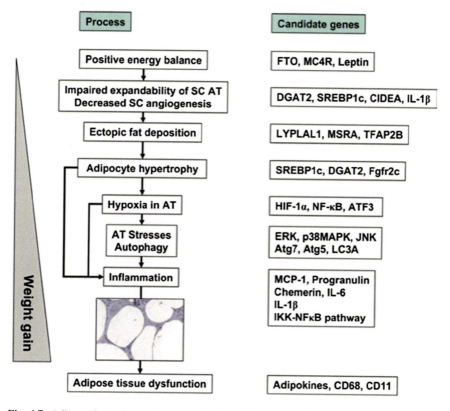

Fig. 4.7 Adipose tissue dysfunction (from Bluher [10], with permission)

References

1. Wilson JR. Harvard University. http://projects.iq.harvard.edu/stigmainshakespeare/falstaff's-obesity.
2. Trayhurn P. Hypoxia and adipocyte physiology: implications for adipose tissue dysfunction in obesity. Annu Rev Nutr. 2014;34:207–36.
3. Lehr S, Hartwig S, Sell H. Adipokines: a treasure trove for the discovery of biomarkers for metabolic disorders. Proteomics Clin Appl. 2012;6:91–101.
4. Bianco P, Robey PG, Simmons PJ. Mesenchymal stem cells: revisiting history, concepts, and assays. Cell Stem Cell. 2008;2:313–9.
5. Gesta S, Bluher M, Yamamoto Y, Norris AW, Berndt J, Kralisch S, Boucher J, Lewis C, Kahn CR. Evidence for a role of developmental genes in the origin of obesity and body fat distribution. Proc Natl Acad Sci. 2006;103:6676–81.
6. Macotela Y, Emmanuelli B, Mori MA, Gesta S, Schulz TJ, Tseng Y-H. Kahn Cr. intrinsic differences in adipocyte precursor cells from different white fat depots. Diabetes. 2012;61:1691–9.
7. Lee YH, Mottillo EP, Granneman JG. Adipose tissue plasticity from WAT to BAT and in between. Biochim Biophy Acta. 2014;1842(3):358–69.
8. Langin D. Recruitment of brown fat and conversion of white into brown adipocytes: strategies to fight the metabolic complications of obesity? Biochim Biophys Acta. 2010;1801:372–6.
9. Dempersmier J, Sul HS. Shades of Brown: a model for thermogenic fat. Front Endocrinol (Lausanne). 2015;8(6):71–80.
10. Bluher M. Adipose tissue dysfunction contributes to obesity related metabolic diseases. Best Pract Res Clin Endocrinol Metab. 2013;27:163–77.
11. Rosell M, Kaforou M, Frontini A, Okolo A, Chan YW, Nikolopoulou E, et al. Brown and white adipose tissues: intrinsic differences in gene expression and response to cold exposure in mice. Am J Physiol Endocrinol Metab. 2014;306(8):E945–64.
12. Carriere A, Jeanson Y, Berger-Muller S, Andre M, Chenouard V, Arnaud E, et al. Browning of white adipose cells by intermediate metabolites: an adaptive mechanism to alleviate redox pressure. Diabetes. 2014;63(10):3253–65.
13. Rosenwald M, Perdikari A, Rulicke T, Wolfrum C. Bi-directional interconversion of brite and white adipocytes. Nat Cell Biol. 2013;15(6):659–67.
14. Blaak EE, Van Baak MA, Kemerink GJ, Pakbiers MT, Heidendal GA, Saris WH. Beta-adrenergic stimulation and abdominal subcutaneous fat blood flow in lean, obese and reduced-obese subjects. Metabolism. 1995;44:184–7.
15. Heinonen I, Kemppainen J, Kaskinoror K, Knuuti J, Boushel R, Kalliokoski KK. Capacity and hypoxic response of subcutaneous adipose tissue blood flow in humans. Circ J. 2014;78:1501–6.
16. Acheson KJ. Influence of autonomic nervous system on nutrient-induced thermogenesis in humans. Nutrition. 1993;9(4):373–80.
17. Yoshikawa T, Naito Y. What is oxidative stress? JMAJ. 2002;45(7):271–6.
18. Sell HH, Habich C, Eckel J. Adaptive immunity in obesity and insulin resistance. Nat Rev Endocrinol. 2012;8:709–12.
19. Lin Q, Yun Z. the hypoxia-inducible factor pathway in adipocytes: the role of HIF-2 in adipose inflammation and hypertrophic cardiomyopathy. Front Endoc. 2015;6(39):1–7.
20. Palmer BF, Clegg DJ. Oxygen sensing and metabolic homeostasis. Mol Cell Endocrinol. 2014;397(1–2):51–8.
21. Netzer N, Gatterer H, Faulhaber M, Burtscher M, Pramsohler S, Pesta D. Hypoxia. Oxid Stress Fat Biomol. 2015;5:1143–50.
22. Goosens GH, Bizzarri A, Venteclef N, Essers Y, Cleutjens JP, Konings E, et al. Increased adipose tissue oxygen tension in obese compared with lean men is accompanied by insulin resistance, impaired adipose tissue capillarization and inflammation. Circulation. 2011;124:67–76.

23. Goosens GH, Blaak EE. Adipose tissue dysfunction and impaired metabolic health in human obesity: a matter of oxygen? Front Endocrinol. 2015;6:1–5.
24. Lecoultre V, Peterson CM, Covington JD, Ebenezer PJ, Frost EA, Schwarz JM, Ravussin E. Ten nights of moderate hypoxia improves insulin sensitivity in obese humans. Diabetes Care. 2013;36:e197–8.
25. Iyengar NM, Hudis CA, Dannenberg AJ. Obesity and inflammation: new insights into breast cancer development and progression. Am Soc Clin Oncol Educ Book. 2013;46–51.
26. Mazzatti D, Lim F-L, O'Hara A, Wood IS, Trayhurn P. A microarray analysis of the hypoxia-induced modulation of gene expression in human adipocytes. Arch Physiol Biochem. 2012;118:112–20.
27. Bluher M. Clinical relevance of Adipokines. Diabetes Metab J. 2012;36:317–27.
28. Van Gaal LF, Mertens IL, DeBlock CE. Mechanisms linking obesity with cardiovascular disease. Nature. 2006;444:875–80.
29. Bluher M. Adipokines-removing roadblocks to obesity and diabetes therapy. Mol Metab. 2014;3:230–40.
30. Margetic S, Gazzola C, Pegg GG, Hill RA. Leptin: a review of its peripheral actions and interactions. Int J Obes Relat Metab Disord. 2002;26:1407–33.
31. Scheer FA, Hilton MF, Mantzoros CS, Shea SA. Adverse metabolic and cardiovascular consequences of circadian misalignment. Proc Natl Acad Sci. 2009;106(11):4453–8.
32. Sinha MK, Ohannesian JP, Heiman ML, Kriauciunas A, Stephens TW, Magosin S, et al. Nocturnal rise of leptin in lean, obese, and non-insulin-dependent diabetes mellitus subjects. J Clin Invest. 1996;97:1344–7.
33. Mantzoros CS, Magkos F, Brinkoetter M, Sienkiewicz E, Dardeno TA, Kim SY, et al. Leptin in human physiology and pathophysiology. Am J Physiol Endocrinol Metab. 2011;301: E567–84.
34. Chan JL, Heist K, DePaoli AM, Veldhuis JD, Mantzoros CS. The role of falling leptin levels in the neuroendocrine and metabolic adaptation to short-term starvation in healthy men. J Clin Invest. 2003;111:1409–21.
35. Rosenbaum M, Goldsmith R, Bloomfield D, Magnano A, Weimer L, Heymsfield S, et al. Low-dose leptin reverses skeletal muscle, autonomic and neuroendocrine adaptations to maintenance of reduced weight. J Clin Invest. 2005;115:3579–86.
36. Heymsfield SB, Greenberg AS, Fujioka K, Dixon RM, Kushner R, Hunt T, Lubina JA, Patane J, Self B, Hunt P, McCamish M. Recombinant leptin for weight loss in obese and lean adults: a randomized, controlled, dose-escalation trial. JAMA. 1999;282:1568–75.
37. Farooqi IS, Bullmore E, Keogh J, Gillard J, O'Rahilly S, Fletcher PC. Leptin Regulates striatal regions and human eating behavior. Science. 2007;317(5843):1355.
38. Banks WA. Leptin Transport across the blood-brain barrier: implications for the cause and treatment of obesity. Curr Pharm Des. 2001;7:124–33.
39. Banks WA, Clever CM, Farrell CL. Partial saturation and regional variation in the blood—to-brain transport of leptin in normal-weight mice. Am J Physiol Endocrinol Metab. 2000;278: E1158–65.
40. Brennan AM, Mantzoros CS. Drug Insight: the role of Leptin in human physiology and pathophysiology-emerging clinical applications. Nat Clin Pract Endocrinol Metab. 2006;2:318–27.
41. Moon HS, Chamberland JP, Diakopoulos KN, Fiorenza CG, Ziemke F, Schneider B, Mantzoros CS. Leptin and amylin act in an additive manner to activate overlapping signaling pathways in peripheral tissues: in vitro and ex-vivo studies in humans. Diabetes Care. 2011;34:132–8.
42. Moon HS, Matarese G, Brennan AM, Chamberland JP, Liu X, Fiorenza CG, et al. Efficacy of metreleptin in obese patients with type 2 diabetes: cellular and molecular pathways underlying leptin tolerance. Diabetes. 2011;60:1647–56.
43. Turer AT, Scherer PE. Adiponectin: mechanistic insights and clinical implications. Diabetologia. 2012;55:2319–26.

44. Sook LE, Park SS, Kim E, Sook YY, Ahn HY, Park CY, et al. Association between adiponectin levels and coronary heart disease and mortality: a systematic review and metaanalysis. Int J Epidemiol. 2013;42:1029–39.
45. Arai Y, Nakazawa S, Kojima T, Takayama M, Ebihara Y, Shimizu K, et al. High adiponectin concentration and its role for longevity in female centenarians. J Gerontol A Biol Sci Med Sci. 2006;6:32–9.
46. Kadowaki T, Yamauchi T, Okada-Iwabu M, Iwabu M. Adiponectin and its receptors: implications for obesity-associated disease and longevity. Lancet Diabetes Endocrinol. 2013;2:8–9.
47. Kwon H, Pessin JE. Adipokines mediate inflammation and insulin resistance. Front Endo. 2013;4(71):1–13.
48. Kershaw EE, Flier JS. Adipose tissue as an endocrine organ. J Clin Endocrinol Metab. 2004;89(6):2548–56.
49. Bluher M, Mantzoros CS. From leptin to other adipokines in health and disease: facts and expectations at the beginning of the 21st century. Metabolism. 2015;64:131–45.

Chapter 5
Obesity-Related Diseases and Syndromes: Insulin Resistance, Type 2 Diabetes Mellitus, Non-alcoholic Fatty Liver Disease, Cardiovascular Disease, and Metabolic Syndrome

Key Message

Understanding the pathophysiology of obesity-related disease will allow providers to better manage the suite of diseases that affect an individual. Fat accumulates within the body of a person who is overweight or obese until many small physiological changes accumulate to a tipping point where adipose tissue becomes "sick." Adisopathy or "sick fat" leads to a host of other obesity-related diseases. In this chapter the development of adisopathy is discussed in detail with an emphasis on insulin resistance and the role of mitochondria, hormones, inflammatory markers and leptin. This chapter also describes the mechanisms of disease for prediabetes and type 2 diabetes and explores the concept of metabolic syndrome. It also explains the pathophysiology of obesity as it relates to non-alcoholic fatty liver disease (NAFLD). This chapter ends with specific discussions about the relationships between obesity and other obesity-related diseases, including hypertension, dyslipidemia, atherosclerosis, coronary heart disease and stroke.

Keeping obesity as the central focus and basis of all treatment strategies for obesity-related diseases is essential. This is important for both the management of current disease as well as the prevention of future disease.

Learning Objectives

1. Identify the key steps in the development of insulin resistance (IR) and the role of cell dysfunction in IR.
2. Summarize the two primary mechanisms of measuring insulin resistance.
3. Define the mechanisms of disease in prediabetes and diabetes.
4. Describe the components of metabolic syndrome (MetS) and define the risk for cardiovascular disease when MetS is present.
5. Understand the pathophysiology of obesity and non-alcoholic fatty liver disease and how it leads to cirrhosis and cancer.

Obesity increases the risk of dying early even in the absence of metabolic disease. The group of people with obesity and no related disease is only 1.6 % in the NHANES III sample, a very rare phenotype. However, their risk of mortality was

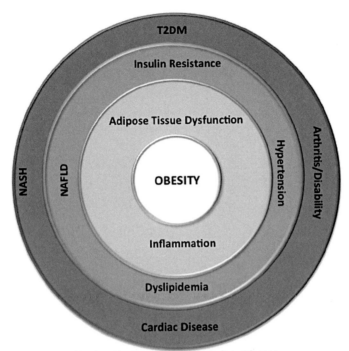

Fig. 5.1 Obesity: the foundation of modern disease

higher than non-obese people even in the absence of insulin resistance or metabolic diseases. This suggests that all patients who are obese, regardless of their metabolic status, should be treated [1].

This chapter will focus on the mechanism of obesity-related disease based on the known biology of obesity. Perhaps the most significant underlying pathophysiology of obesity-related disease is insulin resistance, because it underlies most other pathology. T2DM and the cardiovascular disease it heralds continue to drive concern worldwide, but liver disease and cancers are two new obesity-related diseases that are increasing in incidence. Although all of these diseases are currently treated as individual medical problems, it is important to understand that obesity, inflammation, and insulin resistance are the central problems underlying them all. Weight loss is the one strategy that potentially bridges it all (Fig. 5.1).

Insulin Resistance

Insulin resistance (IR) is one of the most significant side effects of obesity. IR has been recognized as the integral feature of "metabolic syndrome," which includes glucose intolerance, insulin resistance, obesity, hypertriglyceridemia, low HDL cholesterol, hypertension, and accelerated atherosclerosis. To understand IR, the medical practitioner must first have a good working knowledge of both glucose and insulin and the role they play. *The development of IR is a key event that transforms the overweight or obesity state into a health risk.*

Glucose is the fuel that the body uses to drive energy (ATP) production. Glucose is stored in muscle and in the liver as glycogen. Glucose can be derived directly from food ingestion, or it can be made from the glycogen stored in the liver and muscle. In order for glucose to be utilized it must first bind to receptors on cells.

Insulin is a hormone that affects the body's metabolism. Insulin has three basic functions: (1) to help muscle, the liver, and adipose tissue absorb glucose from the bloodstream thereby lowering glucose levels in the blood, (2) to stimulate the liver and muscle to store excess glucose in the form of glycogen, and (3) to decrease the amount of glucose released from the liver. It is clear that insulin and glucose are intimately related and are tightly controlled by the human body under normal circumstances.

When IR occurs, the pancreas can still produce and secrete insulin but target cells are unable to respond effectively to blood concentrations. This, in turn, stimulates beta cells in the pancreas to produce higher and higher levels of insulin, making **hyperinsulinemia** one of the signs of developing IR. Insulin resistance is primarily seen in the liver, muscle and adipose tissue. In some individuals all three organs become insulin resistant within the same time frame although there may be differences in severity.

The liver is responsible for storage of glucose as glycogen after eating and for the production of glucose from glycogen during fasting. Hepatic IR is the impaired ability of the liver to do either of these functions during hyperinsulinemia. Hepatic IR is strongly related to the amount of fat in the liver.

Hyperinsulinemia is a consistent finding in insulin resistance. In a state of hyperinsulinemia, skeletal muscle cells have reduced storage of glucose as glycogen. Individuals with hyperinsulinemia also exhibit impaired fatty acid oxidation and have an impaired ability to switch from oxidation of fatty acids to glucose. The inability of the body to oxidize fuel is known as "metabolic inflexibility." Metabolic inflexibility or incomplete fatty acid oxidation is a critical feature of insulin resistance (IR). Patients with hyperinsulinemia and IR cannot increase their mitochondrial activity or their oxidative capacity thereby causing ongoing and continuous storage of glucose as fat [2].

The key cell organelle involved in IR is the mitochondrion. Variables that control energy (ATP) production in mitochondria are many and complex. In specialized situations, such as during exercise, mitochondrial function may be influenced by calcium release and lactic acidosis [3]. A reduction in the cells' ability to generate energy indicates that the mitochondria in that tissue are not able to meet the energy demands of the cell. Changes in mitochondrial activity due to altered metabolic conditions are termed "mitochondrial plasticity" [4]. Metabolic changes can induce positive or negative changes in plasticity on a short-term basis or on a long term, chronic basis. For example, short-term plasticity might occur in response to acute hyperinsulinemia, whereas long-term plasticity can occur with chronic exercise. *Insulin resistance (IR) is believed to be the initiating defect in T2DM.*

The liver stores glycogen for short-term energy needs and it is activated once the glucose from feeding is consumed or during early fasting. Skeletal muscle accounts for a major portion of glucose storage for use after a meal. During exercise, skeletal muscle determines substrate oxidation for the whole body. Direct measurement by electron microscopy shows that overweight, obese, and insulin resistant (IR) patients with T2DM have 40 % less content in skeletal muscle mitochondria than lean individuals [5]. Mitochondrial content is also reduced in other groups, including elderly patients with IR and the nondiabetic offspring of patients with T2DM with IR [2].

Chronic overeating presents a continuous fatty acid assault on mitochondria until it overwhelms the normal capacity of the mitochondria. This in turn allows excess fatty acids and intermediates (diacylglycerol and ceramide) to accumulate in muscle and in the liver, with export of lipids to fat storage in ectopic locations within the body not designed to store fat.

Insulin resistance (IR) is affected by many body conditions. IR in muscle may be less, for example, in a person who is actively exercising, despite abdominal/visceral obesity [6]. Adiposity is an important variable in establishing insulin resistance but is not sufficient, by itself, to diagnose it. Not all patients with obesity have insulin resistance. However, the groups of patients who do have IR are at the highest risk of cardiovascular disease [7]. The highest levels of IR confer the greatest risk of developing cardiovascular disease. Therefore, it is essential that practitioners identify and communicate as early as possible with patients who are or may become insulin resistant [8, 9].

Insulin resistance and mitochondrial function may be improved through lifestyle interventions such as exercise and/or through pharmaceutical treatment. Unfortunately, the natural history of most people with IR is increasing body weight and worsening hyperinsulinemia [2]. All of the mechanisms outlined above can increase metabolic dysfunction and cause a consistently higher level of hyperglycemia which is clinically diagnosed as prediabetes or intermediate diabetes. Eventually, the beta cells are unable to produce enough insulin to overcome the degree of insulin resistance that is present and the individual eventually develops T2DM.

How to Assess a Patient for Insulin Resistance

In 1985, a seminal paper by D.R. Matthews and colleagues published several different formulae that used fasting insulin and glucose concentrations as simple ways of clinically assessing a patient's level of insulin resistance. The most widely used of those indices is the *homeostasis model assessment for insulin resistance* (HOMA-IR).

Using the HOMA-IR model, a patient's level of insulin resistance and beta cell function can be calculated by measuring the fasting plasma levels of insulin and glucose: HOMA-IR = (fasting plasma insulin mg/dl × fasting plasma glucose mg/dl)/22.5. These calculations correlate with the gold standard euglycemic clamp [10]. The euglycemic clamp measures insulin action by infusing insulin and assessing how much glucose needs to be concurrently infused to hold plasma glucose constant. The euglycemic clamp is a complex research tool and not clinically practical to use. The required level of insulin and glucose used to calculate HOMA-IR is relatively easy to measure, but establishing a standardized reference range has been problematic in widening its use. The cutoff for insulin resistance was first established in 2003 at a HOMA-IR of 2.60 [11], but recent studies show that insulin resistance may span a range: no insulin resistance when HOMA-IR is <2.60 (39.5 % of patients), borderline insulin resistance when HOMA-IR is 2.60–3.80 (21.4 % of patients) and insulin resistance present when HOMA-IR is >3.80 (39.5 % of patients) [12]. These values may be modified by age and by the presence of any metabolic syndrome components [13].

The HOMA-IR seems to correlate best with insulin resistance in liver [6]. Additional studies and improvements in testing have encouraged the replacement of HOMA-IR with a more simple and easily tested measure: plasma insulin levels [14]. In 2004, the American Diabetes Association moved toward standardization of the testing, using pmol/L instead of mIU/ml. Both tests persist and conversion tables are available [15]. Using the American Diabetes Association cutoff points, a fasting insulin level of >9.0 µIU/ml (62.5 pmol/l) identifies prediabetes in 80 % of patients [16]. Using the two-step euglycemic hyperinsulinemic clamp showed that fasting insulin levels of greater than 74 pmol/l (10.66 µIU/ml) indicate insulin resistance in obese men [17]. Smokers have statistically significant higher values of fasting insulin and HOMA-IR, indicating that smokers have a higher risk of insulin resistance [18].

Mechanisms of Insulin Resistance

Although many years of study have gone into trying to understand the mechanisms of insulin resistance, the etiology is still elusive. Many studies have established a relationship between clinically observed pathology but none have established causality. Some studies into the mechanism of IR are promising, giving us insight at the cellular level, but the most promising are studies based on genetic and molecular associations.

Genetic Association: Genetic Predisposition to Obesity

Studies have led to the discovery of obesity gene identification and this has greatly modified our understanding of obesity. By 2011 at least 9 loci involved in various monogenic forms of obesity and 58 loci involved in polygenic obesity had been identified. While there are many more genes to still be discovered, these loci help explain in small part the heritability of obesity. These genetic studies also present evidence that obesity not only predisposes genes, but that obesity also influences the genes' response to treatment relevant to disease progression.

There is evidence of an overlapping continuum between these two forms of obesity (monogenic and polygenic) as demonstrated by the MC4R gene where both rare and common variants occur at the same locus [19]. In addition, the FTO gene, cloned in 1999, was first linked to polygenic human obesity in 2007. Follow-up studies have demonstrated FTO is involved in the development and maintenance of fat tissue. Genetic variations in FTO demonstrate a BMI-dependent association between FTO and T2DM, suggesting a causal relationship [20]. The FTO allele associated with obesity represses the mitochondrial thermogenesis in the precursor adipocyte [21]. The same approach, when applied to other obesity gene variants, confirms that the genetic predisposition to obesity and risk of developing T2DM is mediated by BMI [22]. The FTO genotype has also been used to demonstrate a causal relationship between increased BMI and IR, increased levels of inflammation and lipids and blood pressure, increased risk of atherosclerosis, cardiovascular disease, endometrial, and kidney cancer [23]. A high fat diet amplifies the effect of the FTO genotype on obesity risk [24]. Fortunately, studies show that genetic susceptibility to obesity can be reduced up to 40 % with high intensity physical activity [25].

These genes currently account for only a small percent of inherited obesity, but the complex study of genes and epigenetic influences may explain a causal relationship between obesity genes and BMI-driven disease.

While adiposity is strongly associated with impaired insulin action, there is a distinct movement away from "adipose tissue" centric theories of IR. Endothelial cell dysfunction may be the upstream event that precedes impairment of insulin action. The endothelial cell is ubiquitous throughout the body in all tissues because these cells line blood vessels. Loss of insulin signaling in endothelial cells predisposes the organism to atherosclerotic lesions, thus providing a mechanism to explain the incidence of cardiovascular disease in IR. Endothelial IR may lead to changes in the microcirculation that antagonizes IR by reducing the ability of insulin to reach the target tissue and this may explain some of the progressive decline that is seen in IR. In skeletal muscle, for instance, up to 40 % of insulin-mediated glucose uptake could be the result of microvascular dysfunction due to endothelial IR [26].

Molecular Association: Mitochondria and Hormones

Underlying molecular pathways leading to insulin resistance (IR) are still largely unknown. Studies have established important correlations as well as causative links. Mitochondria are the central focus of much of the research about insulin resistance (IR) because mitochondrial dysfunction is a hallmark of highly prevalent diseases such as obesity, diabetes, cancer, cardiovascular disease, and neurodegenerative diseases. Mitochondria are the primary location of metabolism and energy production and are known to be impaired in metabolic disorders. Epigenetic regulation also plays a role in mitochondria dysfunction. Both obesity and hyperglycemia lead to mitochondrial DNA (mtDNA) instability and decreased ability to generate energy (ATP) [27, 28]. Obesity results in increased free fatty acids flowing into the mitochondria where it overloads the mechanism that allows adequate processing. This results in "oxidative stress" which leads to impairment of insulin action and IR. Oxidative stress also results in the accumulation of reactive oxygen species (ROS) and incompletely oxidized toxic substrates such as diacylglycerol (DAG) and ceramide. Stress-sensitive components of the insulin signaling system lead to impairment in insulin action

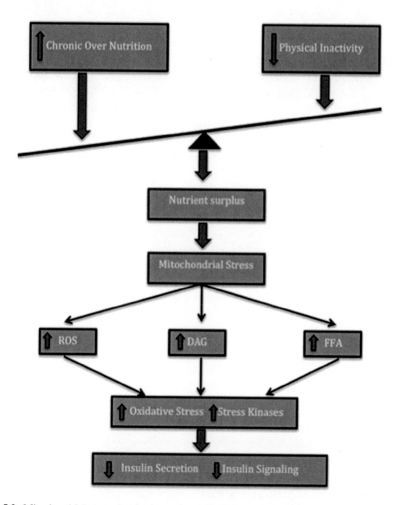

Fig. 5.2 Mitochondrial stress in obesity and type 2 diabetes. Mitochondrial stress occurs when chronic overnutrition and inactivity combine to provide a persistent surplus in nutrient supply. Mitochondrial stress results in accumulation of reactive oxygen species (*ROS*) and an increase in diacylglycerol (*DAG*) and free fatty acid (*FFA*). These in term trigger oxidative stress and promotion of stress-sensitive kinases. Impairment of insulin secretion and signaling result

resulting in IR [29] (Fig. 5.2). Importantly, both calorie restriction and exercise can rescue the mitochondria from the fate of oxidative stress [30].

When a hormone targets a cell, it not only stimulates a specific action in the cell, but it can reset the responsiveness of the cell to require subsequent doses of the same hormone. This process is called homologous desensitization. When insulin rises rapidly it stimulates the cell to take up glucose. However, persistent elevation of insulin over time desensitizes the cell and affects receptors on the cell membrane thereby impairing the cell's ability to respond. This occurs whether the source of insulin is endogenous or exogenous. Down regulation of receptors occurs rapidly [31]. Dysregulation of insulin implements a vicious negative feedback loop. This feedback interrupts and impairs mitochondrial function through dysregulation of the mitochondrial electron transport chain [32]. These epigenetic changes appear to be related to DNA methylation and are seen in obesity and hyperglycemia [33]. DNA methylation is a process by which methyl groups are added to DNA. Methylation modifies the function of the DNA, typically acting to suppress gene transcription. The mechanism of methylation is present in patients with T2DM and non-alcoholic fatty liver disease (NAFLD). It is also related to impaired insulin secretion from the pancreatic beta cells and insulin resistance in the liver [34]. Exercise intervention was found to reduce DNA methylation in humans [35].

Another key etiology of IR focuses on the role of adipokines in insulin resistance. Visceral (belly) fat constitutes about 15 % of total fat. Macrophages are found in higher numbers in visceral fat versus subcutaneous fat depots [36]. Adipocytes (fat cells) and macrophages (large white blood cells) secrete adipokines that play an essential role in the onset and maintenance of IR [37]. New drug therapies designed to mitigate the effect of the adipokines on the system are being tested, but weight loss and preservation of beta cell function are still critical to successful treatment.

Inflammation and Insulin Resistance

Chronic low-grade inflammation of the adipose tissue is one of the primary mechanisms that occur early in the evolution of insulin resistance (IR). Ongoing inflammation is one of the key drivers of metabolic dysfunction leading to IR. Inflammation is detected clinically with elevated blood markers like C-reactive protein (CRP).

Deletion or silencing of genes that influence insulin action tends to diminish inflammation and improve whole body glucose metabolism. A reduction in the level of circulating insulin likewise decreases macrophage expansion and reduces inflammation in adipose tissue [38]. Weight gain and weight loss have an influence on chronic inflammation by changing the levels of adiponectin. With weight loss, increasing levels of adiponectin decrease inflammation.

Impaired Fasting Glucose (IFG), Impaired Glucose Tolerance (IGT), and Prediabetes

Insulin resistance is the underlying pathology of both impaired fasting glucose (IFG) and impaired glucose tolerance (IGT). It is critically important to identify and communicate to patients accurately the status of their glucose metabolism. The earlier abnormalities are identified and communicated, the earlier efforts can be made to correct them, which will help avoid the development of prediabetes. Prediabetes leads to T2DM in 70 % of patients and is accompanied by a marked jump in cardiovascular disease risk [39].

IFG and IGT as indicators of prediabetes are intermediate stages between normal glucose metabolism and T2DM. IFG is defined as having an elevated fasting glucose concentration of ≥ 100 mg/dl and <126 mg/dl. IGT requires a glucose tolerance test for diagnosis. IGT is defined as having a glucose concentration ≥ 140 and <200 mg/dl two hours after the glucose drink is consumed. IFG and IGT identify different populations of patients with separate risks for diabetes [39]. There is substantial concern that the lack of screening in the population will yield future surprises in incidence of diabetes. In a cross-sectional analysis using the Finnish Diabetes Risk Score and HbA1c, the prevalence of undiagnosed IFG was 27.7 %. Similarly, undiagnosed IGT was 10.3 %, and undiagnosed prediabetes was 43.1 % [40].

Patients with intermediate levels of HbA1c (5.7–6.4 mg/dl) are often referred to as "prediabetic" although not all of these patients go on to develop diabetes. Recently, there has been a movement to rename this category "intermediate hyperglycemia" (the World Heath Organization) or "high risk state of developing diabetes" (the American Diabetes Association). Regardless of how the categories are defined, the definitions all have the same HbA1c cutoffs. Currently, it is projected that more than 470 million people will be prediabetic by 2030 [41].

Prediabetes may be diagnosed by IFG, IGT, or based on HbA1c but not every indicator exists in the same individual. For instance, in Caucasian populations the overlap may be as little as 25 % [42]. Individuals with prediabetes have a yearly conversion rate of 5–10 % to diabetes with up to 70 % likely to convert to diabetes without a change in lifestyle. There is also a chance of conversion to normoglycemia which is usually associated with a decrease in weight. Losing weight reduces the risk of conversion to diabetes by 40–70 % [43].

The hallmark of prediabetes is higher blood glucose levels. This has been associated with an increasing need for more insulin to handle the glucose load. With increased glucose production the beta cell's ability to produce the amount of insulin needed to match the level of insulin resistance is inadequate and the patient develops T2DM despite hyperinsulinemia. As the disease progresses, the patient's beta cells fail and the patient requires exogenous insulin therapy to supplement pancreatic production. Early recognition and treatment to stop this progressive loss of the beta cells' ability to produce insulin becomes clinically imperative. Of particular concern is the group of prediabetic patients with insulin resistance, as these patients have a higher risk of conversion to T2DM and cardiovascular disease. Insulin–sensitizing therapy as opposed to therapy that increases insulin may be a more effective treatment for this group of patients [44].

One final group of patients that are considered to have a high risk for conversion to T2DM is the group of women with gestational diabetes. Thirteen percent of mothers with gestational diabetes developed type 2 diabetes after pregnancy versus 1 % of mothers without gestational diabetes [45].

Type 2 Diabetes Mellitus (T2DM)

During times of pestilence and famine, T2DM did not exist. However, in ancient societies where food was in abundance as in Rome or Greece, T2DM was described as being present. Chronic overnutrition in our modern world coupled with a marked decrease in physical activity has allowed epigenetic changes to occur and become a part of the genetic milieu of modern man. T2DM is highly related to cardiovascular disease risk and obesity. For every 1 kg increase in body weight there is a 4.5 % higher risk of developing T2DM [46]. Insulin resistance is observed in 90 % of patients with T2DM and the presence of IR doubles the risk of cardiovascular disease [47]. Despite strong evidence linking T2DM to mortality, 40 % of patients with T2DM do not meet their treatment goals [48]. The treatment paradigm requires weight loss but it is extremely difficult to achieve even with a committed program/patient relationship. Many diabetologists believe weight loss in a diabetic patient is an exercise in futility.

Why is weight loss more difficult to achieve in an obese patient with T2DM? Patients with T2DM who are untreated or sporadically treated for T2DM have a higher than normal energy expenditure. This is due to increased protein turnover and synthesis, increased sympathetic tone, and spillage of calories in urine as glycosuria. Some patients before diagnosis of T2DM may initially lose some weight due to the additional calorie expenditure. Once identification and treatment for T2DM is initiated, the calorie expenditures decrease. Unfortunately, many of the medications that are prescribed for treatment of T2DM may also increase weight. The net result is that patients with T2DM usually gain weight after treatment is begun. *The most important long term treatment strategy for T2DM is weight loss.*

Weight loss trials in obese patients with diabetes show weight loss on average being 4–10 % from baseline. After such weight loss the patient reaches a new set point, with the lower energy expenditure achieved by therapy. At this point the patient's internal stimulus to regain weight begins. The hypothalamic "imprinting" of the original weight set point begins to exert physiologic pressure on the patient's body to return to the higher original weight by increasing hunger and decreasing satiety. Recurrent attempts at weight loss without substantial results have a significantly frustrating psychological effect and can leave the patient and physician feeling that further efforts are futile. Patients often gain additional weight above their initial baseline weight, thereby reinforcing the phenotype and accelerating the progression to cardiovascular disease. Physical activity, which has been shown to have significant weight-independent modulating effects on epigenetic changes that drive insulin resistance in diabetics, is unfortunately rarely emphasized or achieved in these patients [49].

Early identification of IR and treatment can mitigate this paradigm by returning those patients with low to moderate BMI's back to normal weight long before they reach the point of developing prediabetes or T2DM. Once T2DM has occurred the often-competing goal of treatment with weight promoting medications while trying to diet may make weight loss in diabetics even that much harder. Intense, continuous weight loss interventions, perhaps in a clinic specifically devoted to this type of intense treatment rather than traditional treatment which can be sporadic and lack provider follow-up, may be necessary. Treatment may even need to be accelerated to more interventional treatments of obesity (i.e., medication, surgery) if weight loss goals are not met in a reasonable period of time.

There is growing awareness of the importance of the nervous system in obesity-related diseases. Type 2 diabetes mellitus provides one of the best examples of this interrelatedness. One of the unique side effects of T2DM is the functional alteration it generates in the innervation of the gut [50]. Specifically, patients with T2DM have profound loss of autonomic control, resulting in gastroparesis in 50 % of patients [51]. Patients with T2DM also experience prevalence of altered intestinal morphology and an increase in neuropathy and abnormal motility [52, 53].

Insulin normally increases blood flow to both skeletal muscle and subcutaneous adipose tissue. This effect is seen primarily with exercise or after a meal. Increased blood flow facilitates the delivery of insulin to the target tissue. However, when metabolic dysfunction has occurred resulting in IR and T2DM, blood flow decreases through these tissue beds. This reduction in blood flow increases lipolysis and decreases glucose uptake throughout the body, thereby increasing IR in all tissues. This sequence often exists in patients with IR and prediabetes long before hyperglycemia is treated. The delay in treatment exacerbates the associated dyslipidemia and dysglycemia in these patients [54].

Metabolic Syndrome

In 1988, Gerald M. Reaven described "Syndrome X," that proposed a causal relationship between hypertension, insulin resistance, and dyslipidemia. Many believed insulin resistance to be the underlying pathophysiologic problem [55]. Over time, syndrome X became more commonly referred to as "Metabolic Syndrome" and most definitions began to include obesity (usually measured by waist circumference.) More recently, multiple definitions of "Metabolic Syndrome," beginning with the World Health Organization (WHO) definition in 1999, have been proposed and debated. The Internal Federation of Obesity is attempting to establish a consensus definition with adjustments for waist circumference based on ethnicity (Table 5.1). Although there is still some debate about the definition and use of the term "Metabolic Syndrome (MetS)," current research indicates that up to 25 % of adults are predicted to have metabolic syndrome. Most people with MetS are prediabetic with a glycosylated hemoglobin level (HbA1c) between 5.7 and 6.4 % [56]. Whatever the definition is or should be, the clustering of obesity-related diseases in individual patients is not accidental or random.

There continues to be controversy and interdisciplinary debate as to the validity of Metabolic Syndrome even as a screening tool. But as the prevalence of people with clustering of metabolic disease has increased across the world, ways to screen

Table 5.1 The new International Diabetes Federation (IDF) definition of metabolic syndrome

According to the IDF definition, a person defined as having the metabolic syndrome must have:
Central obesity (defined as waist circumference ≥ 102 cm American men and ≥ 88 cm American female)[a]
Plus any two of the following four factors: • **raised TG level**: ≥ 150 mg/dl (1.7 mmol/L) or **specific treatment for this lipid abnormality** • **reduced HDL cholesterol**: <40 mg/dl (1.03 mmol/L) in males and <50 mg/dl (1.29 mmol/L) in females or **specific treatment for this lipid abnormality** • **raised blood pressure**: systolic BP ≥ 130 or diastolic BP ≥ 85 mm Hg, or **treatment of previously diagnosed hypertension** • **raised fasting plasma glucose** (FPG) ≥ 100 mg/dl (5.6 mmol/L), or **previously diagnosed type 2 diabetes**

[a]Waist circumference should be adjusted for ethnicity regardless of where the person lives
Adapted from The International Diabetes Federation Consensus Worldwide Definition of the Metabolic Syndrome, http://www.idf.org/webdata/docs/IDF_Meta_def_final.pdf, with permission

for metabolic disease that requires simple, low technology measurements in areas without many health resources has become a focus of new definitions. One such definition offers one simple and scalable solution. It is known as the Index of Central Obesity (ICO) and it defines metabolic syndrome as: the ratio of waist circumference to height, with a cutoff of >0.50 proposed for all genders and races. The message of the ICO screening tool is simple: "if your waist is more than half your height you should consult your doctor" [57].

Metabolic syndrome is still being researched and debated but there is significant support for the concept in general, and screening will become increasingly important in light of the interrelatedness of these components of metabolic disease.

Central obesity is one of the cardinal features of metabolic syndrome, and waist circumference is the primary measurement-screening tool [58]. Other determinants may be overeating, insulin resistance, chronic stress, and arterial stiffness [59].

Patients within current definitions of metabolic syndrome are likely to be experiencing genetic resetting™ and are at high risk of obesity-related disease. Screening is the key to recognizing and educating patients about their metabolic status and risk of disease. Multidisciplinary committees within a healthcare system may be best suited to review and choose a clinical screening tool they can use for every patient. In the absence of that type of system-wide direction, individual providers of care will need to decide what definition to use and how best to screen their patients for the risk of obesity-related diseases. Currently, each component of metabolic syndrome is treated separately. There is currently no pharmaceutical or therapy that treats all components, except weight loss treatment.

Non-Alcoholic Fatty Liver Disease (NAFLD), Steatohepatitis (NASH) and Cirrhosis

Despite major advancements in fighting certain chronic liver diseases, there is a growing epidemic of liver disease that is directly related to obesity. In the last 20 years, the prevalence of non-alcoholic fatty liver disease (NAFLD) has more than doubled in adolescents as well as in the adult population. Fatty liver disease is now the number one liver disease in the world. There are no drugs currently approved to treat the disease, which causes the liver to swell with fat. The damage is done not by alcohol, but by excess weight. Having a non-alcoholic fatty liver is a strong risk factor for developing T2DM and coronary disease.

In 20–30 % of patients with NAFLD the fat infiltrating the liver leads to inflammation and hepatocellular injury and scarring, which can eventually lead to cirrhosis and liver failure and, in some cases, liver cancer. This more progressive form of NAFLD is known as non-alcoholic steatohepatitis, or NASH. Thus, the spectrum of obesity-related liver disease spans a continuum from non-alcoholic fatty liver disease (NAFLD), to non-alcoholic steatohepatitis (NASH) to cirrhosis. The distinguishing characteristic between NAFLD and NASH is that NASH presents with fibrosis. Fibrosis greatly increases morbidity as it yields a 20 % higher chance of progression to cirrhosis versus a 4 % chance for NAFLD without fibrosis. Patients with NAFLD and NASH are at risk for increased mortality from liver disease, and they are even more at risk for cancer (28 %) and cardiovascular disease (25 %) [60].

NAFLD is currently estimated to affect 100 million people in the United States, increasing in incidence with obesity. Patients with metabolic syndrome are at increased risk for progression to NASH. 66 % of patients 50 years or older who have both diabetes and central obesity show advanced fibrosis on liver biopsies. Progression rates vary widely, with some patients having little change in NAFLD over a decade while others progress rapidly to NASH/fibrosis or cirrhosis within 5 years.

The mechanism for progression from simple steatosis (fatty liver) to NAFLD is not completely understood but generally involves a "multiple hit" hypothesis [61]. The initial accumulation of fat in the liver progresses into mitochondrial dysfunction and oxidative stress, culminating in liver injury and hepatocyte death (Fig. 5.3). Although many changes are taking place internally they often go unnoticed by the patient, or go untreated, until cirrhosis is established.

The Role of Microbiota, Intestinal Dysbiosis, and Metabolic Endotoxemia in NAFLD

Obesogenic food (food that tends to cause obesity), particularly those high in fat and fructose alter gut microbiota, resulting in intestinal dysbiosis. Dysbiosis is commonly associated with inflammatory bowel disease, chronic fatigue syndrome,

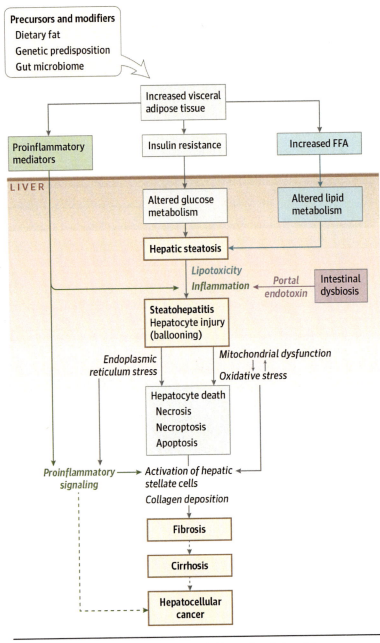

Fig. 5.3 Mechanisms involved in the pathophysiology of nonalcoholic fatty liver disease (NAFLD). From Rinella [60], with permission

obesity, cancer, bacterial vaginitis, and colitis. This disruption of the digestive tract leads to a breakdown in the intestinal barrier, making it more susceptible to the translocation of bacteria to the internal environment of the body. When the bacteria translocates metabolic endotoxemia can result, causing a low-grade inflammation in the liver. This, in turn, results in endoplasmic reticular stress and fatty liver disease. Other mechanisms by which gut bacteria may contribute to NAFLD include interactions between the gut bacteria and signaling compounds that change the usual function of both the liver and adipose tissue. Bacterial lipopolysaccharide (LPS) is a triggering factor of fibrosis of the liver. Significantly, a high fat diet increases the proportion of LPS in the gut resulting in metabolic endotoxemia that stimulates inflammation and fibrosis and sets the tone of insulin sensitivity. It is a precursor to the onset of diabetes and obesity. Similarly, the role of LPS in stimulating fibrosis in the fatty liver may be one of the gateway events in the progression of NASH to cirrhosis [62]. Lowering a patient's LPS concentration could be a potent future strategy for controlling obesity-related metabolic diseases.

Obesity-Related Cardiovascular Disease

The Obesity Paradox

Being overweight or obese puts patients at risk for health complications like diabetes and heart disease, yet there are studies and data suggesting that body fat may, in some cases, impart a kind of protective benefit. This is known as the "obesity paradox" and it refers to the fact that moderately obese people with chronic diseases are often outliving normal weight people with the same health complications. The obesity paradox is responsible for mortality associated with BMI being a "J" shaped curve, with minimum morality close to a BMI of 25 kg/m^2. Mortality increases both below and above a BMI of 25, but many studies show that individuals with overweight and obesity have a lower mortality than normal weight patients in both the incidence and outcomes. Studies in obesity-related diseases including coronary artery disease and acute myocardial infarction show one-year mortality of 9.2 % in normal weight versus 6.1 % in overweight and 4.7 % in obese and clinically severe obesity [63]. This also is shown in patients treated for congestive heart failure and in patients undergoing nonbariatric general surgery procedures. The obesity paradox is sometimes referred to as "reverse epidemiology" [64]. Most of the studies included elderly populations with an average age of >62 years. Gender may also play a role with men but not women showing the effect of the obesity paradox in acute coronary syndrome [65]. In addition, there may be some selection bias in the studies that demonstrates a protective effect of mortality in cardiovascular disease of the "obese" patient with a BMI of 30–34.5 kg/m^2 [66].

The obesity paradox can also be seen in diabetic patients. In a study of diabetic patients with an average age of 63, patients in the overweight group had lower mortality than patients of normal weight [67]. In addition, patients with obesity and diabetes had $1314.00 less healthcare expenditures than normal weight patients with T2DM [68].

It is important to separate overweight from obesity when discussing the obesity paradox. Although in some cases it may be true that obesity (BMI 30–34.5 kg/m^2) shows a protective effect versus normal weight, in most cases it is the overweight category that is most protected.

What is the mechanism behind this seeming protective effect? There is no causal evidence but some observations have been made. Autopsies of individuals with obesity demonstrate less coronary atherosclerosis than would be expected [69]. Part of the protection may be from a greater mobilization of endothelial progenitor cells in patients with obesity. A reduction in endothelial cells that line the vascular system has been proposed as one theory of the etiology of vascular disease [70]. Additional mechanisms of protection may be from a decrease in Thromboxane A2 rendering platelets less active and lowering concentrations of tumor necrosis factor alpha (TNFα) [71, 72].

Given the obesity paradox, the question becomes: what is the optimal weight for health? A BMI of 25 kg/m^2 has the lowest mortality; however a comfortable window of BMI of 25–27 kg/m^2 may be more ideal if it confers the maximum protective effect of adiposity while avoiding inflammation, dyslipidemia and insulin resistance, which are the tipping points into more serious disease. This BMI goal is mitigated by ethnic background. The BMI goal may be lower in people of Asian descent. There are few definitive answers or consensus regarding the obesity paradox. There is, however, no question that if a patient is obese that patient has a higher risk of developing insulin resistance, diabetes, and heart disease. Overweight patients are more likely to be metabolically healthy and may fluctuate in weight 10–30 lb more frequently. On balance, the danger that the overweight individual will continue an upward spiral of weight gain without intervention is strong. Encouraging patients to maintain a healthy weight or to lose that first 20–30 pounds of weight as soon as it is detected remains the optimal approach to prevent chronic disease and to prolong life.

Dyslipidemia

Dyslipidemia is a disorder of lipoprotein metabolism in which there are abnormal amounts of lipids (cholesterol and/or fat) present in the blood. Dyslipidemia is frequently found in patients with obesity and is often one of the first signals that some metabolic dysfunction is taking place. One in three Americans die of heart disease and stroke, and both diseases are related to dyslipidemia.

Dyslipidemia occurs when triglycerides (TG) are elevated and high-density lipoprotein cholesterol (HDL-C) is low. There is some evidence that HDL particles act as anti-inflammatory agents. Thus, low levels of HDL are less desirable and increase the patient's risk for cardiovascular disease [73].

The process of developing dyslipidemia has two major mechanisms. Obesity-related lipolysis increases the volume of free triglycerides going to the liver. The liver attempts to manage this increased flow by increasing storage capacity in the liver, increasing oxidation in liver mitochondria and exporting very low-density lipoprotein (LDL) particles into the blood. This lowers the number of good HDL particles which is associated with increased cardiovascular disease (CVD) risk. Another mechanism by which excess triglycerides are managed by the liver is through the digestive process in the intestine. New guidelines were issued in 2014 regarding treatment of cholesterol abnormalities. These guidelines aim to reduce cardiovascular disease in adults based on best quality evidence using Institute of Medicine principles [74, 75].

Hypertension

Obesity-related hypertension accounts for 65–75 % of hypertension, affecting one out of three Americans. The mechanisms of hypertension in patients with obesity are not completely understood but there is strong evidence that it is related to the kidneys. There is evidence that the increase in incidence of chronic kidney disease (CKD) is closely related to the increase in obesity. Twenty percent of adults over age 20 have CKD. Visceral obesity is closely related to hypertension and diabetes, which are the two main contributors of CKD. In patients with hypertension and no history of smoking, alcohol use, chronic obstructive pulmonary disease (COPD), or cardiovascular disease (CVD), the lowest mortality occurs with BMI of 23.0–26.9 kg/m^2 [76]. End stage renal disease (ESRD) increases as BMI increases with a relative risk of 3.57 for patients with obesity [77].

Proposed mechanisms of obesity-related hypertension include: hyperleptinemia, angiotensin II activation, hyperinsulinemia, impaired baroreceptor sensitivity, and compression of the kidney by fat accumulation around the kidney in a relatively confined space [78] (Fig. 5.4).

The hypothalamus plays a significant role in the development of hypertension associated with obesity [79]. Leptin acts in the hypothalamus and results in hypertension—an effect that may be modulated by gender and the maternal environment during pregnancy [80]. There is also increasing evidence that oxidative stress, lipotoxicity, and inflammation contribute to obesity-related hypertension [81]. Further, adipocytes stimulate renal sodium retention and constriction of arterioles, thereby increasing glomerular hydrostatic pressure. This, too, contributes to obesity-related hypertension. Many patients with hypertension respond to weight loss. Individuals with long-standing hypertension, however, experience escalating damage which makes hypertension eventually resistant to weight loss.

As mentioned earlier, the kidneys are definitely associated with obesity-related hypertension. People with visceral obesity store fat in ectopic locations, including the area around the kidneys. The kidneys may be encased in fat and there may be

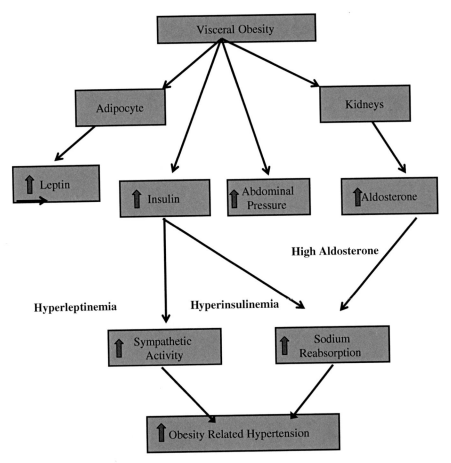

Fig. 5.4 Mechanism of obesity-related hypertension. Adapted from Bueter et al. [78], with permission

invasion of fat into the perirenal sinus. Adipocytes with impaired uptake of glucose stimulate increased salt absorption by the kidneys. The resulting increase in hydrostatic pressure reduces tubular flow and increases sodium reabsorption. The overall intraabdominal pressure in patients with obesity is higher, again adding to compression of the kidneys and creating hypertension [82]. Chronic renal dysfunction is a serious consequence of obesity because of the strong links between visceral adiposity and the two leading causes of chronic kidney disease (CKD): hypertension and diabetes.

Insulin, too, has a number of effects on the reabsorption of sodium in the kidneys. Hyperinsulinemia does not necessarily result in hypertension, but in the setting of insulin resistance in skeletal muscle, it does. It also appears that obesity-related hypertension associated with insulin resistance might be salt-sensitive [83].

Atherosclerosis, Coronary Heart Disease (CHD), and Heart Failure

The obesity paradox seems particularly pertinent to patients with atherosclerosis and coronary artery disease (CAD). The least cardiac mortality is seen in the overweight group and no increased mortality is seen in the obese group or the clinically severe obese group [84]. In a more recent study of patients undergoing coronary angioplasty, optimal medical treatment was more common in obese patients and BMI did not remain an independent predictor of cardiovascular mortality when adjusted for optimal medical treatment [85].

When a patient presents with multiple components of metabolic syndrome the incidence of atherosclerosis and the risk of a cardiovascular event are much more likely. As abdominal fat increases, fat also builds up around the heart. *Evidence is accumulating that an increase in visceral fat, producing increased leptin and reduced adiponectin, may be the signal that accelerates the build up of atherosclerotic plaque and causes plaque to be distributed locally in the coronary arteries* [86]. A low adiponectin level is also shown to be characteristic of metabolic syndrome and independently associated with left ventricular mass [87].

C-reactive protein (CRP) is another well-known marker of inflammation and cardiac risk. CRP is elevated prior to any clinical evidence of atherosclerosis and its presence often foreshadows risk of future cardiac events and sudden death. Elevated CRP seems to correlate with inflammation in the endothelial cells that line arteries [88]. While many of these inflammatory markers signal risk, we now understand they are involved in the pathophysiology of coronary heart disease in a more intimate and influential way. Decreasing levels of these markers may indicate successful treatment of the endothelial dysfunction that underlies coronary heart disease.

Atrial Fibrillation and Stroke

Atrial fibrillation (AF) is increasing in incidence, affecting large populations in China (3.9 million people) and India (5 million people). China has an incidence of 2.5 million new strokes per year [89]. In the United States, there has been a 60 % increase in hospitalizations over the last 20 years for AF with an average increased cost of \$14,875 per patient as compared to people without AF [90]. Similarly, there is a corresponding increase in stroke, with 6 million deaths per year as of 2005. This is primarily due to aging and obesity. Age is a main determinant of AF risk, with AF occurring in only 1 % of 55–59 year olds, but in 11 % of people over age 85 [91]. The relative risk of AF in people aged 75 and above is 5.28 (95 %, CI 4.57–6.09) [92].

Obesity contributes to the risk for both AF and stroke in multiple ways including: insulin resistance, hyperlipidemia, and hypertriglyceridemia, production of inflammatory cytokines, activation of the sympathetic nervous system and increase in sodium absorption with hypertension [93]. From a mechanical standpoint, obesity is associated with atrial enlargement and ventricular diastolic dysfunction. High leptin levels are also associated with increased risk of stroke (RR 1.97, 95 % CI 1.21–3.21) in African-American women, but not in African-American men. The effect in women is related to genetic variability and affects 38 % of African-American women [94].

When measured only by clinical risk factors, obesity appears to increase the risk of developing AF by 50 %, which is a 4 % increase for each 1-unit increase in BMI [95].

Heart Failure

Heart failure remains one of the leading causes of morbidity with mortality. Insulin resistance (IR) has been shown to predict the development of heart failure. Evidence is mounting that IR affects heart muscle and begins a cycle of failure that exacerbates the dysfunctional metabolism, resulting in progression to heart failure. Once heart failure ensues, the increase in sympathetic drive accelerates the heart rate, constricts blood vessels, raises blood pressure and increases the circulation of free fatty acids and cytokines, thereby worsening heart failure [96] (Fig. 5.5).

Fruit fly studies have given us new insights into how heart dysfunction may occur. Flies bred over generations for "starvation resistance" have components of metabolic syndrome. The fat in these flies is preferentially stored in the fat body rather than as lipids within the myocardium. These flies have dilated hearts with

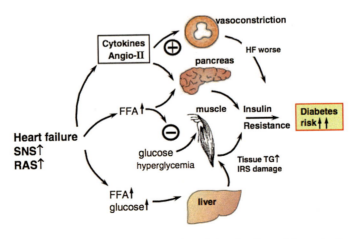

Fig. 5.5 The role of myocardial metabolism in relating insulin resistance to heart failure. Modified from Ashrafian et al. [96], with permission

impaired contractility due to storage of fat along the dorsal cuticle of the heart itself that alters the anatomical position of the heart. Development of models like this help in the investigation of heart dysfunction in the environment of obesity [97].

Diabetes increases the development of cardiomyopathy, leading to a distinct diabetic myocardial phenotype known as "Diabetic Cardiomyopathy" (DCM) [98]. DCM is a progressive disease. Activation of protein kinase C is the early central defect, altering the response of the myocardium to stress. Changes in calcium homeostasis and sensitivity, an increase in reactive oxygen species, suppression of aerobic energy production, and modification of contractile proteins are mechanisms of the pathophysiology of DCM [99].

Conclusion

Obesity is associated with many metabolic diseases, sometimes grouped as "metabolic syndrome," all of which increase the risk for long-term chronic illness and cardiovascular disease.

Evidence is accumulating that the pathophysiological changes that occur with obesity may be causative of these diseases and in some cases bidirectional. The presence of insulin resistance at the level of the endothelial cell may be the tipping factor between simple obesity and obesity that causes related disease, i.e. "sick fat." The progression of mere overweight to obesity with IR is an issue that must concern both patients and medical providers. Early identification of IR and engaging patients in treatment to diminish it may be the most effective way to fight various obesity-related metabolic diseases.

References

1. Kuk JL, Ardern CI. Are metabolically normal but obese individuals at lower risk for all-cause mortality? Diab Care. 2009;32(12):2297–9.
2. Szendroedi J, Phielix E, Roden M. The role of mitochondria in insulin resistance and type 2 diabetes mellitus. Nat Rev Endocrinol. 2012;8:92–103.
3. Messer JI, Jackman MR, Willis WT. Pyruvate and citric acid cycle carbon requirements in isolated skeletal muscle mitochondria. Am J Physiol Cell Physiol. 2004;286(3):C565–72.
4. Hoppeler H, Fluck M. Plasticity of skeletal muscle mitochondria: structure and function. Med Sci Sports Exerc. 2003;35:95–104.
5. Chomentowski P, Coen PM, Radikova A, Goodpaster BH, Toledo FG. Skeletal muscle mitochondria in insulin resistance: differences in intermyofibrillar versus subsarcolemmal subpopulations and relationship to metabolic flexibility. J Clin Endocrinol Metab. 2011;96:493–503.
6. Abdul-Ghani MA, Matsuda M, Balas B, DeFronzo RA. Muscle and liver insulin resistance indexes derived from the oral glucose tolerance test. Diabetes Care. 2007;30:89–94.
7. Reaven GM. Insulin resistance: the link between obesity and cardiovascular disease. Med Clin North Am. 2011;95(5):875–92.

8. Yip J, Facchini FS, Reaven GM. Resistance to insulin-mediated glucose disposal as a predictor of cardiovascular disease. J Clin Endocrinol Metab. 1998;83:2773–6.
9. Reaven GM. All obese individuals are not created equal: insulin resistance is the major determinant of cardiovascular disease in overweight/obese individuals. Diabetes Vasc Dis Res. 2005;2:105–12.
10. Matthews DR, Hosker JP, Rudenski AS, Naylor BA, Treacher DF, Turner RC. Homeostasis model assessment: insulin resistance and beta-cell function from fasting plasma glucose and insulin concentrations in man. Diabetologia. 1985;28(7):412–9.
11. Ascaso JF, Pardo S, Real JT, Lorente RI, Priego A, Carmena R. Diagnosing insulin resistance by simple quantitative methods in subjects with normal glucose metabolism. Diabetes Care. 2003;26:3320–5.
12. Qu H, Li Q, Rentfro AR, Fisher-Hoch SP, McCormick JB. The definition of insulin resistance using HOMA-IR for American of Mexican descent using machine learning. PLoS ONE. 2011;6(6):e21041.
13. Gayoso-Diz P, Otero-Gonzalez A, Rodriguez-Alvarez MX, Gude F, Garcia F, DeFrancisco A, Quintela AG. Insulin resistance (HOMA-IR) cut-off values and the metabolic syndrome in a general adult population: effect of gender and age: EPIRCE cross-sectional study. BMC Endocr Disord. 2013;13:47.
14. Rasmussen-Torvik LJ, Pankow JS, Jacobs DR, Steffen LM, Moran AM, Steinberger J, Sinaiko AR. Heritability and genetic correlations of insulin sensitivity measured by the euglycemic clamp. Diabet Med. 2007;24(11):1286–9.
15. Staten MA, Stern MP, Miller WG, Steffes MW. Campbell SE for the insulin standardization workgroup. Diabetes Care. 2010;33(1):205–6.
16. Johnson JL, Duick DS, Chui MA, Aldasouqi SA. Identifying prediabetes using fasting insulin levels. Endocr Pract. 2010;16(1):47–52.
17. Ter Horst KW, Gilijamse PW, Koopman KE, de Weijer BA, Brands M, Kootte RS, et al. Insulin resistance in obesity can be reliably identified from fasting plasma insulin. Int J Obes. 2015. doi:10.1038/ijo.2015.125.
18. Haj Mouhamed D, Ezzaher A, Neffati F, Douki W, Gaha L, Najjar MF. Effect of cigarette smoking on insulin resistance risk. Ann Cardiol Angeiol (Paris). 2015. doi:10.1016/j.ancard. 2014.12.001.
19. Scherag A, Jarick I, Grothe J, Biebermann H, Scherag S, Volckmar AL, et al. Investigation of a genome wide association signal for obesity: synthetic association and haplotype analysis at the melanocortin 4 receptor gene locus. PLoS ONE. 2010;5(11):e13967.
20. Frayling TM, Timpson NJ, Weedon MN, Zeggini E, Freathy RM, Lindgren CM, et al. A common variant in the FTO gene is associated with body mass index and predisposes to childhood and adult obesity. Science. 2007;316(5826):889–94.
21. Claussnitzer M, Dankel SN, Kyong-Han K, Quon G, Meulemena W, Haugen C, et al. FTO obesity variant circuitry and adipocyte browning in humans. N Engl J Med. 2015. doi:10. 1056/NEJMoa1502214.
22. Li S, Zhao JH, Luan J, Langenberg C, Luben RN, Shaw KT, et al. Genetic predisposition to obesity leads to increased risk of type 2 diabetes. Diabetologia. 2011;54(4):776–82.
23. Choquet H, Meyre D. Genetics of obesity: what have we learned? Curr Genomics. 2011;12:169–79.
24. Ahmad T, Lee IM, Pare G, Chasman DI, Rose L, Ridker PM, Mora S. Lifestyle interaction with fat mass and obesity-associated (FTO) genotype and risk of obesity in apparently healthy U.S. women. Diabetes Care. 2011;34(3):675–80.
25. Li S, Zhao JH, Luan J, Ekelund U, Luben RN, Khaw KT, et al. Physical activity attenuates the genetic predisposition to obesity in 20,000 men and women from EPIC-Norfolk prospective population study. PLoS Med. 2010;7(8):e1000332.
26. Paneni F, Costantino S, Cosentino F. Role of oxidative stress in endothelial insulin resistance. World J Diabetes. 2015;6(2):326–32.

27. Yu T, Robotham JL, Yoon Y. Increased production of reactive oxygen species in hyperglycemic conditions requires dynamic change of mitochondrial morphology. Proc Natl Acad Sci USA. 2006;103:2653–8.
28. Chan DC. Fusion and fission: interlinked processes critical for mitochondrial health. Ann Rev Genet. 2012;46:265–87.
29. Cheng Z, Almeida FA. Mitochondrial alternation in type 2 diabetes and obesity. Cell Cycle. 2014;13(6):890–7.
30. Toledo FG, Goodpaster BH. The role of weight loss and exercise in correcting skeletal muscle mitochondrial abnormalities in obesity, diabetes and aging. Mol Cell Endocrinol. 2013;379:30–4.
31. Shanik MH, Xu Y, Skrha J, Dankner R, Zick Y, Roth J. Insulin resistance and hyperinsulinemia. Diabetes Care. 2008;31(2):S262–8.
32. Sleigh A, Raymond-Barker P, Thackray K, Porter D, Hatunic M, Vottero A, Burren C, Mitchell C, McIntyre M, Brage S, et al. Mitochondrial dysfunction in patients with primary congenital insulin resistance. J Clin Invest. 2011;121:2457–61.
33. Zheng LD, Linarelli LE, Longhua L, Wall SS, Greenawald MH, Seidel RW, et al. Insulin resistance is associated with epigenetic and genetic regulation of mitochondrial DNA in obese humans. Clin Epigentics. 2015. doi:10.1186/s13148-015-0093-1.
34. Sookoian S, Rosselli MS, Gemma C, Burgueno AL, Fernandez Gianotti T, Castano GO, Pirola CJ. Epigenetic regulation of insulin resistance in nonalcoholic fatty liver disease: impact of liver methylation of the peroxisome proliferator-activated receptor γ coactivator 1α promoter. Hepatology. 2010;52:1992–2000.
35. Barres R, Yan J, Egan B, Treebak JT, Rasmussen M, Fritz T, Caidahl K, Krook A, O'Gorman DF, Zierath JR. Acute exercise remodels promoter methylation in human skeletal muscle. Cell Metab. 2012;15:405–11.
36. Coelho M, Oliveira T, Fernandes R. Biochemistry of adipose tissue: an endocrine organ. Arch Med Sci. 2013;9:191–200.
37. Papaetis GS, Papakyriakou P, Panagiotou TN. Central obesity, type 2 diabetes and insulin: exploring a pathway full of thorns. Arch Med Sci. 2014;11(2):463–82.
38. Pedersen DJ, Guilherme A, Danai LV, Heyda L, Matevossian A, Cohen J, et al. A major role of insulin in promoting obesity-associated adipose tissue inflammation. Mol Metab. 2015;4:507–18.
39. Nathan DM, Davidson MB, DeFronzo RA, Heine RJ, Henry RR, Prately R, Zinman B. Impaired fasting glucose and impaired glucose tolerance. Diabetes Care. 2007;30(3):753–9.
40. Zhang Y, Hu G, Zhang L, Mayo R, Chen L. A novel testing model for opportunistic screening of pre-diabetes and diabetes among U.S. adults. PLoS ONE. 2015. doi:10.137/journal.pone.0120382.
41. Tabak AG, Herder C, Rathmann W, Brunner EJ, Kivimaki M. Lancet. 2012;379(9833):2279–90.
42. DECODE Study Group. Age-and sex-specific prevalences of diabetes and impaired glucose regulation in 13 European cohorts. Diabetes Care. 2003;26(1):61–9.
43. Bansal N. Prediabetes diagnosis and treatment: a review. World J Diabetes. 2015;6(2):296–303.
44. Haffner SM, Mykkanen L, Festa A, Burke JP, Stern MP. Insulin-resistant prediabetic subjects have more atherogenic risk factors than insulin–sensitive prediabetic subjects. Circulation. 2000;101:975–80.
45. Bellamy L, Casas JP, Hingorani AD, et al. Type 2 diabetes mellitus after gestational diabetes: a systematic review and meta-analysis. Lancet. 2009;373:1773–9.
46. Ford ES, Williamson DF, Liu S. Weight change and diabetes incidence: findings from a national cohort of US adults. Am J Epidemiol. 1997;146:214–22.
47. Meigs JB, Rutter MK, Sullivan LM, Fox CS, D'Agostino RB, Wilson BW. Impact of insulin resistance on risk of type 2 diabetes and cardiovascular disease in people with metabolic syndrome. Diabetes Care. 2007;30:1219–25.

48. Ali MK, Bullard KM, Saaddine JB, Cowie CC, Imperatore G, Gregg EW. Achievement of goals in U.S. diabetes care, 1999–2010. N Engl J Med. 2013;368:1613–24.
49. Pi-Sunyer FX. Weight loss in type 2 diabetic patients. Diabetes Care. 2005;28(6):1526–7.
50. Uranga-Ocio JA, Bastus-Diez S, Delkader-Palacios D, Garcia-Cristobal N, Leal-Garcia A, Abalo-Delgado R. Enteric neuropathy associated to diabetes mellitus. Rev Esp Enferm Dig. 2015;107(6):366–73.
51. Smith D, Williams C, Ferris C. Diagnosis and treatment of chronic gastroparesis and chronic intestinal pseudo-obstruction. Gastroenterol Clin N Am. 2003;32:619–58.
52. Kopacova M. Small intestinal bacterial overgrowth syndrome. World J Gastroenterol. 2010;16:2978–90.
53. Chandrasekharan B, Srinivasan S. Diabetes and the enteric nervous system. Neurogastroenterol Motil. 2007;19:951–60.
54. Lambadiari V, Triantafyllou K, Dimitriadis GD. Insulin action in muscle and adipose tissue in type 2 diabetes: the significance of blood flow. World J Diabetes. 2015;6(4):626–33.
55. Reaven GM. Banting lecture 1988. Role of insulin resistance in human disease. Diabetes. 1988;37(12):1595–607.
56. American Diabetes Association. Classification and diagnosis of diabetes. Diabetes Care. 2014;38(1):S8–16.
57. Parikh RM, Mohan V. Changing definitions of metabolic syndrome. Indian J Endocrinol Metab. 2012;16(1):7–12.
58. Alberti KG, Eckel RH, Grundy SM, Zimmet PZ, Cleeman JI, Donato KA, et al. Harmonizing the metabolic syndrome: a joint interim statement of the International Diabetes Federation Task Force on Epidemiology and Prevention; National Heart, Lung and Blood Institute; American Heart Association; World Heart Federation; International Atherosclerosis Society; and International Association for the Study of Obesity. Circulation. 2009;120(16):1640–5.
59. Thorpe AA, Schlaich MP. Relevance of sympathetic nervous system activation in obesity and metabolic syndrome. J Diabetes Res. 2015. doi:10.1155/2015/241583.
60. Rinella ME. Nonalcoholic fatty liver disease a systematic review. JAMA. 2015;313(22):2263–73.
61. Zhang XQ, Xu DF, Yu CH, Chen WX, Li YM. Role of endoplasmic reticulum stress in the pathogenesis of nonalcoholic fatty liver disease. World J Gastroenterol. 2014;20(7):1768–76.
62. Kirpich IA, Marsano LS, McClain CJ. Gut-liver axis, nutrition, and non alcoholic fatty liver disease. Clin Biochem. 2015. doi:10.1016/j.clinbiochem.2015.06.023.
63. Buchholz EM, Rathmore SS, Reid KJ, Jones PG, Chan PS, Rich MW, et al. Body mass index and mortality in acute myocardial infarction patients. Am J Med. 2012;125:796–803.
64. Mullen JT, Moorman DW, Davenport DL. The obesity paradox: body mass index and outcomes in patients undergoing nonbariatric general surgery. Ann Surg. 2009;250:166–72.
65. Migaj J, Prokop E, Straburzynska-Migaj E, Lesiak M, Grajek S, Mitkowski P. Does influence of obesity on prognosis differ in men and women? A study of obesity paradox in patients with acute coronary syndrome. Kardiol Pol. 2015. doi:10.5603/KP.a2015.0087.
66. Banack HR, Kaufman JS. Does selection bias explain the obesity paradox among individuals with cardiovascular disease? Ann Epidemiol. 2015. doi:10.1016/j.annepidem.2015.02.008.
67. Costanzo P, Cleland JGF, Pellicori P, Clark AL, Hepburn D, Kilpatirck ES, et al. The obesity paradox in type 2 diabetes mellitus: relationship of body mass index to prognosis: a cohort study. Ann Int Med. 2015;162(9):610–8.
68. Jerant A, Bertakis KD, Franks P. Body mass index and health care utilization in diabetic and nondiabetic individuals. Med Care. 2015. doi:10.1097/MLR.343.
69. Kortelainen MI, Porvari K. Extreme obesity and associated cardiovascular disease verified at autopsy: time trends over 3 decades. Am J Forensic Med Pathol. 2011;32:372–7.
70. Fadini GP, Boscaro E, de Kreutzenberg S, Agostini C, Seeger F, Dimmeler S, et al. Time course and mechanisms of circulating progenitor cell reduction in the natural history of type 2 diabetes. Diabetes Care. 2010;33:1097–102.
71. Graziani F, Biasucci LM, Cialdella P, Lizzo G, Giubilato S, Della Bono R, et al. Thromboxane production in morbidly obese subjects. Am J Cardiol. 2011;107:1656–61.

72. Feldman AM, Combes A, Wagner D, Kadakomi T, Kubota T, Li YY, McTierman C. J Am Coll Cardiol. 2000;35(3):537–44.
73. Savage DB, Petersen KF, Shulman GI. Disordered lipid metabolism and the pathogenesis of insulin resistance. Physiol Rev. 2007;87:507–20.
74. Stone NJ, Robinson JG, Lichtenstien AH, Goff DC, Lloyd-Jones DM, Smith SC, et al. Treatment of blood cholesterol to reduce atherosclerotic cardiovascular disease risk in adults: synopsis of the 2013 American College of Cardiology/American Heart Association cholesterol guideline. Ann Intern Med. 2014;160:339–43.
75. Graham R, Mancher M, Wolman DM, Greenfield S, Steinberg E, editors. Institute of medicine. Clinical guidelines we can trust. Washington, DC: National Academies Press; 2011.
76. Xu W, Shubina M, Goldberg SI, Turchin A. Body mass index and all-cause mortality in patients with hypertension. Obesity. 2015. doi:10.1002/oby.21129.
77. Hsu CY, McCulloch CE, Iribarren C, Darbinian J, Go AS. Body mass index and risk for end-stage renal disease. Ann Intern Med. 2006;144(1):21–8.
78. Bueter M, Ahmed A, Ashrafian H, le Roux CW. Surg Obes Relat Dis. 2009;5(5):615–20.
79. Tanida M, Yamamoto N, Shibamoto T, Rahmouni K. Involvement of hypothalamic AMP-activated protein kinase in leptin-induces sympathetic nerve activation. PLoS ONE. 2013;8(2):e56660.
80. Greenfield JR. Melanocortin signaling and the regulation of blood pressure in human obesity. J Neuroendocrinol. 2011;23(2):186–93.
81. Carmichael CY, Wainford RD. Hypothalamic signaling mechanisms in hypertension. Curr Hypertens Rep. 2015;17:39–47.
82. Hall JE, do Carmo JM, da Silva AA, Wang Z, et al. Obesity-induces hypertension: interaction of neurohumoral and renal mechanisms. Circ Res. 2015;116(6):991–1006.
83. Soleimani M. Insulin resistance and hypertension: new insights. Kidney Int. 2015;87:497–9.
84. Romero-Corral A, Montori VM, Somers VK, Korinek J, Thomas RJ, Allison TG, et al. Association of bodyweight with total mortality and with cardiovascular events in coronary artery disease: a systematic review of cohort studies. Lancet. 2006;368(9536):666–78.
85. Schenkeveld L, Magro M, Oemrawsingh RM, Lenzen M, de Jaegere P, Jan van Geuns R, et al. The influence of optimal medical treatment on the "obesity paradox", body mass index and long-term mortality in patients treated with percutaneous coronary interventions: a prospective cohort study. BMJ Open. 2012;2:e000535.
86. Luna-Luna M, Medina-Urrutia A, Vargas-Alarcon G, Coss-Rovirosa F, Vargas-Barron J, Perez-Mendez O. Adipose tissue in metabolic syndrome: onset and progression of atherosclerosis. Arch Med Res. 2015. doi:10.1016/j.arcmed.2015.05.007.
87. Di Chiara T, Argano C, Scaglione A, Corrao S, Pinto A, Scaglione R. Circulating adiponectin: a cardiometabolic marker associated with global cardiovascular risk. Acta Cardiol. 2015;70 (1):33–40.
88. Berg AH, Scherer PE. Adipose tissue, inflammation and cardiovascular disease. Circ Res. 2005;96:939–49.
89. Wu X, Zhu B, Fu L, Wang H, Zhou B, Zou S, Shi J. Prevalence, incidence, and mortality of stroke in the Chinese island populations: a systematic review. PLoS ONE. 2013;8:e78629.
90. Wu EQ, Birnbaum HG, Mareva M, Tuttle E, Castor AR, Jackman W, Ruskin J. Economic burden and co-morbidities of atrial fibrillation in a privately insured population. Curr Med Res Opin. 2005;21:1693–9.
91. Go AS, Hylek EM, Phillips KA, Chang Y, Henault LE, Selby JV, Singer DE. Prevalence of diagnosed atrial fibrillation in adults: national implications for rhythm management and stroke prevention: the AnTicoagulation and Risk Factors in Atrial Fibrillation (ATRIA) study. JAMA. 2001;285:2370–5.
92. Friberg L, Rosenqvist M, Lip GY. Evaluation of risk stratification schemes for ischemic stroke and bleeding in 182,678 patients with atrial fibrillation: the Swedish Atrial Fibrillation cohort study. Eur Heart J. 2012;33:1500–10.
93. Hajhosseiny R, Matthews GK, Lip GY. The metabolic syndrome, atrial fibrillation and stroke: tackling an emerging epidemic. Heart Rhythm. 2015. doi:10.1016/j.hrthm.2015.06.038.

94. Liu J, Butler KR, Buxbaum SG, Sung JH, Campbell BW, Taylor HA. Leptinemia and its association with stroke and coronary heart disease in the Jackson Heart Study. Clin Endocrinol (Oxford). 2010;72:32–7.
95. Wang TJ, Parise H, Levy D, D'Agostino RB, Wolf PA, Vasan RS, Benjamin EJ. JAMA. 2004;292(20):2471–7.
96. Ashrafian H, Frenneaux MP, Opie LH. Metabolic mechanisms in heart failure. Circulation. 2015. doi:10.1161/Circulationaha.1007.702795.
97. Hardy CM, Birse RT, Wolf MJ, Yu L, Bodmer R, Gibbs AG. Obesity-associated cardiac dysfunction in starvation-selectee drosophila melanogaster. Am J Physiol Regul Integr Comp Physiol. 2015. doi:10.1152/ajpregu.00160.2015.
98. Khavandi K, Khavandi A, Asghar O, Greenstein A, Withers S, Heagerty AM, Malik R. Diabetic cardiomyopathy—a distinct disease? Best Pract Res Clin Endocrinol Metab. 2009;23(3):347–60.
99. Waddingham MT, Edgley AJ, Tsuchimochi H, Kelly DJ, Shirai M, Pearson JT. Contractile apparatus dysfunction early in the pathophysiology of diabetic cardiomyopathy. World J Diabetes. 2015;6(7):943–60.

Chapter 6
Obesity-Related Diseases and Syndromes: Cancer, Endocrine Disease, Pulmonary Disease, Pseudotumor Cerebri, and Disordered Sleep

Key Message

Obesity promotes fundamental pathophysiological changes that permit the development of disease. Diseases associated with obesity do not occur in isolation like diseases in lean individuals, but instead are usually clustered as a group of interrelated problems. For example, psychological barriers may drive avoidance of medical follow-up for routine preventive testing or providers may misinterpret symptoms related to weight, resulting in a lack of focus on signs that might have allowed early detection of a treatable cancer. Poor sleep related to obesity may cause poor job performance that reinforces issues of self-efficacy and value. These interrelated problems are often treated as isolated issues while the more important pathology—obesity—is missed or ignored. Awareness of the interrelationships among these medical problems may alert treating providers to evaluate and communicate with patients and develop a more comprehensive strategy of treatment for specific problems and underlying pathology. This chapter discusses in detail the ways in which obesity relates to and impacts the following diseases and syndromes: cancer, endocrine disease, polycystic ovarian syndrome, infertility, pulmonary disease, asthma, hyperventilation syndrome, venus thromboembolic disease, pseudotumor cerebrii, disordered sleep and sleep apnea.

Learning Objectives

1. Identify mechanisms and pathways by which obesity promotes cancer and recurrent cancer through facilitating preservation of breast cancer stem cells.
2. Define the problems inherent in diagnosing and treating cancer in patients with obesity.
3. Compare the two primary theories of disease regarding polycystic ovarian syndrome.
4. Identify the primary problems you might find in a person with obesity and disordered sleep and define how to diagnose and treat them.

A causal link between inflammation and cancer was described as early as the mid-1800s when Rudolph Virchow suggested that inflammation promotes the type of microenvironment that converts tissue with a normal growth pattern into a malignant tumor. Inflammatory bowel disease resulting in colorectal cancer is one example of just such a causal relationship. The environment of obesity and the state of chronic inflammation that results is the ideal backdrop to promote tumor occurrence and progression. In 2008, it was noted that the tumor microenvironment has the same components and appearance as a healing wound with an influx of immune cells that are molded into the same types of "crown structures" described in white adipose tissue macrophages [1]. In addition, it appears the tumor can co-opt the inflammatory process to promote tumor growth and progression. Inflammation has always been noted to occur when cancer is present. In an obese person inflammation often predates cancer and is a key factor in allowing its development. The stakes for reducing obesity in an individual are high, both in terms of the tertiary prevention of cancer and in the risk of recurrence after diagnosis and treatment of cancer. Obesity has become one of two main risks for cancer second only to tobacco smoking.

The environment of inflammation created by obesity also provides fertile ground for fundamental changes in pulmonary function, incidence and acuity of asthma, pathogenesis of deep venous thrombosis, endocrine problems, infertility, and disordered sleep.

Obesity and Cancer

Most people do not think about obesity as a factor that increases the risk of cancer. Increased BMI ≥ 25 kg/m^2 is correlated with 2.5 % increase incidence of cancer in men and 4.1 % increased incidence of cancer in women. Certain groups of people, including African Americans, Hispanic Americans, and people of lower socioeconomic levels are the least aware and the most affected. Fifteen to twenty percent of total cancers occur in people with obesity and are accompanied by a marked increase in mortality [2]. There is a 75 % increase in mortality in premenopausal women with obesity and cancer, and a 34 % increase in postmenopausal women with obesity and cancer [3]. Men with obesity are known to develop prostate cancer associated with an aggressive phenotype and are often in an advanced stage at diagnosis. Obesity predisposes cancer survivors to higher recurrence rates of previously diagnosed cancer, plus adds the burden on the survivors of potentially developing new primary cancers. Moreover, many of the noncancer-related deaths that occur in cancer survivors are linked to obesity-related disease such as cardiovascular disease and diabetes. Typically, oncologists have not engaged in counseling patients about lifestyle modification as part of the strategy of treatment in cancer care. However, with the recent publication of the American Society of Clinical Oncology (ASCO) Position Statement on Obesity and Cancer, many clinicians are being made aware of the need to do so [4].

The three cancers that correlate most strongly with obesity are colorectal cancer, breast cancer, and endometrial carcinoma. In men who are obese it is generally colon, gallbladder, malignant melanoma, pancreatic and kidney cancers that are most strongly linked. In women who are obese it is generally colon, endometrial, esophageal, gallbladder, leukemia, pancreatic, breast and kidney cancers [5].

Obesity and Cancer

Table 6.1 Relative risk of cancer in patients with obesity BMI ≥ 30 versus BMI ≤ 25

Cancer type	Male	Female
Colorectal	1.95 (1.59–2.39)	1.66 (1.52–1.81)
Breast, postmenopausal		1.58 (1.40–1.79)
Endometrial		3.22 (2.91–3.56)
Ovarian		1.28 (1.20–1.36)
Esophageal	1.21 (0.97–1.52)	1.20 (0.95–1.53)
Kidney	1.82 (1.61–2.05)	2.64 (2.39–2.90)
Pancreatic	2.29 (1.65–3.19)	1.60 (1.17–2.20)
Prostate	1.05 (0.85–1.30)	
Gallbladder	1.47 (1.17–1.85)	1.82 (1.32–2.50)
Thyroid	1.12 (0.72–1.72)	1.03 (0.87–1.23)
Malignant melanoma	1.26 (1.07–1.48)	0.95 (1.84–1.07)
Leukemia	1.16 (0.88–1.52)	1.32 (1.08–1.60)
Non-Hodgkin's lymphoma	1.09 (1.07–1.73)	1.34 (1.22–1.46)

From Refs. [12, 13, 102]

Some cancers have a weak or nonlinear association with obesity. For instance, postmenopausal breast cancer is related to BMI but premenopausal breast cancer is not. In fact, premenopausal breast cancer may actually decrease with increasing BMI. Similarly, malignant melanoma and prostate cancer show a decreased incidence with increasing BMI in men [6]. The diversity and incidence of cancer in persons with obesity reflects the diversity of the etiology of cancer itself. The relative risk for obesity associated cancers has been established (Table 6.1).

Mechanisms of Cancer Growth and Promotion in Patients with Obesity

Obesity creates the perfect environment for cancers to flourish. The exact set of metabolic derangements that are present in obesity, including chronic inflammation, elaboration of adipokines and cytokines (cell signaling proteins), and an increase in the number of receptors for insulin and other hormones all contribute to an environment that promotes the development of cancer. Adipocytes, or fat cells, exhibit a high degree of plasticity and can be thought of as a type of "stem cell." Under the influence of inflammation, the adipocyte can transform into a cancer cell "helper" and create a procancer niche.

Two of the most well-known mechanisms for the development of obesity-related cancer are through the common pathways of chronic inflammation and insulin resistance. The tumor microenvironment includes tumor-associated macrophages (TAMS) that interact with tumor cells to promote the growth of cancer. Insulin-binding proteins and the protein hormones (IGF 1 and IGF 2) promote the development of cancer by favoring tumor cell growth and migration to establish metastasis.

Our understanding about the mechanisms that link obesity to cancers of the digestive system is evolving. Dysbiosis is defined as a microbial imbalance on or inside the body. Intestinal dysbiosis occurs in the digestive tract and is associated with illnesses such as inflammatory bowel disease, chronic fatigue syndrome, obesity, cancer, bacterial vaginosis, and colitis. Dysbiosis may be caused, among other things, by inappropriate diet which in turn can relate to obesity. High-fat feeding induces dysbiosis through the direct microbial activity of bile. Bile secreted during high-fat feeding breaks down insoluble fat molecules into soluble free fatty acids and monoglycerides, which then enter the bloodstream. This process of lipid digestion affects microbial survival and may be related to various illnesses including cancer [7].

Intestinal dysbiosis can create a procancer internal environment and affect the natural immunity that arises from a healthy intestinal system. In colorectal cancer colonic flora converts primary bile acids to secondary bile acids. These secondary bile acids damage DNA and promote apoptosis [8]. These same mechanisms may be active in the pathogenesis of the most common kind of liver cancer, hepatocellular carcinoma [9]. Bacteria in the stomach are linked with the generation of *N*-nitroso compounds that are potent carcinogens [10].

Sex hormones, too, interrelate to obesity and certain diseases, including cancer. Sex hormones have a higher circulating blood volume due to the conversion of androgens to estrogen in visceral (belly) fat. Women with obesity who are postmenopausal have higher levels of estradiol and estrone, making them more likely to develop both breast and endometrial cancer. This is an important clinical point, as postmenopausal women with an increased BMI and vaginal bleeding have a higher likelihood of endometrial cancer and may have to be referred for additional testing such as an endometrial biopsy. Patients with obesity experience changes in their immune function. For example obesity can impair the ability of the natural killer (NK) cells that are part of the surveillance function of the immune system whose mission is to seek out and kill developing cancer cells.

Adipokines, or cell signaling proteins, secreted by adipose (fat) tissue, are implicated in cancer cell progression because they enhance cell proliferation and migration thereby promoting metastasis, inflammation, and immortalizing cancer cells (anti-apoptosis). Leptin is the best-studied adipokine in terms of the magnitude and importance of its effect in promoting a procancer environment (*see* discussion in the breast cancer section below). Adiponectin and adiponectin receptors are at low levels in people with obesity. High adiponectin levels in lean individuals are associated with less cancer progression through improved insulin sensitivity. A higher grade of endometrial cancer is associated with a decreased number of adiponectin receptors. Multiple other adipokines are implicated in cancer (Table 6.2).

Cytokines (small proteins that serve as messengers between cells) are also implicated in the induction and pathogenesis of cancer through their influence on inflammation associated with obesity. The signaling pathway known as transcription factor NF-kB is activated in response to multiple stimuli and is linked to metastasis, angiogenesis, and cell proliferation. IL-6 is the best-studied cytokine relating to cancers of the colon and prostate, where it adopts the role of growth

Table 6.2 The role of adipokines in cancer promotion

Adipokine	Level in obesity	Gene/source/levels	Role in body	Role in cancer
Leptin	↑	OB Gene/Adipocyte Lean: 5–15 ng/ml Obese: 16–250 ng/ml	Energy regulation Food intake	Promote growth, level of aggressiveness in breast and colorectal cancer, marker in esophageal cancer
Adiponectin	↓	AdipQ, Adiopocyte Receptor AdipoR1 (skeletal muscle) and AdipoR2 (Liver) Circulating Levels: 2-20ug/ml	Adipocyte differentiation Insulin sensitivity Decreases inflammation	Cancer expression and progression **High levels in lean persons decrease cancer progression**
Apelin	↑	APLN, expressed by many tissues	Cell signaling Insulin secretion and CV function	LN metastasis and lymphangiogenesis High level, a risk factor for endometrial cancer
Visfatin	↑	Adipocyte Upregulated by hypoxia	Immune cell signaling	Colorectal, breast, and ovarian cancer protecting cancer cells from ROS Induces inflammation
Resistin	↑	RETN gene Produced in macrophage that invade adipose tissue from periphery	Possible link between inflammation and obesity	Active in colorectal, breast, prostate and hepatocellular carcinoma
Chemerin	↑	Adipocytes, spleen, lymph nodes, lung	Proinflammatory, modulates lipolysis	Enhances macrophage response Increased levels in gastric cell cancer
Omentin	↑	Tumor suppressor gene Also called intelectin Made in Adipocyte, higher in visceral adipocytes	Gut immunity pathologic bacteria	Inhibits proliferation of p53

From Booth et al. [103], with permission

promoter. Overall, NF-kB promotes a protumorigenic environment with the stimulation of chronic low-grade inflammation found in obesity [11].

In summary, obesity promotes a tumor microenvironment that promotes cancer progression by extending tumor cell survival, increasing proliferation and angiogenesis, participating with the microbial dysbiosis and promoting the development of inflammatory M1 macrophages [12].

Obesity and Breast Cancer

The breast is 80 % adipose tissue. It increasingly appears that a unique relationship exists between adipose tissue in the breast and breast cancer. Understanding this relationship can shed new light on how adipose tissue in general may be instrumental in cancer's progression elsewhere.

The report on the Women's Health Initiative (WHI) Randomized Clinical Trials recently reported that women with obesity and overweight had an increased risk of invasive breast cancer with the highest risk in women with BMI >35 kg/m^2. This group of women with a BMI >35 kg/m^2 had a 58 % increased risk of invasive breast cancer over women with a baseline BMI of 25 kg/m^2. The WHI trial provided a specific protocol for every woman followed in the trial: every woman underwent repeated measurements of height, weight, and waist circumference. Women with a baseline BMI of 25 kg/m^2 who gained more than 5 % body weight over the 13-year follow-up period had an increased risk of breast cancer, although neither weight gain nor weight loss changed the risk of the women who had been overweight or obese at baseline. For each increment of increased BMI there was an increased risk, suggesting a dose–response relationship. Central adiposity was not more related than subcutaneous adiposity. Obesity was associated with larger tumors, positive lymph nodes, distal metastasis at time of diagnosis, and 2× higher mortality. BMI was also associated with increased mortality for all categories after diagnosis of invasive breast cancer. This data differs from the data reported in the National Surgical Adjuvant Breast and Bowel Project Breast Cancer Prevention Trial (NSABP) where 75 % of those patients were being treated with tamoxifen or raloxifene, both of which decrease risk of breast cancer by as much as 50 % [13].

Obesity causes an increase in inflammation in both the adipose tissue of the breast and throughout the body. Localized and systematic chronic inflammation is believed to contribute to the development and progression of breast cancer.

White adipose tissue within the breast provides an ideal tumor microenvironment for inflammation with elevated levels of adipokines and cytokines, enhanced aromatase expression and increased estrogen receptor gene expression. After menopause, estrogen is made from androgen precursors in white adipose tissue. Obesity is thought to contribute to ER+/PR+ breast cancer after menopause by providing increased androgen substrate, but even with the systemic conversion of androgens to estrogens, the level of estradiol is still much lower than it is prior to menopause [14]. Paradoxically, almost 85 % of breast cancer that occurs after menopause is ER+; implicating the importance the local tumor microenvironment has on creating the ideal niche for the development of cancer [15].

Identifying molecular subtypes of breast cancer using gene expression profiling has resulted in improved treatment strategies and enhanced survival. Identification of unique properties of each subtype allows for specific treatment and provides the basis for improved outcomes. The two most common subtypes, luminal subtypes A and B, express estrogen and progesterone receptors and have improved outcomes due to use of antiestrogen therapy. Human epidermal growth receptor subtype breast cancer expresses Her2 and responds to targeted anti-Her2 therapy. Basal-like breast cancers tend to be triple negative (ER$^-$/PR$^-$/Her2$^-$) and often present with P53 mutations and are more aggressive. A newly described subtype has been found which is also ER and PR negative but low in claudin cell–cell adhesion molecules and basal cytokeratins [16]. Both the basal and claudin subtypes are more difficult to treat. This is related in part, to drug resistance and survival of cancer stem cells that are unique in their ability to repair DNA [17]. Because the tumor microenvironment is a key factor in the activation of cancer stem cell signaling, targeting the microenvironment may be a successful strategy to eliminate stem cell activation and progression [18]. This has been demonstrated in both multiple myeloma and in the use of aromatase inhibitors in postmenopausal breast cancer [19].

Breast cancer stem cell signaling takes place through multiple pathways. The best pathways are (1) activation of the notch receptor, allowing early breast cancer to gain a foothold in the tissue, (2) the Wnt pathway, promoting the invasive edge of tumor growth, and (3) the Oct-4/SOX2/Nanog axis, activating cell self-renewal and conferring pluripotency on a cell. All three means of stem cell signaling are frequently active in breast cancer stem cells. In addition, hypoxia in the tumor microenvironment activates HIF-1 and begins a cascade of events that immortalize cancer stem cells thereby generating the invasive phenotype.

Cancer-associated white adipocytes (fat cells) provide a tumor supportive microenvironment by undergoing changes that promote a specialized tumor "niche" of inflammation [20]. We know that obesity is associated with elevated levels of the "satiety hormone" known as leptin. Leptin acts on tissue through its obesity receptors (OB-R). The leptin receptor, OB-R, mediates the weight regulatory effects of the adipocyte-secreted leptin. In people with obesity leptin can reach up to seven times normal levels. OB-R is upregulated in all breast cancer subtypes and in breast cancer stem cells [21]. Silencing of the OB receptors in triple-negative breast cancer cells inhibited expression of the three means of breast cancer stem cell signaling [22–24]. These data supports the role of leptin in breast cancer initiation and progression as well as stem cell self-renewal.

Adipose tissue produces approximately 33 % of all interleukin 6 (IL-6) found in the blood. IL-6 is one of the major mediators of inflammation, acting as both a proinflammatory cytokine and as an anti-inflammatory myokine. It is secreted by T-cells and macrophages to stimulate an immune response. In healthy adipose tissue macrophages and cells other than adipocytes (fat cells) produce IL-6 [25]. On the other hand, unhealthy adipose tissue (cancer-associated adipocytes) secrete IL-6 through upregulation, with stimulation of invasiveness in ER$^+$ and ER$^-$ breast cancer cells. Breast cancer stem cells secrete up to 1000× more IL-6 than non-stem breast cancer cells [26]. Thus, under certain circumstances both IL-6 and leptin can promote breast cancer stem cell signaling and contribute to cancer progression.

The Challenge of Diagnosing and Treating Cancer in the Patient with Obesity

Women with obesity often do not undergo preventative screening for breast, cervical, and colorectal cancer because of discomfort about their body habitus [27]. This increases the burden on primary care providers to encourage and ensure that women with obesity have safe and accessible screening in a supportive environment. Obese and overweight patients have worse cancer-related outcomes than lean counterparts, with a 33 % increased mortality rate in women with obesity [3, 28]. The endothelial dysfunction present in obesity causes a decrease in blood flow to tissue beds. This may have the effect of decreasing the response of cancers to chemotherapy, especially in the response to targeted biological therapy [29]. Hyperinsulinemia can also affect treatment outcomes by causing a resistance to the death of cancer cells targeted by chemotherapy [30]. Obesity is also associated with higher reoccurrence rates for cancer [31]. Many chemotherapy drugs are lipophilic and accumulate in adipose tissue. Body fat is now being used in the dosage calculation [32]. The ASCO has issued guidelines on dosing in obese patients to ensure that adequate blood and tissue levels are obtained. Both prevention of weight gain with age and weight loss after cancer diagnosis and treatment may be important individual and public health strategies to reduce obesity-related cancer risk.

Obesity and Endocrine Disease

Obesity and Thyroid Hormones

Patients with weight gain often believe they have thyroid disease. Sometimes they do and sometimes they do not. Various glands of the endocrine system secrete hormones that regulate metabolism, growth, development, and reproduction. The thyroid gland is the largest gland in the endocrine system. It produces three hormones: thyroxine (T4), triiodothyronine (T3), and calcitonin. T4 and T3 play significant roles in metabolism and energy regulation in the body. When T4 or T3 are deficient for any reason metabolic function slows and becomes impaired, resulting in hypothyroidism. While weight gain or difficulty losing weight is strongly associated with hypothyroidism, the connection with BMI and obesity is not completely understood.

T4 is generally at normal levels in people with obesity. Thyrotropin, or TSH, is a hormone secreted by the pituitary gland that stimulates the thyroid to produce T4 and T3. TSH is usually in the high normal range, and greater than 2.5 pg/ml in 52 % of people with obesity. TSH levels are usually higher in persons with visceral adiposity [33]. T3 is more variable and, while it is not related to obesity, it may be related to the amount of food consumed This is because it increases with overfeeding and decreases during fasting or weight loss, regardless of the source of calories. T3 levels correlate with total energy expenditure and basal metabolic rate.

There is rarely an increase in body fat with hypothyroidism; weight gain more often is water retention that can often be reversed with thyroid hormone treatment. The water retention is due to the accumulation of hyaluronic acid within body tissues [34]. However, due to the effect of TSH and T3 on energy expenditure, there may be some contribution to weight gain in patients with clinical or subclinical hypothyroidism [35]. Hypothyroidism may impede weight loss efforts and should be considered in people who are employing behavioral methods without adequate response. Weight loss generally restores T3 to normal levels. Thyroid cancer risk increases with increasing BMI in non-Asians and may account for part of the increasing incidence of thyroid cancer [36].

Obesity and Polycystic Ovarian Syndrome

Polycystic ovarian syndrome (PCOS) is a common endocrine system disorder in which a woman has an imbalance of female sex hormones, resulting in various symptoms including irregular or no menstrual periods, excess body and facial hair, acne, difficulty getting pregnant, and patches of thick, dark, velvety skin. One of the reproductive risks of PCOS is infertility. PCOS is caused by a combination of genetic and environmental factors. Risk factors include obesity, lack of physical exercise, and a family history of the condition. PCOS is the most commonly diagnosed endocrine disorder in women. Diagnosis in adult women is made if two of three criteria are met: (1) androgen excess, (2) ovulatory dysfunction, or (3) polycystic ovaries. Disorders that mimic PCOS must also be excluded. PCOS affects 8–10 % of females of reproductive age, with 73 % of those women being overweight (38 %), or obese (53 %). Signs of the underlying pathology, including acanthosis nigricans (thick, dark, velvety skin), are identified in 62 % of female patients who are overweight and 21 % of female patients with obesity [37].

PCOS is often regarded as a reproductive issue but it is also associated with strong cardiometabolic risk factors. Many women with obesity, whether they have PCOS or not, have additional cardiometabolic risk factors. Lean women with PCOS also have additional cardiometabolic risk factors. PCOS should therefore be viewed as having both reproductive and cardiometabolic aspects. The pathophysiology of the cardiometabolic issues are linked to a low-grade chronic inflammatory state with hyperinsulinemia, hyperandrogenism and dysregulation of the sympathetic nervous system [38].

The Endocrine Society has developed guidelines for the diagnosis and treatment of PCOS, endorsing the Rotterdam criteria. It is acknowledged that the diagnosis is more problematic in adolescents and menopausal women [39]. PCOS can also create a state of anxiety in many women leading to mood disorders and depression. Consideration of quality of life issues and psychological consequences of PCOS should be taken into account when working with women of reproductive age who are overweight or obese [40].

Obesity and Infertility

Infertility is a disease of the reproductive system and is defined as the failure to achieve pregnancy after 12 months or more of regular sexual intercourse. One in seven couples in the United States is affected by infertility and the rate of infertility continues to rise. Men and women with obesity have an increased incidence of infertility. The conception rate for the fertile population is approximately 30 % per cycle with a cumulative conception rate of 84 % within one year. There are similar rates with assisted reproductive technology. Rates of conception for both groups in patients with uncomplicated obesity are significantly lower [41].

The biochemical effect of obesity on fertility includes hormone-related changes that increase the levels of estradiol and testosterone. Luteinizing hormone (LH) and increased androgen along with the changes in estrogens and sex hormone binding globulin (SHBG) cause impaired follicular development and atresia. In addition, the patient with obesity will often have insulin resistance, hypertension, dyslipidemia and metabolic syndrome, all of which independently affect fertility. The presence of inflammation, measured by C-reactive protein (CRP), IL-6 and TNFα, has additional deleterious effects on the reproductive cycle [42].

Women with obesity have increased rates of miscarriage [relative risk of 1.67 (95 % CI; 1.25–2.25)]. Following fertility manipulations to achieve pregnancy, miscarriage has a relative risk of 5.11 (95 % CI: 1.76–14.83) [43]. The risk of recurrent miscarriage is also higher. Guidelines in the United Kingdom suggest that pregnancy is best achieved at a BMI of <30 kg/m^2, although strict restrictions have not been implemented and decisions are based on individual situations. The chance of having a child with serious birth defects is also higher in obesity, with the risk being highest for spina bifida [44].

Infertility in men accounts for approximately 30 % of all cases of infertility and is primarily due to reduced semen quality. Sub-fertile men generally have higher BMI. The odds of infertility increase by 10 % for every 20 lb over ideal body weight [45].

Despite many reports of the relationship of leptin and adiponectin to infertility, a critical analysis suggests that the effects of both are minor and nonessential to human reproductive function [46]. Although semen quality may be lower in terms of sperm concentration and total sperm count, it appears that higher BMI is not associated with a higher level of DNA damage to sperm [47].

The primary hormonal defect in men is hypotestosteronaemia, leading to impaired spermatogenesis. The mechanisms of infertility in men include impaired semen quality, sexual dysfunction, endocrinopathy, and aromatization in peripheral tissues, sleep apnea, and psychological effects. Many of these mechanisms of infertility in men are reversible [48]. When working with couples facing infertility, reversal of risk factors including repletion of testosterone and weight loss may be important strategies.

Obesity and Pulmonary Disease

Abnormalities of Pulmonary Function

The most consistently reported effect of overweight and obesity on lung function is a reduction in functional residual capacity (FRC) of the lung with preservation of forced expiratory volume (FEV1) and forced vital capacity (FVC). In other words, the major effect of obesity is on lung volume. This is worse in visceral obesity and the mechanism is primarily mechanical. In obesity there is a stiffening of the total respiratory system which manifests as a rapid, shallow breathing pattern of reduced volumes. Ventilation/perfusion mismatch also occurs in a pattern opposite that of people who are lean, which means that the ratio of air (ventilation) and the amount of blood (perfusion) reaching the alveoli do not match, thus potentially causing type 1 respiratory failure. Although breathlessness often occurs in patients with obesity, an increase in ventilation can be enough to avoid high CO_2 levels from accumulating. Obesity and asthma affect the respiratory system through different mechanisms and obesity may increase the severity of asthma. The mechanisms of breathlessness in patients with obesity are still not well understood but we do know they are not related to lower blood oxygen concentrations [49]. Risk assessment for respiratory failure of the person with obesity could include clinic oximetry, V/Q scanning, and testing for sleep-disordered breathing, especially obstructive sleep apnea (OSA).

Asthma

Obesity is acknowledged as a risk factor for asthma and although they are associated the exact mechanism of the relationship is unknown. Many investigators are looking closely at the inflammatory pathways generated in obesity as a causal link [50]. Studies have linked low adiponectin levels and high leptin levels with asthma in both mice and humans, although exact causality in humans has not been firmly established [51]. As BMI increases there is an increasing incidence of asthma in women, especially if they gained their excess weight after 18 years of age [52]. There is also evidence that obesity exacerbates asthma reflected in increased asthma-related hospitalizations (OR 4.6, 95 % CI 1.4–14.4), poorer control (OR 2.8, 95 % CI 1.7–4.3), and worse quality of life (OR 2.8, 95 % CI 1.6–4.9) [53]. Weight loss from behavioral programs or bariatric surgery improves asthma [54–56].

Obesity Hyperventilation Syndrome

Obesity Hyperventilation Syndrome (OHS) is defined as the combination of obesity (BMI >30 kg/m^2), hypoxemia (falling oxygen levels in the blood) during sleep, and hypercapnia (increased CO_2 levels in the blood during the day), all resulting in hyperventilation. The exact cause of OHS is not known. Patients with obesity generally compensate for the increased respiratory load by breathing more rapidly but more shallowly, a response that is missing in those with OHS. In OHS, severely overweight patients fail to breathe rapidly enough or deeply enough, resulting in less ventilation with low blood oxygen levels and high carbon dioxide (CO_2) levels. Many patients with this condition also frequently stop breathing altogether for short periods of time during sleep. This is a secondary condition known as obstructive sleep apnea (OSA). The OHS puts strain on the heart and causes leg swelling and other symptoms. OHS may exist in 30 % of patients with obesity along with OSA. Both syndromes may predispose them to respiratory failure.

Venous Thromboembolic Disease

Venous thromboembolism (VTE) occurs when a blood clot breaks loose and travels within a vein. VTE disease includes both deep vein thrombosis (DVT) and pulmonary embolism (PE) and is the third leading cause of cardiovascular mortality. VTE results from a combination of hereditary and acquired risk factors. Deep venous thrombosis (DVT) is associated with obesity and it increases in incidence with increasing BMI (Table 6.3). For obese individuals in high-risk groups (i.e., patients age >60 years and presenting with Leiden Factor V) the 10-year relative risk increased 35 % in individuals with obesity versus 18 % in normal weight individuals [57]. Leiden Factor V is an inherited blood clotting disorder and is a genetic risk factor for VTE.

Obesity-related genes such as FTO may be highly associated with VTE but the presence of obesity genes account for a small percent of the people who have VTE, indicating that other factors promoting VTE should be considered [58]. Other factors in the etiology of VTE that are associated with obesity include elevated levels of proteins produced by the liver that help blood to clot. There is also often a change in platelet biology in these patients, which can include an increase in platelet counts, volume, and aggregation. The hormone leptin, too, induces both venous and arterial thrombosis through promotion of platelet aggregation [59]. Leptin is also implicated in worse 30-day outcomes of patients with PE independent of BMI. The average level of leptin was 10.1 ng/ml with lower levels of leptin associated with a 38 % increase in a complicated post-PE course of recovery and worse probability of survival [60].

Table 6.3 Risk of deep venous thrombosis (DVT) and pulmonary embolus (PE) with increasing BMI

	Overweight BMI 25–29.9 kg/m²	Obese BMI 30–34.5 kg/m²	Severe obesity BMI >35 kg/m²
DVT	1.3 (1.1–1.6)	1.8 (1.4–2.2)	3.4 (2.6–4.6)
PE	1.2 (0.8–1.8)	2.1 (1.3–3.5)	5.1 (2.8–9.2).

Data from Klovaite et al. [57], with permission

Some common conditions associated with obesity such as insulin resistance have not been shown to be independent of the effect of BMI [58].

Awareness of the impact increasing BMI may have on the development of VTE is important. Many dysfunctional metabolic mechanisms associated with obesity impact risk for cardiovascular mortality. In addition to addressing the underlying issue of excessive weight, pharmaceutical treatment may need to be adjusted in order to be effective.

Obesity and Pseudotumor Cerebrii

Pseudotumor cerebrii, also known as Idiopathic Intracranial Hypertension (IIH), is a condition in which pressure inside the skull increases and the brain is affected in a way that the condition may appear to be caused by a tumor, but is not. Pseudotumor cerebrii or IIH occurs more often in women than men, and is particularly prevalent in women with obesity who fall in the 20–40 year-old age group. IIH is a chronic disorder that often presents with headache, blurred vision, tinnitus, dizziness, nausea, papilledema, and vision loss. IIH is increasing in incidence with the increase in obesity. IIH has a relative risk of 8.0 (95 % CI, 2.29) for patients who are obese. Women of childbearing age 16–24 years have the highest relative risk of 17 (95 % CI: 5.62). Clinically severe obesity defined as a BMI of >40 kg/m^2 was associated with poor visual outcome [61]. Diagnosis of IIH is most common in women of childbearing age with obesity. Up to 25 % of severely obese patients with pseudotumor cerebrii or IIH suffer severe and permanent vision loss [62].

The etiology of IIH continues to be elusive. New evidence shows a link between IIH and OSA. The mechanism for this link is believed to be related to hypoxia (lack of oxygen in the body) and hypercapnia (elevated CO_2 in the body) that causes increased cerebral perfusion pressure from cerebral venous dilation [63].

The only proven therapy for pseudotumor cerebrii or IIH at this time for overweight and obese patients is weight loss. In a review of 62 patients treated with bariatric surgery, 56 of 62 patients (92 %) had resolution of their IIH symptoms. Patients with pre and postoperative testing had remission of papilledema (97 %), resolution of visual field defects (92 %), and an average decrease of 254 mm H_2O in cerebrospinal fluid pressures [64]. This is the best result of weight loss reported in commercially administered or primary care administered weight loss programs [65].

Disordered Sleep

There are many inputs to the brain that have not traditionally been considered as being connected to weight and metabolic disturbances. Now, however, many of the pathways that cause physical responses, including key signaling to the brain, are better understood. Disruption of circadian rhythms, sleep disorders, and stress are some of these inputs to the brain that are linked to weight and metabolic processes.

Sleep-disordered breathing (SDB) is a term that encompasses various forms of sleep apnea, hypopneas, and respiratory effort-related arousals that occur during sleep. SDB is associated with adverse effects on overall health. SDB affects an estimated 18 million Americans. Obesity is one of the most significant risk factors for the development of SDB. Over 70 % of patients with SDB are obese, and 40 % of persons with obesity suffer from SDB. Patients with SDB appear to be predisposed to weight gain and have abnormalities in plasma, leptin, ghrelin, and other mediators involved in regulating weight gain. The relationship between obesity and SDB may be bidirectional, with SDB actually contributing to obesity and vice versa [66].

Circadian Rhythm

Most living things have an internal clock or "circadian rhythm" that is in charge of life processes. Circadian rhythms are based upon 24-h intervals, and respond primarily to light and darkness within the environment. These 24-h rhythms tell our bodies when to sleep and these rhythms regulate many other essential processes including metabolism, hormone secretion, body temperature, sleep/wake cycles, waste elimination and arousal. These molecular clocks exist in every cellular system governed by direct exposure to the sun [67]. In mammals, the Suprachiasmatic Nucleus (SCN) is a tiny region in the brain that connects our bodies to the sun. The SCN is essential for behavioral rhythmicity. Complex, interconnected and interdependent signaling from robust clocks located around the body synchronize the entire system. In this way, the SNC is able to coordinate the activities of the organism as a whole [68].

The disruption of circadian rhythms occurs throughout the lifespan of humans and can result in disease. Circadian rhythm disorders can be caused by various factors, including shift work, pregnancy, time zone changes, medications, changes in routine, and various medical problems including dementia, Alzheimer's, Parkinson's disease, and mental illness [69–71]. Moreover, disruptions in the circadian rhythm have been associated with clinical impairments in metabolic processes and physiology. There is also evidence that disruption of circadian rhythms can result in cardiovascular disease, obesity, and cancer. This is because many hormones are affected by the disruption of the circadian clock and the disruption of sleep, including growth hormone, melatonin, thyroid stimulating hormone, cortisol, ghrelin, and leptin. In addition, circadian rhythm regulates glucose and lipid metabolism, so the disruption of the circadian rhythm can disrupt these levels as well [72].

Sleep

Humans spend about 30 % of their life sleeping. Breathing disorders during sleep along with disruptions in the duration and quality of sleep have been studied as contributors to obesity and obesity-related disease. Sleep disturbances have both personal and societal impact. Quality of life is affected when sleep habits such as excessive snoring disturb those around you. There are more serious life-threatening aspects of sleep disturbances as well, such as sleep deprivation and falling asleep while operating machinery or while at the wheel of a motor vehicle. Up to 20 % of accidents occur in drivers that fall asleep at the wheel, with major peaks at 0200, 0600 and 1600 h [73]. Recently, sleep disturbance has been associated with interfering with complex decision making required of leaders in stressful situations [74].

Owl or Lark?

Chronotype is defined as a trait determining individual circadian preference in rhythm relative to external light/dark cycles. An individual's chronotype can be determined by using a simple Q & A test to determine whether he/she is a morning person, an evening person, or an intermediate type [75]. Studies of chronotype reveal that larks and night owls are a part of the "circadian phenotype" of individuals. Chronotype can vary not only between individuals, but also within an individual's lifespan. Determining the "clock characteristics" of an individual can assist in identifying the connection between their individual circadian chronotype and potential disease. For example, studies of a person's fibroblast tissue correlate with that individual's chronotype and may help us understand why there is variability in who develops metabolic disorders and cancer and who does not [76].

Delayed sleep phase disorder in adolescents, where adolescents stay up very late at night and sleep late into the morning, is estimated at an incidence of 7–16 % [77]. Teenagers who do not meet the diagnostic criteria for deep sleep phase disorder nevertheless still have the chronotype of the "night owl." Night owl chronotype can be linked to depression and obsessive-compulsive disorder [78, 79]. Adapting the life schedule to account for the "night owl" chronotype may successfully treat the depression in some cases [80]. Beyond the chronotype, new data shows that it is not the habitual sleep duration pattern in adolescents that is significant vis-a-vis their food consumption, but rather the *variability* of their sleep duration pattern that is related to increased food consumption. Sleep variability of even one hour was associated with a 65–94 % increase in the consumption of snacks after dinner [81]. Maintaining regular sleep patterns may decrease the risk of obesity in adolescents.

There are gender differences between men and women who exhibit "night owl" chronotype. Night owl men are associated with an increased risk ratio of diabetes

(Odds ratio (OR) 3.89, 1.33–11.33) while night owl women have a higher risk for developing metabolic syndrome [OR 2.22(1.11–4.43)] [82].

Chronic exposure to light that does not allow us to get consistent quality of sleep may relate to incidence of obesity. Excess exposure to light caused weight gain in groups of animals that had consistent caloric intake and physical activity. This was studied again in a group of over 100,000 women in the United Kingdom from 2003 to 2012. In that study, obesity assessed through BMI and waist circumference increased with increased exposure to light at night. These data were adjusted for confounding variables such as alcohol intake, smoking, and activity levels [83].

Lack of sleep has been shown to increase inflammation. Both acute loss of sleep for three consecutive days or sleep reduction by 25–50 % across consecutive days increases interleukin-6 (IL-6) and CRP. Sleep disturbances, inflammation, and body pain often occur together. The optimal amount of sleep is 7 h in a dark and noiseless room. When a person gets 4 h as opposed to 8 h of sleep it leads to increases in IL-6 and CRP [84]. There are gender differences in the amount of inflammation that occurs with sleep disturbance. Men exhibiting both obesity and sleep disturbance have more inflammation than obese controls without sleep disturbance [85].

Rapid eye movement (REM) sleep is a highly prized period of sleep that occurs in humans more than other mammals. It is associated with random movement of the eyes, low muscle tone, dreaming and is associated with a physiological "fast". The average human spends about 90–120 min in REM. Early in the sleep cycle the periods of REM are short, increasing in time through the sleep period. A newborn baby spends about 80 % of their sleep in REM. REM decreases in childhood and throughout adulthood. One of the unique qualities about REM is that it resembles "wakefulness" more than sleep. The brain emits oscillations similar to wakefulness. During REM many of the physiological functions of the body that are normally under autonomic regulation, such as heart rate, cardiac pressure and breathing rate, become irregular. The final REM period just prior to wakefulness may have unique properties that specifically impact obesity. This final period of REM sleep acts as an appetite suppressant and may be integral to developing food preferences and dislikes. It may also induce energy balancing effects with respect to body heat retention [86].

The issue of sleep duration has become a central research question. In a 7.5-year sleep study conducted on 815 non-obese adults the incidence of obesity was 15 %. Uniquely, this study examined each person for emotional stress and subjective sleep disturbance as well as sleep duration. Self-reported short sleep duration in non-obese persons was a surrogate marker for emotional stress and subjective sleep disturbance. Measured short sleep duration was not associated with the risk of incident obesity. These findings have raised important questions regarding emotional stress and whether the person's perception that they have short sleep is the root cause of sleep-related obesity rather than actual duration of sleep itself [87].

Insomnia and Stress

Insomnia is the most common sleep disorder. Over 60 % of patients who suffer from insomnia are never asked about it and they never complain of insomnia during discussions with their physicians. Many think of insomnia as a loss of sleep but it is, in fact, a *state of hyperarousal* during the night, and also during the day [88]. Positron emission tomography (PET) scanning of the brain has shown enhanced cerebral glucose metabolism in people with insomnia vs. those with sleep deprivation or normal sleepers [89]. Insomnia is more common in aging individuals, with an incidence of 50 % in people over age 65. Insomnia is also more frequently found in women, in people of lower education and/or lower socioeconomic status, and in separated, widowed or divorced individuals [90]. Insomniacs do not show increased sleepiness as compared to normal sleepers. In fact, insomniacs are more alert which lends support to the concept that insomnia is a 24-h hyperalert state [91]. Markers of stress such as increased adrenocorticotropic hormone (ACTH) and increased cortisol are often significantly higher in patients with insomnia. Proinflammatory cytokines, interleukin-6 (IL-6), and tumor necrosis factor (TNF) are also often elevated in patients with insomnia [92].

It appears that disordered sleep of multiple varieties plays a key role in the resulting phenotypic expression of people with obesity. The concept of "subtyping" obesity based on different biological drivers and evaluating their relationships to different treatments may be one way to sort out the relative contribution of each subtype and enable more targeted therapy to be developed [93].

We often think of stress as the situation in which we feel discomfort or anxiety. People can experience stress from external or internal factors. External sources of stress include adverse physical triggers such as pain, or hot or cold temperatures. External sources of stress can also include adverse psychological triggers such as poor working conditions or a verbally abusive relationship. Internal sources of stress include physical triggers like infections, disease or inflammation, as well as internal psychological triggers like worrying about the future or the fear of snakes. Feelings of stress, regardless of cause, translate directly into the physiological system that governs metabolism, caloric intake, and energy expenditure. In terms of biology, stress is often the direct result of chemical interactions and signaling in the body that require biological systems to act in ways that override normal function.

No discussion of the biological drivers of obesity is complete without a discussion of the hypothalamic–pituitary–adrenal (HPA) axis of the brain. It is an integral part of almost everything we have discussed and is governed by one's circadian rhythm and sleep. The HPA is often used as a marker for general circadian and sleep-related health. As we have seen, many internal and external signals from the body impact this same area of the hypothalamus of the brain. Stress results in the pituitary's production of ACTH which in turn influences the adrenal glands to produce steroid hormones. This process emits both circadian patterns as well as rhythmic pulses every 80–110 min that are not related to the SCN. White adipose tissue is a direct target of the circadian clock process in the sense that the brain's processing of stress generates leptin, adiponectin, lipogenesis and lipolysis, all of which affect a person's weight. Leptin acts directly on the hypothalamus and is implicated in the dysregulation of the HPA, which contributes to higher levels of glucocorticoids [94]. While glucocorticoids are generally beneficial in reducing inflammation throughout the body, moderate to high levels of glucocortoids actually suppress, instead of amplify, the body's ability to fight the effects of stress. In addition, high levels of glucocortoids can affect metabolism by stimulating the liver to release more sugar. This may lead to an excess of sugar in the blood and ultimately diabetes [95, 96].

Obstructive Sleep Apnea

Sleep Disordered Breathing (SDB) is associated with morbidity and increased mortality. In a population-based study of people without a known diagnosis of SDB, the median apnea–hypopnea index (AHI) was 6.9 events per hour in women and 14.9 events per hour in men with a prevalence of 23.4 % in women and 49.7 % in men. The upper 25 % of HPI was associated with hypertension, diabetes, metabolic syndrome, and depression [97]. One of the most common types of disordered sleep is Obstructive Sleep Apnea (OSA). In 1993 it was estimated that 4 % of men and 2 % of women had OSA [98]. Currently, the rates are 23.4 % in women and 49.7 % in men (AHI > 15) with the increased incidence associated with rising rates of obesity [97]. OSA occurs due to a mechanical collapse of the pharyngeal airway. Obesity worsens this mechanism. It appears that a simple diagnosis of OSA based on AHI is naïve as the mechanisms that underlie apnea may be broader. Suspicion of OSA can be established by measuring neck circumference Diagnostic testing has shifted from the sleep lab environment to home testing [99].

Sleep apnea is strongly associated with both obesity and increased cardiovascular risk factors including inflammation, insulin resistance, hyperlipidemia and hypertension. A 10 % reduction in body weight reduces the AHI by 26–32 %. The link between OSA and cardiovascular risk may be through the effect of OSA on endothelial dysfunction by creating an environment of oxidative stress and inflammation [100].

A recent randomized prospective trial reported on the success of CPAP treatment alone versus CPAP and lifestyle intervention. CRP, insulin and triglyceride levels were reduced after lifestyle intervention with or without CPAP. The group with CPAP alone (no lifestyle intervention) experienced no impact with respect to cardiovascular risk factors [101]. A secondary finding of the trial was that both OSA and obesity had an independent causal relationship with hypertension.

Conclusion

Inflammation and dysfunction of adipose tissue underlies much of the pathology that we see in obese patients. The only comprehensive strategy for treatment is through weight loss. Comprehensive evaluation of patients and treatment of each related disease in the context of recognizing obesity as the primary problem makes the most sense for a treatment paradigm. In addition, consistent and persistent encouragement of the patient to participate in preventive screening is critical. Educating the patient on how to best address the problem of obesity can vastly improve their health and their quality of life. This is an important role for the provider to play.

Chapter 5 and this chapter have reviewed many of the mechanisms by which obesity can be a central underlying pathology for many related disorders and diseases. It is easy to understand why weight loss is a powerful and important treatment goal.

References

1. Mantovani A, Allavena P, Sica A, Balkwill F. Cancer-related inflammation. Nature. 2008;454:436–44.
2. Flegal KM, Carroll MD, Kit BK, Ogden CL. Prevalence of obesity and trends in the distribution of body mass index among U.S. Adults, 1999–2010. JAMA. 2012;307:491–7.
3. Calle EE, Rodriguez K, Walker-Thurmond K, Thun MJ. Overweight, obesity and mortality from cancer in a prospectively studied cohort of U.S. adults. N Engl J Med. 2003;238(17):1625–38.
4. Ligibel JA, Alfano CM, Courneya KS, Demark-Wahnefried W, Burger RA, Chlebowski RT, et al. American Society of Clinical Oncology position statement on obesity and cancer. J Clin Oncol. 2014;32(31):3568–74.
5. Dobbins M, Decorby K, Choi BC. The association between obesity and cancer risk: a meta-analysis of observational studies from 1985 to 2011. ISRN Prev Med. 2013;680536.
6. Bhaskaran K, Douglas I, Forbes H, dos-Santos-Silva I, Leon DA, Smeeth L. Body-mass index and risk of 22 specific cancers: a population—based cohort study of 5.24 million UK adults. Lancet. 2014;384:755–65.
7. Chan YK, Estaki M, Givson DL. Clinical consequences of diet-induced dysbiosis. Ann Nutr Metab. 2013;63(2):28–40.
8. Pearson JR, Gill CI, Rowland IR. Diet, fecal water, and colon cancer-development of a biomarker. Nutr Rev. 2009;67:509–26.
9. Ohtani N, Yoshimoto S, Hara E. Obesity and cancer: a gut microbial connection. Cancer Res. 2014;74(7):1885–9.
10. Wang LL, Yu XJ, Zhan SH, Jia SH, Tian ZB, Dong QJ. Participation of microbiota in the development of gastric cancer. World J Gastroenterol. 2014;20(17):4948–52.
11. Karin M. Nuclear factor-kb in cancer development and progression. Nature. 2006;441:431–6.
12. Ungefroren H, Gieseler F, Fliedner S, Lehnert H. Obesity and cancer. Horm Mol Biol Clin Invest. 2015;21(1):5–15.
13. Neuhouser ML, Aragaki AK, Prentice RL, Manson JE, Chlebowski R, Carty CL, et al. Overweight, obesity, and the postmenopausal invasive breast cancer risk. JAMA Oncol. 2015. doi:10.1001/jamaoncol.2015.1546.

14. Iyengar NM, Judis CA, Dannenberg AJ. Obesity and inflammation: new insights into breast cancer development and progression. Am Soc Clin Oncol Educ Book. 2013;46–51.
15. Lorinez AM, Sukumar S. Molecular links between obesity and breast cancer. Endocr Relat Cancer. 2006;13:279–92.
16. Wolfson B, Eades G, Qun Z. Adipocyte activation of cancer stem cell signaling in breast cancer. World J Biol Chem. 2015;6(2):39–47.
17. Dean M, Fojo T, Bates S. Tumor stem cells and drug resistance. Nat Rev Caner. 2005;5:275–84.
18. Quail DF, Joyce JA. Microenvironmental regulation of tumor progression and metastasis. Nat Med. 2013;19:1423–37.
19. Brodie A, Long B. Aromatase inhibition and inactivation. Clin Cancer Res. 2001;7:4343–49s.
20. Dirat B, Bochet L, Dabek M, Daviaud D, Dauvillier S, Majed B, et al. Cancer-associated adipocytes exhibit and activated phenotype and contribute to breast cancer invasion. Cancer Res. 2011;71:2455–65.
21. Feldman DR, Chen C, Punj V, Tsukamoto H, Machida K. Pluripotency factor-mediated expression of the leptin receptor (OB-R) links obesity to oncogenesis through tumor-initiating stem cells. Proc Natl Acad Sci USA. 2012;109:829–34.
22. Zheng Q, Banaszak L, Fracci S, Basali D, Dunlap SM, Hursting SD, et al. Leptin receptor maintains cancer stem-like properties in triple negative breast cancer cells. Endocr Relat Cancer. 2013;20:797–808.
23. Guo S, Liu M, Gonzalez-Perez RR. Role of Notch and its oncogenic signaling crosstalk in breast cancer. Biochim Biophys Acta. 2011;1815:197–213.
24. Gillespie C, Quarshie A, Penichet M, Gonzalez-Perez RR. Potential role of leptin signaling in DMBA induced mammary tumors by non-responsive C57BL/6J mice fed a high fat diet. J Carcinogene Mutagene. 2012;3:132.
25. Galic S, Oakhill JS, Steinberg GR. Adipose tissue as an endocrine organ. Mol Cell Endocrinol. 2010;316:129–39.
26. Yang L, Han S, Sun Y. An Il6-STAT3 loop mediates resistance to PI3K inhibitors by inducing epithelial-mesenchymal transition and cancer stem cell expansion in human breast cancer cells. Biochem Biophys Res Commun. 2014;435:582–7.
27. Cohen SS, Palmieri RT, Nyante SJ, Koralek DO, Kim S, Bradshaw P, Olshan AF. Obesity and screening for breast, cervical and colorectal cancer in women: a review. Cancer. 2008;112(9):1892–904.
28. Protani M, Coory M, Martin JH. Effect of obesity on survival of women with breast cancer: systematic review and meta-analysis. Breast Cancer Treat. 2010;123:627–35.
29. Guiu B, Petit JM, Bonnetain F. Visceral fat area is an independent predictive biomarker of outcome after first-line bevacizumab-based treatment in metastatic colorectal cancer. Gut. 2010;59:341–7.
30. Chen J, Katsifis A, Hu C, Huang XF. Insulin decreases therapeutic efficacy in colon cancer cell line HT29 via the activation of the P13K/Akt pathway. Curr Drug Discov Technol. 2011;8:119–25.
31. Jones DH, Nestore M, Henophy S, Cousin J, Comtois AS. Increased cardiovascular risk factors in breast cancer survivors identified by routine measurements of body composition, resting heart rate and arterial blood pressure. SpringerPlus. 2014;3:150.
32. Griggs JJ, Mangu PB, Anderson H, Balaban EP, Dignam JJ, Hryniuk WM, et al. Appropriate chemotherapy dosing for obese adult patients with cancer: American Society of Clinical Oncology Clinical Practice Guideline. J Clin Oncol. 2012;30:1553–61.
33. Muscogiuri G, Sorice GP, Mezza T, Prioletta A, Lassandro AP, Pirronti T, et al. High-normal TSH values in obesity: is it insulin resistance or adipose tissue's guilt? Obesity. 2013;21(1):101–6.
34. Weaver JU. Classical endocrine diseases causing obesity. Front Horm Res. 2008;36:212–28.
35. Kokkoris P, Pi-Sunyer FX. Obesity and endocrine disease. Endocrinol Metab Clin N Am. 2003;32:895–914.

36. Zhao AG, Guo XG, Ba CX, Wang W, Yang YY, Wang J, Cao HY. Overweight, obesity and thyroid cancer risk: a meta-analysis of cohort studies. J Int Med Res. 2012;40:2041–50.
37. Baer TE, Milliren CE, Waills C, DiVasta AD. Clinical variability in cardiovascular disease risk factor screening and management in adolescent and young adult women with polycystic ovary syndrome. J Pediatr Adolesc Gynecol. 2014. doi:10.10161/j.jpag.2014.09.101.
38. Shorakae S, Teede H, de Courten B, Lambert G, Bovle J, Moran LJ. The emerging role of chronic low-grade inflammation in the pathophysiology of polycystic ovary syndrome. Semin Reprod Med. 2015;33(4):257–69.
39. Legro RS, Arslanian SA, Ehrmann DA, Hoeger KM, Hassan-Murad M, Pasquali R, Welt CK. Diagnosis and treatment of polycystic ovary syndrome: an Endocrine Society Clinical Practice Guideline. J Clin Endocrinol Metab. 2013;98(12):4565–92.
40. Podfigurna-Stopa A, Luisi S, Regini C, Katulski K, Centini G, Meczekalski B, Petraglia F. Mood disorders and quality of life in polycystic ovary syndrome. Gynecol Endocrinol. 2015;31(6):431–4.
41. Wilkes S, Murdoch A. Obesity and female fertility: a primary care perspective. J Fam Plan Reprod Health Care. 2009;35(3):181–5.
42. Talmor A, Dunphy B. Female obesity and infertility. Best Pract Res Clin Obstet Gynecol. 2015;29:498–506.
43. Metwally M, Ong KJ, Ledger WL, et al. Does high body mass index increase the risk of miscarriage after spontaneous and assisted conception? A meta-analysis of the evidence. Fertil Steril. 2008;90(3):714–26.
44. Stothard KJ, Tennant PW, Bell R. Maternal overweight and obesity and the risk of congenital anomalies: a systematic review and meta-analysis. JAMA;2009;301:636–50.
45. Sallmen M, Sandler DP, Hoppin JA, Blair A, Baird DD. Reduced fertility among overweight and obese men. Epidemiology. 2006;17:520–3.
46. Kawwass JF, Summer R, Kallen CB. Direct effects of leptin and adiponectin on peripheral reproductive tissues: a critical review. Mol Hum Reprod. 2015;21(8):617–32.
47. Bandel I, Bungum M, Richtoff J, Malm J, Axelsson J, Pedersen HS, et al. No association between body mass index and sperm DNA integrity. Hum Reprod. 2015;30(7):1704–13.
48. Katib A. Mechanisms linking obesity to male infertility. Cent European J Urol. 2015;68:79–85.
49. Salome CM, King GG, Berend N. Physiology of obesity and effects on lung function. J Appl Physiol. 2010;108:206–11.
50. Papoutsakis C, Priftis KN, Drakouli M, et al. Childhood overweight/obesity and asthma: is there a link? A systematic review of recent epidemiologic evidence. J Acad Nutr Diet. 2013;113(1):77–105.
51. Sood A, Shore SA. Adiponectin, leptin and resistin in asthma: basic mechanisms through population studies. J Allergy. 2013;785835.
52. Camargo CA, Weiss St, Zhang S, Willett WC, Speizer FE. Prospective study of body mass index, weight change, and risk of adult-onset asthma in women. Arch Intern Med. 1999;159 (21):2582–8.
53. Mosen DM, Schatz M, Magid DJ, Camargo CA. The relationship between obesity and asthma severity and control in adults. J Allergy Clin Immunol. 2008;122(3):507–11.
54. Stenius-Aarniala B, Poussa T, Kvarnstrom J, Gronlund EL, Yikahri M, Mustajoki P. Immediate and long term effects of weight reduction in obese people with asthma: randomized controlled study. BMJ. 2000;320(7238):827–32.
55. Eneli IU, Skybo T, Camargo CA. Weight loss and asthma: a systematic review. Thorax. 2008;63(8):671–6.
56. Dixon AE, Pratley RE, Forgione PM, Kaminsky DA, Whittaker-Leclair LA, Griffes LA, et al. Effects of obesity and bariatric surgery on airway hyper responsiveness, asthma control and inflammation. J Allergy Clin Immunol. 2011;128(3):508–15.
57. Klovaite J, Benn M, Nordestgaard BG. Obesity as a causal risk factor for deep venous thrombosis: a Mendelian randomization study. J Intern Med. 2015;277(5):573–84.

58. Van Schouwenburg IM, Mahmoodi BK, Veeger NK, Bakker SJ, Kluin-Nelemans HC, Meijer K, Gansevoort RT. Insulin resistance and risk of venous thromboembolism: results of a population-based cohort study. J Thromb Haemost. 2012;10(6):1012–8.
59. Schafer K, Konstantinides S. Adipokines and thrombosis. Clin Exp Pharmacol Physiol. 2011;38(12):864–71.
60. Dellas C, Lankeit M, Reiner C, Schafer K, Hasenfuß G, Konstantinides S. BMI-independent inverse relationship of plasma leptin levels with outcomes in patients with acute pulmonary embolism. Int J Obes (Lond). 2013;37(2):204–10.
61. Rowe FJ, Sarkies NJ. The relationship between obesity and idiopathic intracranial hypertension. Int J Obes. 1999;23(1):54–9.
62. Mollan SP, Markey KA, Benzimra JD, Jacks A, Matthews TD, Burdon MA, Sinclair AJ. A practical approach to, diagnosis, assessment and management of idiopathic intracranial hypertension. Pract Neurol. 2014;14:380–90.
63. Fraser CL. Obstructive sleep apnea and optic neuropathy: is there a link? Curr Neurol Neurosci Rep. 2014;14(8):465.
64. Fridley J, Foroozan R, Sherman V, Brandt ML, Yoshor D. Bariatric surgery for the treatment of idiopathic intracranial hypertension. J Neurosurg. 2011;114:34–9.
65. Jolly K, Lewis A, Beach J, Denley J, Adab P, Deeks JJ, Daley A, Aveyard P. Comparison of range of commercial or primary care led weight reduction programmes with minimal intervention control for weight loss in obesity: lighten up randomized controlled trial. BMJ. 2011; 343:c6500.
66. Leinum C, Dopp J, Morgan B. Sleep disordered breathing and obesity: pathophysiology complications and treatment. Nutr Clin Prac. 2009;24(6):675–87.
67. Underwood H, Steele CT, Zivkovic B. Circadian organization and the role of the pineal in birds. Microsc Res Tech. 2001;53(1):48–62.
68. Bedont JL, Newman EA, Blackshaw S. Patterning, specification and differentiation in the developing hypothalamus. Interdiscip Rev Dev Viol. 2015. doi:10.1002/wdev.187.
69. Tranah GJ, Blackwell T, Stone KL, Ancoli-Israel S, Paudel ML, Ensrud KE, et al. Circadian activity rhythms and risk for incident dementia and mild cognitive impairment in older women. Ann Neurol. 2011;70:722–32.
70. Morton AJ, Wood NI, Hastings MH, Hurelbrink C, Barker RA, Maywood ES. Disintegration of the sleep-wake cycle and circadian timing in Huntington's disease. J Neurosci. 2005;25:157–63.
71. Harper DG, Stopa EG, McKee AC, Satlin A, Fish D, Volicer L. Dementia severity and Lewy bodies affect circadian rhythms in Alzheimer disease. Neurobiol Aging. 2004;25:771–81.
72. Kim TW, Jeong JH, Hong SC. The Impact of sleep and circadian disturbance on hormones and metabolism. Int J Endocrinol. 2015; PMID 591729.
73. Horne JA, Reyner LA. Sleep related vehicle accidents. BMJ. 1995;210(6979):565–7.
74. Harrison Y, Horne JA. The impact of sleep deprivation on decision-making: a review. J Exp Psychol Appl. 2000;6(3):236–49.
75. Horne JA, Ostberg O. A self-assessment questionnaire to determine morningness-eveningness in human circadian rhythms. Int J Chronobiol. 1976;4(2):97–110.
76. Saini C, Brown SA, Dibner C. Human peripheral clocks: applications for studying circadian phenotypes in physiology and pathophysiology. Front Neurol. 2015;6(95):1–8.
77. Bartlett DJ, Biggs SN, Armstrong SM. Circadian rhythm disorders among adolescents: assessment and treatment options. Med J Aust. 2013;199(8):S16–20.
78. Reid KJ, Jaksa AA, Eisengart JB, Baron KG, Lu B, Kane P, et al. Systematic evaluation of Axis-I DSM diagnoses in delayed sleep phase disorder and evening—type circadian preference. Sleep Med. 2012;13:1171–7.
79. Schubert JR, Coles ME. Obsessive-compulsive symptoms and characteristics in individuals with delayed sleep phase disorder. J Nerv Ment Dis. 2013;201:877–84.
80. Miller NL, Tvaryanas AP, Shattuck LG. Accommodating adolescent sleep-wake patterns: the effects of shifting the timing of sleep on training effectiveness. Sleep. 2012;35:1123–36.

References

81. He F, Bixler EO, Berg A, Imamura KY, Vgontzas An, Fernandez-Mendoza J, Ynosky J, Liao D. Habitual sleep variability, not sleep duration, is associated with caloric intake in adolescents. Sleep Med. 2015;16(7):856–61.
82. Yu JH, Yun CH, Ahn JH, Suh S, Cho HJ, Lee SK, et al. Evening chronotype is associated with metabolic disorders and body composition in middle-aged adults. J Clin Endocrinol Metab. 2015;100(4):1494–502.
83. McFadden E, Jones ME, Schoemaker MJ, Ashworth A, Swerdlow AJ. The relationship between obesity and exposure to light at night: cross-sectional analyses of over 100,000 women in the breakthrough generations study. Am J Epidemiol. 2014;180(3):245–50.
84. Haak M, Sanchez E, Mullington JM. Elevated inflammatory markers in response to prolonged sleep restriction are associated with increased pain experience in healthy volunteers. Sleep. 2007;30(9):1145–52.
85. Gaines J, Vgontzas An, Fernandez-Mendoza J, Kritikou I, Basta M, Bixler EO. Gender differences in the association of sleep apnea and inflammation. Brain Behav Immun. 2015;47:211–7.
86. Horne JA. Human REM sleep: influence on feeding behavior, with clinical implications. Sleep Med. 2015;S138909457(15):00706-6.
87. Vgontzas AN, Fernandez-Mendoza J, Miksiewicz T, Kritikou I, Shaffer ML, Liao D, Basta M, Bixler EO. Unveiling the longitudinal association between short sleep duration and the incidence of obesity: the Penn State Cohort. Int J Obes. 2014;38(6):825–32.
88. Basta M, Chrousos GP, Vela-Bueno A, Vgontzas AN. Chronic insomnia and stress system. Sleep Med Clin. 2007;2(2):279–91.
89. Nofzinger EA, Buysse DJ, Germain A, Price JC, Miewald JM, Kupfer DJ. Functional neuroimaging evidence for hyperarousal in insomnia. Am J Psychiatry. 2004;161:2126–9.
90. Ohayon MM. Epidemiology of insomnia: what we know and what we still need to learn. Sleep Med Rev. 2002;6:97–111.
91. Vgontzas AN, Zoumakis E, Bixler EO, Lin HM, Follet H, Kales A, et al. Adverse effects of modest sleep restriction on sleepiness, performance and inflammatory cytokines. JCME. 2004;89:2119–26.
92. An Vgontzas, Bixler EO, Lin HM, Prolo P, Mastorakos G, Vela-Bueno A, et al. Chronic insomnia is associated with nyctohermeral activation of the hypothalamic-pituitary-adrenal axis: clinical implications. J Clin Endocrinol Metab. 2001;86:3878–94.
93. Vgontzas AN, Bixler EO, Chrousos GP, Pejovic S. Obesity and sleep disturbance: meaningful sub-typing of obesity. Arch Physiol Biochem. 2008;114(4):224–36.
94. Kolbe I, Dumbell R, Oster H. Circadian clocks and the interaction between stress axis and adipose function. Int J Endocrinol. 2015. doi:10.1155/2015/693204.
95. Berthoud HR. The neurobiology of food intake in an obesogenic environment. Proc Nutri Soc. 2012;71(4):478–87.
96. Munck A, Guyre PM, Holbrook NJ. Physiological function of glucocortoids in stress and their relation to pharmacological actions. Endocr Rev. 1984;5(1):25–44.
97. Heinzer R, Vat S, Margques-Vidal P, Marti-Soler H, Andreis D, Tobback N, et al. Prevalence of sleep-disordered breathing in the general population: the HypnoLaus study. Lancet Respir Med. 2015;3(4):210–8.
98. Young T, Palta M, Dempsey J, Skatrud J, Weber S, Badr S. The occurrence of sleep-disordered breathing among middle-aged adults. N Engl J Med. 1993;32:1230–5.
99. Malhotra A, Orr JE, Owens RL. On the cutting edge of obstructive sleep apnea: where next? Lancet Respir Med. 2015;3(5):397–403.
100. Budhiraja R, Parthasarathy S, Quan SF. Endothelial dysfunction in obstructive sleep apnea. J Clin Sleep Med. 2007;3(4):409–415.
101. Chirinos JA, Gurubhagavatula I, Teff K, Rader DJ, Wadden TA, Townsend R, et al. CPAP, weight loss or both for obstructive sleep apnea. N Engl J Med. 2014;370(24):2265–75.

102. Guh DP, Zhang W, Bansback N, Amarsi Z, Birmingham CL, Anis AH. The incidence of co-morbidities related to obesity and overweight: a systematic review and meta-analysis. BMC Public Health. 2009;9:88–108.
103. Booth A, Magnuson A, Fouts J, Foster M. Adipose tissue, obesity and adipokines: role in cancer promotion. Horm Mol Biol Clin Invest. 2015;219(1):57–74.

Chapter 7
Pediatric Obesity

Key Message

Obesity now affects 1 in 6 children and adolescents in the United States. Sixty million American preschoolers are expected to be overweight or obese by 2020. Rates of childhood and adolescent obesity are increasing globally, as well. We blame the parents, the schools, the environment, computers, and cell phones – the list is endless. Obesity has a profound effect on the self-esteem of both children and adolescents.

Parents, some of whom suffer from obesity themselves, are often unaware of the dire consequences of childhood obesity and may be defensive about their children's weight. Nonetheless, as good practitioners we must engage in nonjudgmental communication with parents not only about their children's weight but about the risks of obesity-related disease. Forecasting the child's future health and educating the parents about obesity may energize the parents and family as a whole to rectify poor choices they may be inadvertently making. Medical practitioners, teachers and the many other people who work with, encourage and advise children must seek to help all children overcome the bias and stigma of obesity. It will require a collaborative effort on everyone's part, including the patient's, to achieve the goal of optimum physical and mental health for this group of children. The question is: what will it take to reverse the trend? The future is dim unless we can answer this crucial question.

This chapter explains in detail why epigenetics and fetal/metabolic programming are strong risk factors for obesity in children and adolescents. It describes how the "body mass index (BMI) for age" growth charts are used to evaluate changes in the health status of children and adolescents. This chapter also discusses how childhood obesity can lead to the emergence during childhood of specific adult obesity-related diseases. The unique challenges of managing childhood obesity are explored and the four stages of obesity intervention that all practitioners can use to diagnose and treat childhood and adolescent obesity are explained.

Learning Objectives

1. Explain why epigenetics and metabolic programming are strong risk factors for obesity in children and adolescents.
2. Describe the influence of the *in utero* environment on obesity and chronic disease.
3. Describe how "body mass index (BMI) for age" growth charts are used to evaluate changes in health status during childhood and adolescence.
4. Explain the concept of "early adiposity rebound" and its utility in assessing pediatric obesity.
5. Explain how childhood obesity can lead to the emergence of adult obesity-related diseases during childhood.
6. Describe the unique challenges for managing childhood obesity.
7. Describe the four stages of obesity intervention for childhood and adolescent obesity.

Childhood obesity has more than doubled in children and quadrupled in adolescents over the past 30 years. Obesity now affects 1 in 6 children/adolescents in the United States. Although there are specific inherited types of pediatric obesity, most obesity in the pediatric age group is "common" obesity. The causes of "common" obesity in children is similar to those causes found in adult obesity: a transgenerational epigenetic inheritance of obesity susceptible genes, the interaction of the child with the environment through their behavior (i.e., dietary patterns, inactivity, medications, depression) and other contributing factors including lack of education, decreased physical activity, socioeconomic conditions, and the unrelenting marketing, promotion and availability of unhealthy foods.

Parents, schools, and healthcare professionals and children themselves all have an impact on childhood obesity. Education about the importance of making healthy food and lifestyle choices has been somewhat abandoned to peers and mass marketing. Health education is missing from the curriculum of many schools. Some schools provide hot meals for their students via popular food vendors, but those meals consist largely of unhealthy fast food that is high in fat, endocrine disrupting chemicals, and high glycemic carbohydrates. Diet staples in the United States and increasingly around the globe include fast food, soda, candy, chips, and snacks, all often super sized. To make matters worse, these empty calories are enticingly and continuously promoted in the media and are addictive when consumed on a regular basis. The pediatric patient is vulnerable to all of these influences and the result is devastating.

Scope of the Epidemic

"Overweight" is defined in children as a body mass index (BMI) between the 85th and 94th percentile. "Obesity" is defined as a BMI greater than the 95th percentile for sex and age. The effect of being obese upon entering kindergarten is profound. 75 % of children who are obese between 5 and 14 years of age were above the 70th percentile for BMI upon entering kindergarten. Overweight 5-year olds are four

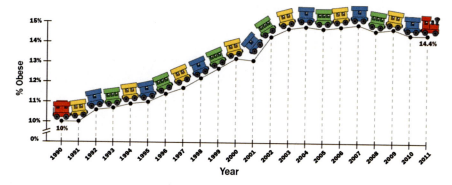

Fig. 7.1 Obesity rates among low-income preschoolers (from pediatric nutrition surveillance 2011 report www.cdc.gov.ped)

times as likely as normal weight children to become obese. Children with overweight at age 5 have a cumulative incidence of 31.8 % for obesity versus 7.9 % for kids that are normal weight upon entering kindergarten [1].

Prevalence of obesity in the US is currently 12.5 % in 2–5-year olds, 18 % in 6–11-year olds and 18.4 % in 12–19-year olds, with an overall prevalence rate of 17.3 %. Sixty million American preschoolers are expected to be overweight or obese by 2020. Rates of childhood and adolescent obesity are increasing globally, as well. Prevalence of childhood obesity in developed countries increased substantially from 1980 to 2013, with 23.8 % of boys and 22.6 % of girls being defined as overweight or obese. In developing countries the prevalence increased from 8.1 to 12.9 % in boys and from 8.4 to 13.4 % in girls [2].

Data compiled in 2013 suggested a slight leveling off or decrease in the prevalence of childhood obesity [3] (Fig. 7.1). Despite this good news, many experts are skeptical of the data because the representation among different age groups was not consistent and the focus was only on BMI and did not take into account waist circumference, which may show a general increase in obesity [4]. In any event, the current generation of children is not expected to outlive their parents due to the burden of chronic obesity-related disease [5]. Enlisting every parent, teacher, health care provider and child in this battle is required to stem the tide.

Genetic Influence on Childhood Obesity

Obesity is a heritable disease. If both parents are obese there is a 75 % chance that the child will be obese. 80 % of obese adolescents remain obese as adults. Up to 70 % of human obesity is inherited as a polygenic trait [6].

Hales and Barker first posited the "thrifty gene" hypothesis in 1992, proposing that susceptibility to certain adult chronic diseases, including insulin resistance and type 2 diabetes, occurred due to under-nutrition in the fetal and infant environment.

The hypothesis was that in order to adapt, the fetus and the infant had to be nutritionally "thrifty." If nutrition increased at a later point in time the ability of the pancreas to maintain homeostasis was theoretically exceeded, resulting in insulin resistance and diabetes [7]. The origins of the "thrifty gene" hypothesis started with the idea that the bodies of our prehistoric ancestors harbored calorie-hoarding "thrifty" genes to survive long stretches of near starvation, relying on inner reserves of adipose tissue. This has been a dominant theory for the evolutionary origins of obesity and, by extension, for obesity-related diseases such as insulin resistance and diabetes. Support for this "thrifty gene" hypothesis, as an explanation by itself for obesity, is eroding in scientific circles. However, the cause of obesity definitely has a genetic component and "thrifty genes," if they exist, are part of a complex genetic picture that is contributing to the obesity epidemic.

The genetic component of obesity has been demonstrated in multiple studies. The studies describe distinct processes by which epigenetic changes can influence an individual's propensity for obesity. Both pre and postnatal epigenetic changes can occur and can lead to an increased risk for obesity and type 2 diabetes (T2DM) [7].

Epigenetic changes do not change the DNA gene sequence, but they alter the transcription of genes, resulting in a different expression of the genes. In obesity this is often seen in genes that regulate energy balance. Postnatal epigenetic changes can also routinely occur in response to aging, diet, ingested drugs, or environmental chemicals. Epigenetic changes manifest as DNA methylation and histone modifications and can lead to strong associations with chronic disease.

Prenatal epigenetic changes and genetic imprinting can occur during the development of the fetus in response to its unique environmental influences. Imprinting can occur *in utero* when certain genes are silenced which affects fetal growth and results in changes to organ structure and function.

Some genetic imprinting is related to a parent's own health. For example, a pregnant woman can pass on epigenetic changes to her offspring. A pregnant woman with obesity and poorly or uncontrolled type 2 diabetes has chronically high levels of glucose circulating in the placenta. This excess glucose can cause epigenetic changes in leptin, insulin, and growth factor genes, resulting in large-for-gestational-age (LGA) babies. Conversely, women who smoke and/or who are malnourished with high levels of stress experience changes in the genes that control cortisol production, resulting in small-for-gestational-age (SGA) babies [8]. Both pathways, LGA and SGA, lead to an increased risk for obesity and T2DM.

The external environment to which parents are exposed also can have a physical effect on their offspring. Exposure to hazardous chemicals is one such example. Daughters of Danish women exposed to the chemical perfluorooctanoate (PFOA) *in utero* were three times more likely to be obese at age 20, even after controlling for other risk factors [9]. PFOA alters lipid metabolism and has been associated with cancers, thyroid disease, high cholesterol, and hypertension of pregnancy. In 2012, scientists at Emory University showed that workers in a chemical plant in West Virginia with high exposure to PFOA had roughly $3\times$ the risk of dying from mesothelioma or chronic kidney disease and roughly $2\times$ the risk of dying of diabetes [10].

Paternal imprinting and epigenetic alterations in the sperm of fathers also contribute to SGA babies with an increased risk for obesity and type 2 diabetes [11].

Both the mother and father have a critical role in influencing the future of their children through the imprinting of epigenetic changes, through their own health and lifestyle choices, and through their own exposure to environmental influences.

In the postnatal period obesity susceptibility genes interact with dietary fats, carbohydrates, physical inactivity, and social and psychological factors to establish individual physiology that promotes obesity. This is an area of medicine called "nutritional genomics" [12]. *Parents should be made aware of these pre and postnatal contributions to the future health of their offspring.*

There are important signs that can be observed by healthcare providers and parents that signal an increased risk for obesity in children. Early infancy is a period of rapid growth. Body weight doubles during the first 4–6 months of life and this weight gain should be carefully monitored. One study of 19,397 infants followed from birth to age 7 showed that too rapid weight gain in the first four months increased the risk of obesity at age 7. The study further showed that "catch up growth" between ages 0 and 2 resulted in heavier children with higher body fat by 5 years of age [13].

Body mass index (BMI) in children normally declines to a nadir between ages 2 and 6 before increasing again into adulthood. This nadir followed by a subsequent increase is called adiposity rebound (AR). This is the normal pattern of growth that occurs in children. The mean age of adiposity rebound is 5.5 years. Recent research indicates that the age at which adiposity rebound occurs may signal a critical period in childhood for the development of obesity as an adult. Children with *early* adiposity rebound occurring between ages 3 and 5 are likely to become obese adults. Early adiposity rebound increased the risk of developing obesity to 25 % versus a 5 % risk of developing obesity with normal adiposity rebound, with an odds ratio of 6.0 (95 % CI, 1.2–26.6) [14].

In summary, specific risk factors present during the period prior to the father and mother becoming pregnant as well as during the pre and postnatal period can have a profound effect on whether an individual child will become obese as an adult (Table 7.1).

Types of Childhood Obesity

When evaluating a child with either overweight or obesity it is helpful to consider how genetics are contributing to their obesity. Three classifications can be made based on both genetic and physical findings.

Table 7.1 Modifiable early life risk factors for pediatric obesity

Preconception/parental traits	Pre-pregnant BMI in mother of >30 kg/m^2
Pregnancy	Excess gestational weight gain Smoking Low vitamin D status in mother (<64 nmol/L)
Infancy	Short duration of breastfeeding (none or <1 month)

Data from Robinson et al. [67]

Common Obesity

For most children, *common obesity* results from epigenetic changes in several genes. At least 16 genes that are designated as "susceptibility genes," including FTO and MC4R, have been identified. This type of inheritance of obesity is "polygenic," meaning that many genes act together to promote obesity in the child. This type of inheritance is transmitted with codominance of the genes involved and each has a small or modest effect on its own. These genes can be influenced by the environment to magnify or minimize their effect.

Syndromic Obesity

The other two classifications of childhood obesity are monogenic and are not easily confused with common obesity because they present with obvious and serious early signs, symptoms, and complications. Approximately 30 (with some as yet to be identified) genes are estimated to be responsible for rare but significant monogenic forms of *syndromic obesity*. Syndromic obesity is characterized in general by extreme adiposity, congenital physical malformations, and intellectual disabilities. Clinically, the parent and child will often report *hyperphaga* or abnormally increased appetite/consumption of food. The most commonly identified form of syndromic obesity is Prader–Willi disease (1/25,000 births). The neonate is hyptotonic with a weak sucking reflex and failure to thrive. Hyperphagia is usually apparent by age 6 years but may be absent earlier in the child's life. Short stature, undersized genitals, mild to moderate intellectual impairment, narrow forehead, almond-shaped eyes, and small hands and feet characterize this disease. The onset of puberty may be delayed. Insatiable appetite is usually noted by 6 years of age, resulting in chronic overeating (hyperphaga) and obesity. There are different forms of this single gene disorder therefore the severity and timing of clinical presentation can vary. Some people with a mild presentation may not be identified until adulthood.

Additional types of syndromic obesity include Laurence–Moon (Bardet–Biedl) syndrome (LMBBS) and Beckwidth–Weiderman syndrome (BWS). LMBBS is characterized by vision loss, developmental delay, learning disabilities, abnormalities of the genitalia and kidneys, multiple digits of the hands and feet (polydactyly), retinitis pigmentosa, and obesity. LMBBS occurs in 1/140,000 newborns with key gene mutations that affect cilia, which are the finger-like projections involved in cell movement and chemical signaling. Beckwidth–Weiderman syndrome (BWS) is characterized most often by a large tongue and omphalocele, which is a birth defect in which the intestines and abdominal organs are outside the abdomen at birth. Infants with BWS are usually larger than normal and their growth is asymmetrical and slows by age 8. Children with BWS do not usually have developmental delay. These children are at higher risk of developing both cancerous and noncancerous tumors particularly of the kidney and liver, with 10 percent of children developing these tumors.

Non-syndromic Obesity

The final type of childhood obesity is *non-syndromic obesity*. Eight susceptibility genes define rare monogenic forms of obesity. Mutations in the LEP gene, for example, result in profound leptin deficiency. In these cases administering leptin reverses obesity. These children also experience hyperphagia and a lack of satiety. A case was recently reported in which the leptin mutation led to biologically inactive leptin with high levels of circulating but inactive hormone. These levels of leptin appeared to be normal but were not effective in controlling energy homeostasis. The patient responded to metreleptin (synthetic leptin) which rresulted in normalized weight and lower levels of circulating inactive leptin. Patients with early onset, severe obesity and with high levels of leptin that appear to correlate with BMI and body fat may have biologically inactive leptin which could obscure the diagnosis of leptin deficiency [15].

Children who possess a variation in the Melanocortin 4 Receptor (MC4R) exhibit hyperphagia but have accelerated linear growth. They eat large volumes of food even from an early age. Both of these characteristics distinguish them from children with Prader–Willi. Specific mutations in the Melanocortin 4 Receptor account for at least 6 % of severe early onset obesity in children. In the evaluation of a severely obese child there are specific items in the history that are important to solicit in order to distinguish the type of obesity and to eliminate syndromic forms of pediatric obesity (Tables 7.2 and 7.3).

Clinical Consequences of Childhood Obesity

Childhood obesity is associated with the same obesity-related diseases we used to think of as occurring only in adults (Fig. 7.2). These may include disordered sleep, respiratory problems, gastrointestinal issues, and a variety of endocrine disorders,

Table 7.2 Evaluation of the obese child

Age of onset	Early onset at less than 5 years of age suggests a genetic cause
Duration of obesity	Short history suggests endocrine or central cause (hypothalamus)
Frequent infections and fatigue	ACTH deficiency due to POMC mutations
Hyperphagia	Does the child wake at night to eat or demand food too soon after a meal?
Developmental delay	Milestones, educational history, behavioral disorders may be due to structural causes or genetic ones
Visual impairment and deafness	Suggests genetic cause, Bardet–Biedl syndrome
Onset and tempo of puberty	Genetic disorders associated with hypogonadism
Family history	Consanguineous relationships, other children affected, refer to a family reunion photograph, increased severity may be due to the interaction with the environment

From Faroogi and O'Rahilly [68] with permissions

Table 7.3 The differential diagnosis in pediatric obesity

General	Endocrine disorder	Genetic syndrome	Acquired lesion of the hypothalamus	Single gene mutation
Over-nutrition	Hypothyroidism	Down's	Tumor or post surgery damage	Melanocortin 4-receptor
Idiopathic/familial obesity	Glucocorticoid excess—endogenous or exogenous	Prader–Willi	Head trauma	Leptin
	Growth Hormone deficiency	Bardet Biedel (also called Lawrence–Moon)	Meningitis	Leptin receptor
		Alstrom	Anoxic brain injury	
		Cohen		
		PTH resistance with Albright's Hereditary osteohystrophy		
		Rapid-onset obesity with hypothalamic dysfunction, hypoventilation and autonomic dysregulation		

Data from Siebert et al. [45]

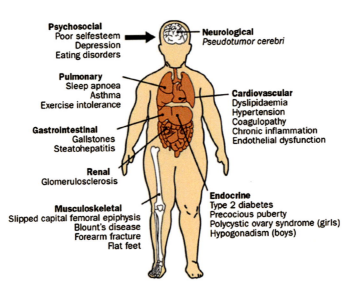

Fig. 7.2 The major complications associated with childhood obesity (from Garver et al. [66], with permission)

Table 7.4 Recommended hours of sleep required by age

Age	Recommended sleep (h)
0–1 months	12–18
3–11 months	14–15
1–3 years	12–14
3–5 years	11–13
5–10 years	10–11
10–17 years	8.5–9.25

From Matricciani et al. [69] with permission

all of which are discussed in more detail below. The two most effective screening tools for childhood obesity-related health issues and disease are a thorough review of systems and a physical exam.

Disordered Sleep

Disordered sleep can affect the level of steroid hormones in the body and can be a contributing factor to childhood obesity. Many children are not getting enough sleep in a sleep friendly environment for a variety of reasons. The recommended hours of sleep for children from infancy to age 17 ranges from 18 h for infants to 9.25 h for 17 year olds [16] (Table 7.4).

Poor sleep quality also contributes to childhood obesity with the onset of obstructive sleep apnea characterized by loud snoring, pauses in breathing, daytime sleepiness, and waking with a headache. Sleep apnea affects as many as 50 % of adolescents [17]. On physical exam the patient may have enlarged tonsils and adenoids. Evaluation by a pulmonologist may be indicated if the tonsils and adenoids are not enlarged. Untreated sleep apnea can lead to right ventricular hypertrophy, pulmonary hypertension, enuresis, and poor academic performance. Screening through the ROS may also reveal enuresis or poor academic performance. A strong current recommendation is not to allow a television or computer in the child's bedroom.

Obesity Hypoventilation Syndrome (OHS) is another sleep disorder that manifests when excess weight on the chest and abdomen impairs ventilation in children who have very severe obesity. The main symptoms of OHS mimic the symptoms of obstructive sleep apnea and may include depression, headaches, and daytime sleepiness. Polysomnography is necessary to distinguish OHS from sleep apnea and the test may reveal high carbon dioxide levels. Lab work may reveal elevated hemoglobin and hematocrit levels. In addition, the patient may manifest rapid shallow breathing with normal oxygen levels.

Respiratory Problems in Children with Obesity

Asthma is the most common chronic disease in childhood and obesity is a risk factor for asthma. In 2014, the causal link between obesity and asthma was demonstrated using a Mendelian randomization study showing that the effect of BMI on asthma had a relative risk of 1.55 per kg/m^2. Every one-unit increase in BMI increases the risk of asthma by 55 %. The rise in obesity toward the end of the twentieth century may largely account for the increase in the prevalence of asthma [18].

Gastrointestinal Problems in Children with Obesity

Non-alcoholic fatty liver disease (NAFLD) in children encompasses all the pathology that accompanies liver disease associated with adult obesity. NAFLD affects 1 % of 2–4-year olds and 17 % of 15–19-year olds. Overall, NAFLD is present in 38 % of children with obesity. Currently NAFLD is the third leading cause for liver transplantation in the United States. Children with obesity have the potential to have the disease far longer than a patient with adult-onset NAFLD. These children may be at unique risk for future liver failure and need for transplantation. The immediate importance of NAFLD is the relationship it has with insulin resistance and promotion of T2DM. Liver biopsy is the standard of diagnosis but it is rarely indicated in pediatric-age patients. However, an ALT/AST liver enzyme screening every two years is indicated in children with obesity. If enzymes are elevated over 2× normal, referral to a pediatric gastroenterologist is recommended. Weight loss generally leads to improvement in liver function.

Gastroesophageal reflux disease (GERD) is more common in children with obesity than in normal weight children. The prevalence of GERD is estimated to be 3–5 % among all children [19] as reported by Marek Lukacik, MD at Digestive Disease Week in 2015. He estimated a prevalence of GERD in 25–30 % of children who are overweight or obese. The management of GERD in children with overweight and obesity is managed the same as it is managed in normal weight children.

The risk of cholelithiasis or gallstones increases as BMI increases. Boys with moderate and extreme obesity have an adjusted odds ratio for developing gallstones of 1.83(1.17–2.85) and 3.10(1.99–4.83). Girls with moderate and extreme obesity have an adjusted odds ratio for developing gallstones of 5.75(4.62–7.17) and 7.71 (6.13-9.71), respectively [20]. Gallstones may occur more frequently in children undergoing weight loss. In one study, children with weight loss greater than 10 % had a prevalence of 5.9 %, with the highest prevalence found in those children losing more than 25 % of their weight. Of those children with gallstones, 22 % required cholecystectomy. The relative risk of developing gallstones was 3.26 (95 % CI: 1.60–6.65) for each change in BMI z score [21].

Endocrine Disorders in Children with Obesity

Insulin Resistance and Type 2 Diabetes in Children with Obesity

For many years type 1 diabetes was the most prevalent form of diabetes in children. With the increase in childhood obesity, T2DM has now become more prevalent, especially in children that are overweight or obese. Prediabetes prevalence in children with obesity is 19.5 and 27.3 % for those with clinically severe obesity (BMI >99th percentile). Prevalence for T2DM is 39.8 % in children who are obese and 52.4 % for those with clinically severe obesity [22]. Children with T2DM present differently than adults and require laboratory screening. Risk factors for T2DM in children include obesity (BMI > 85th percentile), family history of diabetes, special ethnic group including Black, Latino or Native American, polycystic ovarian syndrome (PCOS), acanthosis nigricans, NAFLD, or other cardiovascular risk factors. Biyearly screening beginning at age 10 using a fasting blood glucose is recommended by the American Diabetes Association if the child is overweight and has two additional risk factors. Fasting blood glucose levels of ≥ 100 mg/dL indicate prediabetes, whereas ≥ 126 mg/dL indicate diabetes. Referral to a pediatric endocrinologist should be in made in cases where childhood diabetes is proven.

Metabolic Syndrome in Children with Obesity

Four different diagnostic criteria for metabolic syndrome (MetS) in children have been established by four different medical groups based on different risk factors, resulting in different prevalence rates. The World Health Organization published their definition and criteria for MetS in 1999. Two years later the National Cholesterol Education Program and Adult Treatment Panel III for Adults published their criteria. In 2005, the Brazilian Cardiology Society proposed the I Guideline for Prevention of Atherosclerosis in Infancy and Adolescent.

In an attempt to standardize the diagnostic criteria for children and adolescents, the International Diabetes Federation (IDF) in 2007 released a definition of MetS for children and adolescents between the ages of 10 and 19, according to age groups [23].

In these criteria the reference values are the same as those proposed for adults except that waist circumference percentiles (rather than absolute values) are used. This compensates for varying degrees of development and ethnicity. Central obesity *plus* two or more other risk factors is an essential condition to diagnosing MetS [24] (Table 7.5).

In 2015, a new definition of MetS for children ages 6–18 emerged. It was tested on 15,794 youth aged 6–18, using specific risk factors. The results of this study showed that more youth had clustering of cardiovascular disease (CVD) compared to the number selected by existing MetS definitions. In the 2015 study BMI and waist circumference were interchangeable, but an insulin resistance homeostasis model assessment (HOMA) instead of fasting glucose was used, which increased the MetS scores. The scores also increased when cardiorespiratory fitness

Table 7.5 A comparison of requirements for metabolic syndrome

Risk factors	IDF	WHO	NCEP	I DPAIA
Age	10 to <16 years		12–19 years	
MS diagnosis	Obesity plus 2 or more RF	3 or more RF	3 or more RF	
Obesity	WC ≥90th percentile or adult cut off if lower	BMI >95th percentile	WC ≥90th percentile	BMI >85th percentile according to sex and age
Glycemic homeostasis	Fasting glucose ≥5.6 mmol/L (100 mg/dL) or known diabetes mellitus type 2	Hyperinsulinemia prepubertal >15 mU/L; [29] pubertal >30 mU/L; [29] (stage 1 tanner) (stages 2–4 tanner) post pubertal ≥20 mU/L (stage 5 tanner) fasting glucose ≥6.1 mM/L glucose intolerance glucose at 120 min ≥7.8 mM/L	Fasting glucose ≥110 mg/dL	Plasma insulin >15 μm/L
Elevated arterial pressure	Systolic BP ≥130 mmHg or diastolic BP ≥85 mmHg	SBP >95th percentile for age, sex and stature NHBPEP [44]	SBP/DBP ≥90th percentile for age and sex and stature NHBPEP [43]	SBP and/or DBP in >90th and >95th percentiles or always that BP >120/80 mmHg
Dylsipidemia	TG ≥1.7 mmol/L (150 mg/dL) HDL <1.03 mmol/L (40 mg/dL)	TG >105 mg/dL for <10 years, >136 mg/dL for ≥10 years HDL <35 mg/dL TC >95th percentile	TG ≥110 mg/dL HDL ≤40 mg/dL	TC <150 mg/dL LDL <100 mg/dL HDL ≥45 mg/dL TG <100 mg/dL

MS metabolic syndrome; *RF* risk factors; *IDF* International Diabetes Federation; *WHO* World Health Organization; *NCEP* National Cholesterol Education Program-Adult Treatment Panel III; *I DPAIA* Guidelines for the Prevention of Atherosclerosis in Childhood and Adolescence; *BMI* body mass index; *WC* waist circumference; *TC* total cholesterol; *TG* triglycerides; *HDL* high density lipoprotein; *SBP* systolic blood pressure; *mmHg* millimeters of mercury; *mg/dL* milligrams per deciliter; *mM/L* millimoles per liter
From Silveira et al. [24] with permission

(CRF) and leptin levels were included. A score greater than 0.85 indicated a cluster of risk factors suggestive of MetS in this cohort. Approximately 6.2 % of youths in the 2015 study showed a clustering of CVD risk factors, thereby suggesting the presence of MetS, as opposed to the <1 % selected by existing MetS definitions, specifically the IDF criteria [25].

Hypothyroidism in Children with Obesity

Thyroid function is closely related to regulation of basal metabolism and thermogenesis. The thyroid plays an important role in glucose metabolism and fat oxidation. Hypothyroidism can be associated with weight gain and a decrease in both thermogenesis and basal metabolic rate. In children the most common thyroid abnormality is hyperthyrotropinemia, which is defined as a high TSH and normal T4. However, this normalizes with weight loss and no specific other treatment is necessary. It is unclear whether this is bidirectional, i.e., a result of obesity in children or a potential cause of obesity in children. High levels of TSH may be the result of high circulating levels of leptin or may be due to the inflammation that exists in patients with obesity [26]. Routine testing of thyroid hormones is not recommended if the child has normal linear growth[27].

Polycystic Ovarian Syndrome in Adolescents with Obesity

Polycystic Ovarian Syndrome (PCOS) affects 5–10 % of reproductive-age females. PCOS is highly related to insulin resistance and its presence may indicate the adolescent is at risk for MetS. PCOS, originally thought of as a syndrome that affected the risk for infertility, is now known to be an important sign of general metabolic dysfunction and may indicate the development of serious cardiometabolic risk factors.

PCOS is characterized primarily by menstrual cycle dysfunction. In addition, adolescents may exhibit cutaneous signs such as acanthosis nigricans, acne, hirsutism, and alopecia that can be a signal of hyperandrogenism. Obesity is a frequent finding in PCOS. Ultrasonography may reveal multiple cysts in the ovaries and laboratory evaluation may reveal abnormalities in luteinizing hormone (LH) and follicle-stimulating hormone (FSH) [28].

Primary Cushing Disease in Children with Obesity

Cushing's disease is rare in children but is heralded by violaceous striae on the abdomen different from those seen in obesity due to rapid weight gain. The patient may also exhibit "moon facies" and a "buffalo hump," but these are also findings in obesity in general. When Cushing Disease is present it leads to short stature, thus it is extremely unlikely to be diagnosed in a tall child with obesity. If Cushing Disease in a child with obesity is suspected, referral to a pediatric endocrinologist is recommended [27].

Idiopathic Intercranial Hypertension in Children with Obesity

Evaluation for Idiopathic Intercranial Hypertension (IIH) is prompted by a child's complaint of severe headaches with photophobia. The child may also complain of blurred or double vision if they have an impairment of Cranial Nerve VI. On ophthalmologic exam the optic disk may appear blurred. The diagnosis is made by elevated intracranial pressure without etiology. The cerebrospinal fluid is normal in appearance and the patient will have normal contrast-enhanced computerized tomography. Magnetic resonance imaging of the brain may show subtle signs of elevated intracranial pressure [29]. The presentation and demographics of IIH in the pediatric age group differ slightly from adults. IIH in general tends to be associated with the female gender, but in prepubertal patients an equal sex distribution is found [30]. Adolescents with IIH under age 10 tend to be overweight but not obese [31]. Other etiologies for IIH should be eliminated, including otitis media, dural sinus thrombosis, systemic lupus erythematosus, neck injury, metastatic disease, nephrotic syndrome, and arteriovenous malformations [32].

If IIH in a child with obesity is suspected, urgent referral to a pediatric neurologist is advised due to the possibility of vision loss. Weight loss is effective treatment but often not rapid enough to treat IHH and so alternative methods may need to be employed urgently as weight loss is achieved. Bariatric surgery has shown efficacy in adult IHH.

Cardiovascular Disease in Children with Obesity

The possibility of hypertension in children with obesity should be considered and assessed. Three or more readings with an appropriate-sized blood pressure cuff are required to establish a diagnosis of high blood pressure in children. The National Heart, Lung and Blood Institute have tables defining elevated blood pressure by age, gender, and height percentile: https://www.nhlbi.nih.gov/files/docs/guidelines/child_tbl.pdf. Causality between obesity and hypertension in children has not been established and the mechanism of hypertension in children with overweight and obesity is similar to the pathophysiology in adults. This includes increased activity of the sympathetic nervous system with elevated levels of corticosteroids, oxidative stress, and inflammation from obesity, endothelial dysfunction, disturbance in sodium homeostasis and increased levels of adipokines [33].

Dyslipidemia has been a particular focus for all ages of patients with obesity over the past few years due to the role it plays in CVD. The availability of statins for therapy and the significant risk reduction they represent in heart disease has increased that focus. The prevalence of dyslipidemia in children is also high and the current recommendations are for a fasting lipid profile when BMI is in the 85th percentile, whether additional risk factors exist or not. Total cholesterol levels of <170 mg/dL and low-density lipoprotein levels (LDL) of <110 mg/dL are acceptable while levels above ≥ 200 mg/dL for total cholesterol or ≥ 130 mg/dL for LDL are considered high. The transition from pediatric criteria for dyslipidemia to adult criteria for the 17–21-year-old group indicates that although 2.5 % of the National Health and Nutrition Examination Survey (NHANES) population would qualify for treatment in this age group, only 0.4 % would qualify using adult criteria. Pediatric participants had higher rates of hypertension, smoking, and obesity compared to those who met adult guidelines. Based on this representative NHANES population and extrapolating to the US population, 483,000 adolescents age 17–21 would qualify for treatment [34].

In terms of treatment, supervision of dietary changes by the primary care provider is appropriate. However, if high levels do not respond to dietary therapy then referral to a pediatric cardiologist may be advisable. Implementing the kinds of pharmaceutical treatments used in the adult population may not be advisable or approved for use in the pediatric age group.

Numerous longitudinal studies have demonstrated risk factors in children for future CVD as adults. These risk factors include: LCL cholesterol, non-HDL cholesterol and serum apolipoproteins, obesity, hypertension, tobacco use, and T2DM. A tiered approach to the diagnosis and monitoring of children with hyperlipidemia or other risk factors has been proposed [35].

In a cohort of adolescents undergoing bariatric surgery as part of the Teen Longitudinal Assessment of Bariatric Surgery Study, 74 % had CVD risk factors. C reactive protein levels increased for each 5-unit increase in BMI. Overall 75 % of the adolescents in the study had high-sensitivity C-reactive protein levels. There was a high incidence of impaired fasting glucose (26 %) and T2DM (14 %). Dyslipidemia (50 %) and hypertension (49 %) showed a gender bias toward boys. These patients were in the 99th percentile for BMI with a mean BMI of 50 kg/m^2 [36].

Orthopedic Disorders in Children with Obesity

In addition to the orthopedic abnormalities associated with Blount's disease (bowed lower leg and slipped capital femoral epiphysis), pediatric patients with overweight and obesity have a higher incidence of fractures and musculoskeletal discomfort. The most common complaint is knee pain reported in 21.4 % of children who are overweight or obese, and a decrease in mobility when compared to normal weight children. Misalignment of the lower extremity, detected on Dual-Energy X-Ray Absorptiometry (DXA), is also seen more commonly [37]. Musculoskeletal problems may hamper exercise and contribute to weight gain.

Depression, Discrimination, and Stigma in Children with Obesity

Children and adolescents who are overweight or obese often experience obesity stigma and discrimination in various forms, including peer victimization and bullying (directly or indirectly through digital means) and teasing. It may even take the form of physical abuse [38]. In grades 3–6, the incidence of bullying is 63 % higher for children who are overweight or obese compared to normal weight children in the same grade [39]. Victimization increases in middle school and is worse for children in a higher BMI range. Victimization is reportedly worse for girls than boys [40]. Victimization toward children and adolescents with obesity often takes the form of rumor and innuendo, social isolation, and avoidance. Students and teachers may observe the bullying and victimization without actively or effectively intervening. It is unclear whether either the observers or the victims themselves know how to effectively address these issues. In one study, 92 % of children reported observing teasing of peers with obesity, 57 % saw them being verbally threatened, and 54 % saw them being physically harassed [41].

A lesser-known problem is that many children who are overweight or obese suffer the same stigmatization at the hands of family members. This poor treatment of those who are overweight or obese often extends into adulthood with friends (60 %) and spouses (47 %) being the bullies. Weight discrimination and stigmatization is more common among girls (29 %) versus boys (16 %) [42, 43].

Creating an atmosphere of sensitivity and acceptance while at the same time trying to encourage and establish better health habits is a difficult goal to achieve. Organizations like the National Education Association, with its "Bully Free—It Starts With Me" campaign, are starting to take notice of issues related to bullying, but we need to educate everyone in the school environment about bullying and good nutrition. Social interaction is the quintessence of puberty. It is during these formative years that many of our future expectations about relationships are established. Adolescents are subject to scrutiny and sanctioning by their peers. The social networks they form are largely motivated by the security that comes with a sense of belonging. Many of these interactions are developed around sexuality and subject to specific rules of social network development. Social networks have power outside of interpersonal relationships. In fact, social networks form in large part the basis for diffusion of disease including obesity [44]. Education about the issues and a commitment to stand up against bullying and abuse can become strong medicine within a peer group. Leveraging the right peer members to act in a better way may change the rules enormously for all children who are overweight or obese and who suffer needless discrimination.

Clinical Assessment of Children with Overweight/Obesity

A thorough clinical assessment of any pediatric patient with overweight or obesity should encompass several factors: a physical assessment, a family and social history assessment, a drug assessment, a nutritional assessment, a physical exercise assessment and an individual risk assessment for obesity-related health issues and disease. Each type of assessment specifically designed for the pediatric patient is discussed in more detail below.

A routine physical assessment of each child for overall health, including BMI, should be done annually starting at age 2. The child's BMI should be charted on the WHO charts from age 0 to 2 and then on the CDC growth charts after age 2 (Fig. 7.3) (http://www.cdc.gov/growthcharts/). Even pediatric specialists are unable

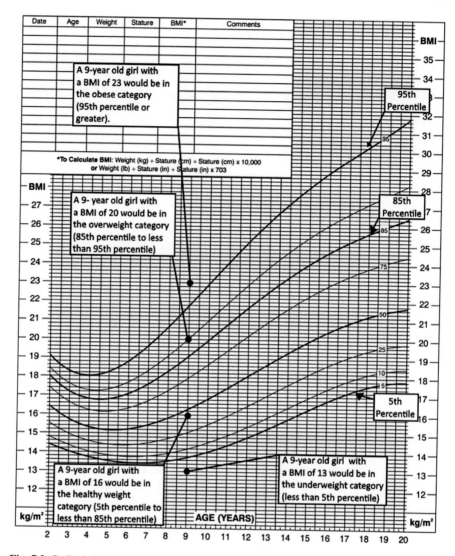

Fig. 7.3 Pediatric body mass index for age percentile, girls, 2–20 years old (from http://www.cdc.gov/growthcharts/)

to know from just observing a child whether his/her height is appropriate for their age, much less whether their weight, at that particular moment in the childhood growth continuum, is appropriate for his/her age. Therefore it is crucial to take the measurements of height, weight, and BMI and to chart the results at the patient's annual well visits. Children coming in for other reasons between the annual visits should again be charted, as these opportunities may allow the provider to notice changes in growth that are the harbinger of increasing overweight and obesity. Unfortunately parents do not always bring their children for annual well visits

Table 7.6 Physical exam findings in childhood obesity

General observations	Body fat distribution, psychosocial affect and facial features, relationship to family
Anthropometric measurements	Calculation of BMI and BMI percentile based on growth curve, changes in growth velocity—note waist circumference is not recommended due to lack of standardization data
Vital signs	Blood pressure adjusted for gender, age, and height percentile on more than one occasion
Eyes	CN VI paralysis and/or papilledema (pseudotumor cerebrii), abnormally shaped eyes (syndromic obesity)
Skin	Acanthosis nigricans (insulin resistance), keratosis pilaris, skin tags, intertrigo, acne, hirsutism (PCOS), violaceous striae
Neck/thyroid	Enlarged tonsils causing obstruction, thyromegaly, goiter
Chest	Heart rhythm, wheezing
Abdomen	Tenderness, palpation of a enlarged liver
Extremities	Abnormal gait, joint tenderness especially hips and knees (slipped capital femoral epiphysis), foot pain, bowing of tibia (Blount's disease), edema, polydactyly
Secondary sexual characteristics	Tanner stage, gynecomastia, thelarche, testicular enlargement, hypogonadism, precocious puberty

Data from Sibert et al. [24] and Eisenmann and Subcommittee on Assessment [46]

(particularly between age 6 and 12 years when immunizations are not required) if nothing is "wrong" with them. *Measurement and charting are best done whenever the child appears for any reason.*

The physical exam goes beyond physical measurements and the growth chart. It should include an evaluation of physical abnormalities indicating fixable problems like Blount's disease (a bowing of usually the lower legs associated with a disorder of the tibial growth plate), slipped capital femoral epiphysis (diagnosed by a limp and complaints of knee and hip pain), and acanthosis nigricans which is a skin condition characterized by dark discoloration in body folds and creases. Blood pressure, too, should be taken with an appropriate-sized blood pressure cuff and should be adjusted for age, gender and height percentile [45, 46] (Table 7.6).

If the pediatric patient is noted to 1) have increasing weight out of proportion to height or to previous exams, 2) is crossing percentile thresholds, or 3) shows signs of obesity-related disease, then a separate appointment should be made for a more thorough evaluation. Prior to that next evaluation, informed consent should be obtained to discuss the child's history of weight and any related problems and to perform a more thorough physical exam. Ideally, educational information should be provided for the parents and child prior to any extensive discussion of weight-related issues, but certainly such information should be made available at the time of the evaluation. Education and communication can help establish an environment of trust and safety in the discussion of these difficult issues.

An assessment of the pediatric patient should include any family history of obesity and obesity-related diseases in the first and second-degree relatives, especially for CVD and T2DM. The personal history of weight from birth, information about any weight loss attempts and results, and a thorough social history should be obtained, including school attendance and performance, whether the patient is a victim of stigma and bias by peers, socioeconomic factors, whether any cultural factors exists, and the patient's extracurricular activities both at school and in the community. The patient's home environment and a sense of the family's attitude and level of support for the patient should also be assessed, as well as the overall quality of the patient's life. Does the patient feel he/she is living and going to school in a safe and blameless environment? A complete lifestyle assessment of customary diet, physical activity, and sleep habits is also required. A comparison to national sleep recommendations should be made.

A history of the child's current use and need for medication should be included in the clinical evaluation. An assessment of the patient's use of any antipsychotic drugs, selective serotonin reuptake inhibitors (SSRI) or other antidepressants, anticonvulsants, prednisone, oral contraceptives, or stimulants should be obtained and the reason for their use discussed.

The nutritional assessment determines what foods are actually being consumed on a regular basis. Data is very strong linking consumption of sweetened beverages with increased eating and obesity. Fruit juice is a frequent snack or breakfast food that many parents do not realize contains large amounts of sugar. Other important questions to ask in the nutritional assessment include whether the patient regularly eats breakfast and what they eat, whether fast food or "eating out" is a regular event and what is usually ordered, how often meals are prepared and eaten as a family and a description of those meals, the patient's portion sizes and whether they have "seconds," how many servings of fruits and vegetables are eaten daily, how many and what kind of snacks are consumed on a daily basis by the patient, and what items of the food pyramid are not eaten by the patient. Quite often a significant amount of food is being consumed in between meals in the form of "grazing" or snacking. In addition, the assessment should determine exactly what foods the child eats at school and whether sweetened beverages are served at school, and whether the patient has access to and uses food vending machines at school.

Levels of physical activity should be assessed for the duration, frequency, intensity and type of activity, and whether there are specific types of exercise or activities the child particularly enjoys. Consideration should be given to the environment the child lives in and whether bike paths, walking paths, parks, recreation centers, sports teams, activity groups, or other sources and means of physical activity are available, safe, and affordable. Family activities as well as individual activities should be encouraged for the pediatric patient.

The attitude of the patient and family members, the patient's readiness to change, and an assessment of the patient's motivation to become more physically active are critical goals to establish with the patient and the parents. The attitude of parents and other family members is important. Children often feel singled out if other siblings or parents do not have similar weight issues. The child cannot be successful without changes being made in the home environment.

An individual risk assessment for obesity-related health issues and disease should also be done during screening of the pediatric patient with obesity.

The recommendations for testing are based upon expert opinion. Routine blood pressure monitoring and universal lipid screening are recommended every two years in children who are overweight and obese. At age 10 the expert committee recommends adding ALT/AST and fasting glucose tests for children with obesity and no other risk factors, as well as for children who are overweight with risk factors. Risk factors include history of T2DM in a first or second degree relative, ethnicity with an increased risk for diabetes (Native American, African American, Latino, Asian American) and signs of insulin resistance or conditions associated with insulin resistance. The American Diabetes Association recommends diabetes screening in all children classified as overweight or obese once every 3 years beginning at age 10, or at onset of puberty when risk factors are present. Fasting glucose is the most common test used in asymptomatic children although technically a 2-h glucose test would be the most sensitive. HbA1c, which does not require fasting, should be used if they are symptomatic.

This type of comprehensive clinical assessment of the pediatric patient who is overweight or obese takes time and requires sensitivity. Questions by the provider may be viewed as confrontational or as a negative judgment of the child, the parents, and/or the family. All efforts to avoid an atmosphere of blame should be made. Careful communication is imperative and no derogatory, judgmental, or blameful comments should be made. The health care provider must at all times demonstrate a commitment to the pediatric patient's welfare and best interest, and make every attempt to engage the child's family in the long-term working relationship that will be necessary to address the issues. Obesity is a chronic disease. Establishing a long-term working relationship that is supportive and not overly aggressive in short-term expectations is critical to success.

Biobehavioral Susceptibility Model of Child Obesity

The emerging biobehavioral susceptibility model provides a tool for explaining childhood obesity, and suggests that prevention and treatment strategies should acknowledge the powerful, but modifiable, influences of genetics and biology on a child's eating behavior. Understanding this complex interaction is the key to treating childhood obesity in general.

Our culture of parental/family/peer feeding of a child is responsible for a large part of the child's early appetitive training. There is often pressure to eat certain foods and easy access to or promotion of certain foods versus restriction or absence of other foods. This "food culture" establishes appetitive traits of satiety sensitivity and food cues that, together with an obesogenic food environment, result in physiologic cues that influence eating habits and can result in excess body weight. The "food culture" overlies a foundation of family genetics that can create a propensity to obesity in the child. These cultural and genetic tendencies can override efforts by the provider to impact obesity in the child and undermine any

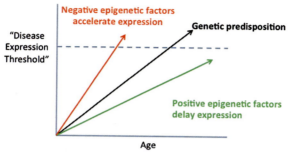

Fig. 7.4 Impact of genetics on expression of obesity and related disease. Courtesy of Joy Bunt, MD, PhD)

reasonable attempts to change eating patterns. Education is paramount to changing these cultural norms and altering the genetic propensity [47].

Overcoming these cultural norms once they are established is very difficult. Prevention is preferable to treatment. Management of maternal and paternal health, education and prevention during pregnancy, and mindful feeding and activity from infancy on up will have a positive impact on the child's future health, resulting in lower risk trajectories over time (Fig. 7.4).

Treatment Recommendations for Children with Obesity

Weight loss goals are somewhat different in children and adolescents than in adults in part because the child is still experiencing linear growth. The current recommendations pertaining to weight management for children depend upon age, weight percentile and the presence or absence of risk factors. Children 2 to 18 years old in the 5th to 84th percentile for weight (healthy weight) are advised to simply maintain their weight. Overweight youth in the 85th to 94th percentile of weight *without* cardiovascular risk factors also receive the same advice: to maintain their weight. Overweight youth in the 85th to 94th percentile <u>with</u> cardiovascular risk factors in the 2 to 5 year-old age group are advised to slow their weight gain; the 6 to 11 year-old age group is advised to maintain their weight; the 12 to 18 year-old age group is told to maintain or gradually lose weight. Children and adolescents that are obese (in the 95th to 99th percentile) are advised as follows: to maintain weight (2 to 5 year-olds), to gradually lose 1 lb per month (6 to 11 year olds) or 2 lbs per month (12 to 19 year olds). Finally, those youth who are severely obese (in the ≥ 99th percentile) are advised to lose up to 1 lb per month (2 to 5 year olds) or 2 lbs per month (6 to 18 year olds) [48].

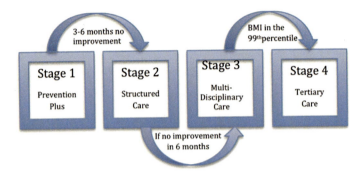

Fig. 7.5 American academy of pediatrics structured plan for intervention in pediatric obesity (data from Barlow [27])

While these goals may satisfy the requirement for safety in terms of not having accelerated massive weight loss, it may do little to help overweight or obese pediatric patients who are stigmatized at school, suffering psychologically, struggling with peer relationships or losing opportunities due to obesity. The goals of weight loss need to be a collaborative choice with the best interest of the patient and the patient's own goals taken into consideration. Education of the family members and patients provides a critical foundation. As part of that foundation all parents and children should be taught the 5-2-1-0 rule:

5 or more fruits and vegetables
2 h or less of recreational screen time

No screen time under age 2
Keep computer/TV out of the bedroom

1 h or more of physical activity
0 Sugary drinks.

The American Academy of Pediatrics Expert Committee suggests that intervention in pediatric obesity take the form of a Structured Plan. That Plan outlines a set of progressive recommendations in 4 stages (Fig. 7.5). Each Stage is discussed in detail below.

These recommendations invoke specific stages of increasing interventional treatment [27] (Fig. 7.6).

Stage 1: Prevention Plus

Stage 1 is Prevention Plus and is usually delivered in the primary care setting. The primary care pediatric office is the ideal setting to establish the patient's expectation of having height and weight measured at every appointment as part of their weight-related health indicators (WRHI). This will also allow the practitioner to

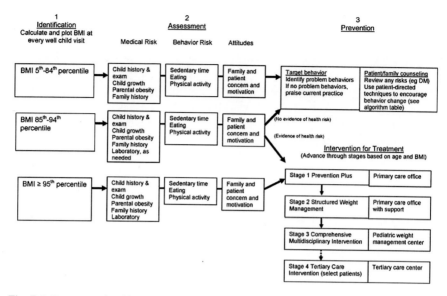

Fig. 7.6 Treatment algorithm for childhood obesity (from Barlow [27])

establish communication regarding the pediatric patient's BMI and, when indicated, schedule a more thorough evaluation of factors related to overweight and obesity.

A large part of the initial work with a pediatric patient and their family in Stage 1 is designed to gain their respect and trust. The provider will need to establish a good working relationship to encourage and support the patient and the family through a series of behavioral interventions for weight control/reduction.

In Stage 1 the focus is on the food: reduce or eliminate sweetened beverage consumption, reduce portion size, reduce saturated fat consumption, and increase fruit/vegetable consumption. Meal replacements should not be included in the primary strategy of Stage 1. Consider sending the patient and family to a live, local presentation focused on pediatric obesity to enhance their education. Moving on to Stage 2 is warranted if goals have not been achieved after 3 to 6 months of Stage 1 strategy.

Stage 1 Recommendations
Goal: improve health through lifestyle change
Patient Goals:

≥ 5 servings of fruits and vegetable
≤ 2 h of screen time
≥ 1-h activity per day
0 sugar-containing drinks
Eat healthy breakfast daily

1. More meals at home
2. Family meals 5–6 times per week
3. Involve whole family.

Stage 2: Structured Weight Management

Stage 2 builds on the recommendations of Stage 1. Stage 2 is distinguished by the level of support given the patient and family regarding weight reduction with an emphasis on planned supervision or recording of activities. This may include keeping ongoing food journals, logs of activities/exercise, supervised exercise, and structured meals and snacks via daily eating plans. Providing specific meals and lists of healthy foods that are "allowed" may be a better approach than putting foods on a "never eat" list. The meal plans should be created by a registered dietician or clinical provider with training in the nutritional requirements of children and adolescents. Training in motivational interviewing and teaching is invaluable for the staff who work with this patient group and their families. Referral to an exercise professional or a wellness coach trained in both nutrition and exercise may be warranted. The family may also need a counselor to facilitate conflict resolution or to provide additional motivation and education on how to achieve change in the family as a whole.

Curtailment of screen time may be difficult to implement and enforce with children and adolescents. Incorporating positive screen time that includes or requires some kind of physical activity may be possible. Many parenting models recommend that screen time be used as a positive reward for good behavior.

Stage 2 Recommendations
Focus on same behaviors but with more support and structure

1. Planned diet or daily eating plan with the input of dietitian
2. Further screen time reduction to ≤ 1 h/day
3. 60 min of activity daily (ex: pedometers)
4. Use of logs to track adherence to goals
5. Planned reinforcement with check-ins/nonfood rewards
6. Monthly visits appropriate at this level.

Stage 3: Comprehensive Multidisciplinary Program

Stage 3 builds on the recommendations of Stages 1 and 2. The pediatric patient should progress to Stage 3 when Stages 1 and 2 have failed to provide significant return to health after 3–6 months of effort. Comprehensive support for behavior change in Stage 3 requires extensive engagement of the family, pediatric bariatric specialist, exercise specialist, registered dietician, and behavioral specialist. This Stage is more extreme in that it requires whole family involvement with parental training to improve the home environment in regards to (1) food and behavior modification, (2) negative energy balance counseling, (3) portion control, and (4) the physical removal of junk/unhealthy food from the home.

Stage 3: Comprehensive Multidisciplinary Program

Intensive weight management program including all of the former elements of Stages 1 and 2 management plus:

1. Behavior Modification
2. Negative energy balance (nutrition and activity goals)
3. Parents trained on improvement of home environment
4. Systemic evaluation of body measurements
5. Weekly visits for 8–12 weeks, then monthly.

Stages 1, 2, and 3 represent traditional therapy in the approach to childhood overweight and obesity. This approach has some troubling secondary affects and outcomes. When this approach works to decrease weight and increase exercise there is evidence that, compared to controls, it increases endothelial progenitor cells and decreases endothelial microparticles which contribute to the early microvascular changes that result in adult atherosclerosis [48]. Another aspect that is troubling with this approach is the ability of the health care team to provide the long-term follow-up necessary to maintain weight loss. Long-term follow-up often requires scheduling during school and work hours, requiring the patient and parent not only to miss school/work, but to also incur the cost of service and transportation. The family must also meet the challenge of finding comprehensive, affordable programs. Perhaps most discouraging is the fact that in most comprehensive programs the average weight loss of 5 lb (3 %) is not maintained even for 7 months. Two recent studies have confirmed that the overall net positive effect of this approach is unfortunately small [49, 50].

Stage 4: Tertiary Care

Tertiary care intervention is advised for the adolescent with severe obesity (99th percentile) after at least 6 months of Stage 3 intervention has been completed. Stage 4 involves progressive intervention using meal replacements with very low calorie diets, pharmaceuticals, and bariatric surgery when indicated.

When considering an adolescent for Stage 4 intervention, it is critical they understand the fundamentals of behavior modification and be committed to the aspects of behavior change that will improve long-term outcomes, including physical activity. These extreme interventions have the potential to result in fundamental changes to their anatomy. The adolescent patient must understand the risks and be able to give informed consent for treatment. The parents must be involved and give informed consent as well. Many of these interventions require long-term vitamin regimens and/or abstinence from alcohol use in order to maintain health after weight loss. These requirements may be difficult for the adolescent to understand and commit to at such a young age. All candidates for Stage 4 intervention should have participated in at least six months of structured multidisciplinary care (Stage 3) prior to referral for these advanced interventions.

The use of very low calorie diets in youth has not been studied and should only be used in residential programs or with very close follow-up in tertiary care settings. The most common diet prescribed is the 300–800 cal Protein-Sparing Modified Fast or a variation of that diet. Dehydration is a concern with this diet, therefore fluid, vitamin, and mineral supplementation is mandatory. It is also reportedly important that adolescents receive a minimum of 1 g protein/kg IBW/day in order to maintain positive nitrogen balance [51].

Many experts believe that medication use for treatment of obesity in adolescents should be reserved for those with high BMI (99th percentile) or obesity-related medical problems like dyslipidemia, hypertension, insulin resistance, fatty liver disease, or obstructive sleep apnea. When the Federal Drug Administration approves a medication for use in adults the lower age limit is usually 16 years of age [52]. Weight loss is higher in groups that adhere to lifestyle modification while taking the medications [53]. No weight loss medications are approved below age 12. However, two weight loss medications are approved for use in adolescents: Orlistat and Metformin.

In 2003, the FDA approved use of Orlistat for use in adolescents (12–16 years of age) at a dose of 120 mg three times per day. Orlistat prevents the absorption of fat in the intestines. The largest randomized trial compared a group receiving Orlistat (3:1) to a group receiving a multivitamin, with both groups instructed to follow a hypocaloric diet and engage in physical activity. Both groups demonstrated a 35 % drop out rate. At 52 weeks there was a decrease of 0.55 kg/m^2 in BMI with Orlistat versus a 0.31 kg increase in BMI in the placebo group. Participants experienced oily stools, spotting and evacuation with abdominal pain, and fecal urgency. Seven participants in the Orlistat group developed gallstones [54]. To date, there is little evidence that Orlistat is effective in adolescents with severe obesity.

Metformin is an oral medication that lowers blood glucose by inhibiting intestinal glucose absorption, increasing insulin sensitivity in peripheral tissue, and decreasing hepatic glucose production. It is approved for the treatment of T2DM in children over age 10, but not for the treatment of obesity. Small trials have been done in children and adolescents that show a modest reduction in BMI (-0.9 kg/m^2 to -1.47 kg/m^2) and weight loss averaging 3 kg over 6 months, compared to the placebo groups [55, 56]. Gastrointestinal complaints and fatigue were the most significant reported side effects. It appears metformin has a relatively small but statistically significant effect on BMI in adolescents when added to a lifestyle intervention program.

All other medications used in children would be "off label," meaning the FDA has not approved them for use in children and adolescents. In general, besides the unknown long-term effects, the limiting factor in prescribing medications for obesity in children and adolescents is the frequent dosing and negative side effects [57].

Bariatric Surgery in Adolescents

Multiple factors are driving the increasing use of bariatric surgery in the end stage management of obesity in adolescents. It is known that adolescents who are obese generally remain obese into adulthood and develop obesity-related diseases at a younger age that threaten to shorten their lifespan. Adolescents suffer from significant social and psychological impairment affecting life choices, including career and partnering/sexual choices. The limited efficacy of nonsurgical options in the group of severely obese adolescents (BMI > 99th percentile) utilizing low calorie diets, physical activity, or pharmaceutical approaches is increasingly evident. The use of very low calorie diets is not supported by data. Bariatric surgery in certain adolescent patients is proving to be safe and effective, not only for weight loss, but to improve obesity-related disease in adolescent patients.

The emotional, cognitive and social development of the adolescent patient are the most important components to evaluate when assessing whether the adolescent with obesity is a good candidate for bariatric surgery. Serious consideration has to be given to the long-term nutritional consequences of surgery, the possible effects on reproduction, and the patient's ability to comply with a vitamin regimen and long-term monitoring [58]. All candidates for surgery are required to have learned sound behavior management gleaned from participating in traditional weight management treatment programs at the Stage 3 multidisciplinary approach for at least six months. They must also have the consent and involvement of the parents and family. The adolescent patient must have completed at least 95 % of linear bone growth and attained Tanner stage 4 or 5 in physical development. This usually occurs at approximately 13 years of age in girls and 15 years of age in boys. Adolescent candidates for bariatric surgery are usually at the extremes of BMI (>99th percentile) and have one or more obesity-related diseases.

Contraindications for surgery in adolescents include (1) a medically correctable cause of obesity, (2) active substance abuse, including nicotine, (3) medical, psychiatric, or cognitive disability that impairs adherence or impairs understanding of consequences, (4) current pregnancy, planned pregnancy within a year of surgery or breastfeeding, and (5) the inability or unwillingness of the patient or parents to understand the procedure or its consequences. Adolescents without adequate social support or who suffer abuse or neglect are not candidates. If a psychiatric condition is present it must be under management. Often, the adolescent may have parents or other family members that have undergone surgery and their understanding of the procedure may be based on that experience. Compliance with office visits is often a good indicator of the adolescent patient's willingness and ability to comply with long-term follow-up.

Bariatric Surgery Procedures

The three most commonly performed bariatric procedures offered to adolescents are: adjustable gastric band (AGB), sleeve gastrectomy (VSG) and roux-en-y

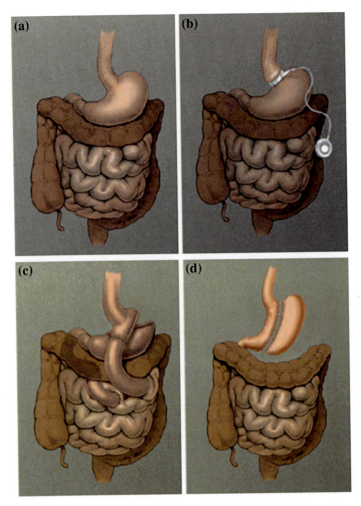

Fig. 7.7 a Normal gastrointestinal anatomy; **b** Adjustable gastric band; **c** Roux-en-Y gastric bypass; and **d** Vertical sleeve gastrectomy (from Thakkar and Michalsky [59] with permission)

gastric bypass (RYBP) [59] (Fig. 7.7). More detailed descriptions and discussions of these procedures are in Chap. 11 Bariatric Surgery. There is no consensus on the best operation for any given individual however, FDA approval for the AGB is for age 18 and older. The more complex duodenal switch/biliopancreatic diversion is not recommended because of the protein and nutrient malabsorption that often accompanies this procedure. *The two procedures most commonly performed on adolescents are the vertical VSG and gastric bypass, both usually performed from a laparoscopic approach.*

The National Institute of Health funded a multicenter trial of bariatric surgery in adolescent patients. Of the initial 277 enrolled patients, 13 declined participation and 22 do not meet the study deadline for operation. The final analysis included a cohort of 242 subjects with a mean age of 17.1 years of age, median BMI of 50.5 kg/m^2, and a median waist circumference of 145.9 cm. Almost a quarter of the patients had a BMI greater than 60 kg/m^2 at the time of enrollment and micro albuminuria was present in 17.7 %. The surgical procedures performed were gastric bypass (RYBP) (66.5 %), sleeve gastrectomy (VSG) (27.7 %), and adjustable gastric band (ABG) (5.8 %). Within 30 days of surgery, 7.9 % experienced major complications and 14.9 % had minor complications, without mortality. The major complication rate by procedure within 30 days was 9.3 % for RYBP, 4.5 % for VSG, and 7.1 % for AGB. Major complications included intestinal obstruction, bleeding, and confirmed or suspected gastrointestinal leak [60].

A recent meta-analysis of six studies which included 131 adolescent patients with gastric bypass surgery (RYGB) and 1 to 6.3 years follow-up, showed significant and sustained weight loss with improvement in obesity-related T2DM and hypertension [61].

Sleeve gastrectomy has recently surged in popularity in adults and is being increasingly used in adolescents. A report at 12 months demonstrates a reduction of BMI from 49.6 to 32.4 kg/m^2 [62] and a study reported at 12 and 24 months demonstrates a reduction of BMI from 38.5 to 26.3 kg/m^2 [63]. All studies also showed improvement in insulin resistance, dyslipidemia, and obstructive sleep apnea.

Access to bariatric surgery is a significant barrier to improving the health of severely obese adolescents. Attitudes among primary care providers are mixed about the appropriateness for surgery. Even if referred, the adolescent patient may not have an insurance benefit for surgery. Less than 50 % of adolescent patients are being approved by their insurance companies even when a benefit is technically available. Multiple appeals are sometimes necessary. Recent data shows that delay in surgery exacts a steep penalty, as adolescent patients with a BMI $\geq$ 65 kg/m^2 have a lower probability of attaining non-obese status, (i.e., BMI < 30 kg/m^2) [64].

Overall, the surgical data for adolescents who undergo surgical therapy demonstrates a 5 % rate of major inpatient morbidity, a 2.9 % reoperation rate, and an 11.5 % readmission rate [65].

The perioperative education and follow-up of the adolescent patient and parents/family is critical to positive outcomes and the avoidance of adverse events after surgery. Ideally, the adolescent undergoes the operation in a nationally accredited adolescent bariatric program, the Metabolic and Bariatric Surgery Accreditation and Quality Improvement Program (MBSAQIP). This program is offered jointly by the American College of Surgeons and the American Society for Metabolic and Bariatric Surgery. Approved sites are required to have the participation of pediatric specialists within a multidisciplinary structure and participating surgeons must demonstrate adequate volume to ensure current proficiency. In addition, every case is reported to a national registry. The adolescent program will often reside within an adult program, with the ongoing collaboration of a multi-disciplinary pediatric bariatric clinic.

Conclusion

Obesity now affects 1 in 6 children and adolescents in the United States. Childhood obesity is a complex health issue caused by genetics, behavior and the environment. Against the background of their genetic inheritance the odds in a child's disfavor are magnified by the ever-present seduction of readily available high calorie/high fat/high sugar food and drink, and lack of exercise. This sets the child up for becoming overweight or obese and increases the risk for developing CVD and multiple other obesity-related diseases at a young age that will undoubtedly impact longevity and promote physical and mental disability.

Obesity erodes self-esteem and breeds insecurity in children and adolescents via the discrimination and bias that exists in schools, in peer groups, and perhaps in their own families. Even when this occurs due to a lack of education, which may be the case most often, as opposed to any malicious intent, the resulting long term effects may be similar. Obesity robs these children and these adolescents not only of their physical health, but it can also detrimentally affect their social lives, productivity, and career opportunities.

The medical community must search for the best way to work with children and their parents around the issue of childhood obesity. The point for concern and action should perhaps be set at a lower BMI threshold, perhaps treatment recommendations for children and adolescents should begin at the onset of the overweight category, BMI in the 85th percentile, *with or without* cardiovascular risk factors. This is when traditional weight management techniques may have more impact. Parents and teachers need targeted education to advance their knowledge. Schools and healthcare systems should take leadership roles in promoting not only safe environments for children and adolescents free of bias and bullying, but also free of unhealthy food. Immediate action could include sensitivity training as part of a core curriculum for teachers, administrators and students, having no tolerance for discrimination or bullying, and reducing the availability of sugary, fatty, salty, high calorie food and drinks in our schools. Global efforts have already begun and are perhaps having some positive effect. Time will tell. In any event, traditional approaches to weight management are falling short. Action must be taken on all fronts.

References

1. Cunningham SA, Kramer MR, Narayan V. Incidence of childhood obesity in the United States. N Engl J Med. 2014;370(5):403–11.
2. Ng M, Fleming T, Robinson M, Thomson B, Graetz N, Margono C, et al. Global, regional, and national prevalence of overweight and obesity in children and adults during 1980–2013: a systematic analysis for the global burden of disease study 2013. Lancet. 2014;384(9945):766–81.
3. Ogden CL, Carroll MD, Kit BK, Flegal KM. Prevalence of childhood and adult obesity in the United States, 2011–2012. JAMA. 2014;311(8):806–14.

References

4. Visscher TL, Heitmann BL, Rissanen A, Lahti-Koski M, Lissner L. A break in the obesity epidemic? Explained by biases or misinterpretation of the data? Int J Obes. 2015;39(2):189–98.
5. Olshansky SJ, Passaro DJ, Hershow RC, Layden J, Carnes BA, Brody J, et al. A Potential decline in life expectancy in the United States in the 21st century. N Engl J Med. 2005;352:1138–45.
6. Ravussin E, Bogardus C. Energy balance and weight regulation: genetics versus environment. Br J Nutr. 2000;83(1):S17–20.
7. Smith CJ, Ryckman KK. Epigenetic and developmental influences on the risk of obesity, diabetes, and metabolic syndrome. Diab Metab Syndr Obes Targets Ther. 2015;8:295–302.
8. Stevenson T, Symonds ME. Maternal nutrition as a determinant of birth weight. Arch Dis Child Fetal Neonatal Ed. 2002;86:F4–6.
9. Halldorsson TI, Rytter D, Haug LS, Bech BH, Danielsen I, Becher G, Henriksen TB, Olsen SF. Prenatal Exposure to perfluorooctanoate and risk of overweight at 20 years of age: a prospective cohort study. Environ Health Perspect. 2012;120(5):668–73.
10. Steenland K, Woskie S. Cohort mortality study of workers exposed to perfluoroctanoic acid. Am J Epidemiol. 2012;176(10):909–17.
11. Frayling TM, Hattersley AT. The role of genetic susceptibility in the association of low birth weight with type 2 diabetes. Br Med Bull. 2001;60(1):89–101.
12. Garver WS, Newman SB, Gonzales-Pacheco DM, Castillo JJ, Jelinek D, Heidenriech RA, Orlando RA. The genetics of childhood obesity and interaction with dietary macronutrients. Genes Nutr. 2013;8(3):271–87.
13. Krebs NF, Himes JH, Jacobson D, Nicklas TA, Guilday P, Styne D. Assessment of child and adolescent overweight and obeisty. Pediatrics. 2007;120(4):S193.
14. Whitaker RC, Pepe MS, Wright JA, Seidel KD, Dietz WH. Early adiposity rebound and the risk of adult obesity. Pediatrics. 1998;101(3):E5.
15. Wabitsch M, Funcke J, Lennerz B, Kuhnle-Krahl U, Lahr G, Debatin KM, et al. Biologically inactive leptin and early-onset extreme obesity. N Engl J Med. 2015;372(1):48–54.
16. National Sleep Foundation. Sleep in American poll; 2006. https://sleepfoundation.org/sites/default/files/2006_summary_of_findings.pdf.
17. Kalra M, Inge T, Garcia V, et al. Obstructive sleep apnea in extremely overweight adolescents undergoing bariatric surgery. Obes Res. 2005; 13:1175–79.
18. Granell R, Henderson AJ, Evans DM, Smith GD, Ness AR, Lewis S, Palmer TM, Sterne JAC. Effects of BMI, fat mass and lean mass on asthma in childhood: a mendelian randomization study. PLOS Med. 2014;. doi:10.137/journal.pmed.1001669.
19. Koebnick C, Getahun D, Smith N, Porter AH, Der-Sarkissian JK, Jacobsen SJ. Extreme childhood obesity is associated with increased risk for gastroesophageal reflux disease in a large population-based study. Int J Pediatri Obes. 2011;6(202):2257–63.
20. Koebnick C, Smith N, Black MH, Porter AH, Richie BA, Hudson S, et al. Pediatric obesity and gallstone disease. JPGN. 2012;55(3):v328–33.
21. Heida A, Koot BG, vd Baan-Slootweg OH, Pels Rijcken TH, Seidell JC, Makkes S, Jansen PL, Benninga MA. Gallstone disease in severely obese children participating in a lifestyle intervention program: incidence and risk factors. Int J Obes. 2014; 38(7):950–3.
22. Propst M, Colvin C, Griffin RL, Sunil B, Harmon CM, Yannom G, et al. Diabetes and pre-diabetes significantly higher in morbidly obese children compared to obese children. Endocr Pract. 2014;. doi:10.4158/EP14414.OR.
23. Zimmet P, Alberti G, Kaufman F, Tajima N, Silink M, Arslanian S, Wong G, Bennett P, Shaw J, Caprio S. On behalf of the international diabetes federation task force on epidemiology and prevention of diabetes. The metabolic syndrome in children and adolescents: the IDF consensus. Diab Voice. 2007: 52(4):29–32.

24. Silveira LS, Buonani C, Monteiro PA, Mello Antunes BM, Freitas Junior IF. Metabolic syndrome: criteria for diagnosing in children and adolescents. Endocrinol Metab Synd. 2013; 2:118.
25. Andersen LB, Lauersen JB, Brand JC, Anderssen SA, Sardinha LB, Steene-Johannessen J, et al. A new approach to define and diagnose cardiometabolic disorder in children. J Diab Res. 2015;. doi:10.1155/2015/539835.
26. Longi S, Radetti G. Thyroid function and obesity. J Clin Res Pediatr Endocrinol. 2013;1:40–4.
27. Barlow SE, The Expert Committee. Expert committee recommendations regarding the prevention, assessment, and treatment of child and adolescent overweight and obesity: summary report. Pediatrics. 2007;120(4):S164–92.
28. Bremer AA. Polycystic ovary syndrome in the pediatric population. Metab Syndr Relat Disord. 2010;8(5):375–94.
29. Brodsky MC, Vaphiades M. Magnetic resonance imaging in idiopathic intracranial hypertension. Ophthalmology. 1998;105:1686–93.
30. Babikian P, Corbett JJ, Bell W. Idiopathic intracranial hypertension in children: the Iowa experience. J Child Neurol. 1994;9:144–9.
31. Baker RS, Baumann RJ, Buncic JR. Idiopathic intracranial hypertension (idiopathic intracranial hypertension) in pediatric patients. Pediatr Neurol. 1989;5:5–11.
32. Jiraskova N, Rozsival P. Idiopathic intracranial hypertension in pediatric patients. Clin Opthalmol. 2008;2(4):723–36.
33. Wirix AJ, Kaspers PJ, Nauta J, Chinapaw JM, Kist-van Holthe JE. Pathophysiology of hypertension in obese children: a systematic review. Obes Rev. 2015;. doi:10.1111/obr.12305.
34. Gooding HC, Rodday Am, Wong JB, Gillman MW, Lloyd-Jones DM, Leslie LK, de Ferranti DS. Application of pediatric and adult guidelines for treatment of lipid levels among US adolescents transitioning to young adulthood. JAMA Pediatr. 2015; 169 (6):569–74.
35. Kavey REW. Expert panel on integrated guidelines for cardiovascular health, risk reduction in children and adolescents. Summary report. Pediatrics. 2011;128(5):S213–56.
36. Michalsky MP, Inge TH, Simmons M, Jenkins TM, Buncher R, Helmrath M, For the Teen-LABS Consortium, et al. Cardiovascular risk factors in severely obese adolescents: the teen longitudinal assessment of bariatric surgery (Teen-LABS) study. JAMA Pediatr. 2015; doi:10.1001/jamapediatrics.2014.3690.
37. Taylor ED, Thei KR, Mirch MC, Ghorbani S, Tanofsky-Kraff M, et al. Orthopedic complications of overweight in children and adolescents. Pediatrics. 2006;117(60):2167–74.
38. Puhl RM, King KM. Weight discrimination and bullying. Best Pract res Clin Endocrinol Metab. 2013;27:117–27.
39. Lumeng JC, Forrest P, Appugliese DP, Kaciroti N, Corwyn RF, Bradlesy RH. Weight status as a predictor of being bullied in third through sixth grades. Pediatrics. 2010;125:e1301–7.
40. Neumark-Sztainer D, Falkner N, Story M, Perry C, Hannan PJ, Mulert S. Weight-teasing among adolescents: correlations with weight status and disordered eating behaviors. Int J Obes Relat Metab Disord. 2002;26(1):123–31.
41. Puhl RM, Leudicke J, Heuer C. Weight-based victimization toward overweight adolescents: observations and reactions of peers. J Sch Health. 2011;81:696–703.
42. Eisenberg ME, Neumark-Sztainer D, Story M. Associations of weight-based teasing and emotional well being among adolescents. Arch Pediatr Adolesc Med. 2003;157:733–8.
43. Puhl RM, Brownell KD. Confronting and coping with weight stigma: an investigation of overweight and obese adults. Obesity. 2006;14:1802–15.
44. Bearman PS, Moody J, Stovel K. Chains of affection: the structure of adolescent romantic and sexual networks. AJS. 2004;110(1):44–91.

45. Seibert TS, Allen DA, Carrel AL. Adolescent obesity and its risks: how to screen and when to refer. J Clin Outcomes Manag. 2014;21(2):87–96.
46. Eisenmann JC. Subcommittee on assessment in pediatric obesity management programs, national association of children's hospital and related institutions. Pediatrics. 2011;128(2):351–8.
47. Carnell S, Kim Y, Pryor K. Fat brains, greedy genes, and parent power: a biobehavioural risk model of child and adult obesity. Intl Rev Psychiatry. 2012;24(3):189–99.
48. Bruyndonckx L, Hoymans VY, de Guchtenaere A, Van Helvoirt M, Van Craenenbroeck EM, Frederix G, et al. Diet, exercise and endothelial function in obese adolescents. Pediatrics. 2015;135(3):e653–61.
49. Luttikhuis HO, Baur L, Jansen H, Shrewsbury VA, O'Malley C, Stolk RP, Summerbell CD. Interventions for treating obesity in children (review). Cochrane Database Syst Rev. 2009;3:1–7.
50. Muhlig Y, Wabitsch M, Moss A, Hebebrand J. Weight loss in children and adolescents. Dtsch Arztebl Int. 2014;111:818–23.
51. Widhalm KM, Zwiauer KF. Metabolic effects of a very low calorie diet in obese children and adolescents with special reference to nitrogen balance. J Am Coll Nutr. 1987;6(6):467–74.
52. United States Food and Drug Administration. Guidance for industry; 2005. Web page http://www.fda.gov/downloads/drugs/guidancecomplianceregulatoryinformation/guidances/ucm079756.pdf.
53. Berkowitz RI, Wadden TA, Tershakovec AM, Cronquist JL. Behavior therapy and sibutramine for the treatment of adolescent obesity: a randomized controlled trial. JAMA. 2003;289(14):1805–12.
54. Chanoine JP, Hampl S, Jensen C, Boldrin M, Hauptman J. Effect of orlistat on weight and body composition in obese adolescents: a randomized controlled trial. JAMA. 2005; 293(23):2873–83.
55. Wilson DM, Abrams SH, Aye T, Lee PD, Lenders C, Lustig RH, et al. Metformin extended release treatment of adolescent obesity: a 48-week randomized, double-blind, placebo-controlled trail with 48-week follow-up. Arch Pediatr Adolesc Med. 2010;164(2):116–23.
56. Yanovski JA, Krakoff J, Salaita CG, McDuffie JR, Kozlosky M, Debring NG, et al. Effects of metformin on body weight and body composition in obese insulin-resistant children: a randomized clinical trial. Diabetes. 2011;60(2):47–85.
57. Sherafat-Kazemzadeh R, Yanovski SZ, Yanovski JA. Pharmacotherapy for childhood obesity: present and future prospects. Int J Obes. 2013;37(1):1–15.
58. Nogueira I, Hrovat K. Adolescent bariatric surgery: review on nutrition considerations. Nutr Clin Pract. 2014;29(6):740–6.
59. Thakkar RK, Michalsky MP. Update on bariatric surgery in adolescents. Curr Opin Pediatr. 2015;27:370–6.
60. Inge TH, Zeller MH, Jenkins TM, Helmrath M, Brandt ML, Michalsky MP, et al. Perioperative outcomes of adolescents undergoing bariatric surgery: the Teen-61. Longitudinal assessment of bariatric surgery (Teen-LABS) study. JAMA Pediatr. 2014; 168:47–53.
61. Treadwell JR, Sun F, Schoelles K. Systematic review and meta-analysis of bariatric surgery for pediatric obesity. Ann Surg. 2008; 248:763–76.
62. Alqahtani AR, Antonisamy B, Alamri H, Elahmedi M, Zimmerman VA. Laparoscopi sleeve gastrectomy in 108 obese children and adolescents aged 5–21 years. Ann Surg. 2012;256:266–73.
63. Boza C, Viscido G, Salinas J, Crovari F, Funke R, Perez G. Laparoscopic sleeve gastrectomy in obese adolescents: results in 51 patients. Surg Obes Relat Dis. 2012;8:133–7.
64. Inge TH, Jenkins TM, Zeller M, et al. Baseline BMI is a strong predictor of nadir BMI after adolescent gastric bypass. J Pediatr. 2010;156:103–8.
65. Jen HC, Rickard DG, Shew SB. Trends and outcomes of adolescent bariatric surgery in California, 2005–2007. Pediatrics. 2010;126(4):e746–53.
66. Garver WS, Newman SB, Gonzales-Pacheco DM, Castillo JJ, Jelinek D, Heidenriech RA, Orlando RA. The genetics of childhood obesity and interaction with dietary macronutrients. Genes Nutr. 2013;8(3):271–87.

67. Robinson SM, Crozier SR, Harvey NC, Barton BD, Law CM, Godfrey KM, et al. Modifiable early-life risk factors for childhood adiposity and overweight: an analysis of their combined impact and potential for prevention. Am J Clin Nutr. 2015;101(2):368–75.
68. Farooqi IS, O'Rahilly S. New advances in the genetics of early onset obesity. Int J Obes. 2005;29:1149–52.
69. Matricciani L, Blunden S, Rigney G, et al. Children's Sleep needs: Is there sufficient evidence to recommend optimal sleep for children? Sleep. 2013;36(4):527–34.

Chapter 8
Fundamentals of Diet, Exercise, and Behavior Modification

Key Message

Most people are able to lose weight. Their frustration comes from regaining it. The way you eat, what you eat, and the amount of physical activity have to be consistent day to day to maintain a stable body weight. Even when a person is consistent, the metabolism naturally slows with age and weight gain often occurs. Vigilance about diet, exercise and weight gain is important because it is far easier to keep from gaining weight than to lose it.

As explained in previous chapters, excessive weight gain causes epigenetic changes that modulate the genes that control metabolism, hunger and satiety. These changes become hard wired in the individual with obesity, thereby genetically resetting^{tm} the individual to a new set point of excessive weight. It is partly this genetic resetting^{tm} that makes losing weight in the individual with obesity so difficult and the inevitable regaining of the weight so frustrating.

Food is a source of energy. Humans have manipulated food to feed large groups of people as well as to create culinary magic. In the end all food, whether mundane or magical, breaks down into chemicals that signal the brain, direct metabolism, and affect weight. Therefore, understanding the science of food is important. Understanding the science of exercise and the value of behavior modification is also important.

This chapter describes the mechanics of eating and the science of digestion. It defines the essential nutrients of a healthy diet and describes the roles of essential macronutrients including protein, carbohydrates, amino acids, fiber, fat, water, vitamins and minerals. The three components of energy expenditure are defined and discussed. The effects of depression and anxiety on eating and obesity are also addressed. Finally, the controversy over categorizing obesity as a "food addiction" is explained.

Learning Objectives

1. Define the nutritional components of a healthy diet, describe the mechanics of eating and the science of the digestive process.
2. Outline the types of energy expenditure and how to maximize them in a weight loss or weight maintenance program.
3. Discuss the impact of categorizing obesity as a "food addiction."

The facts about nutrition, exercise, and behavior modification are key fundamentals that medical practitioners should be able to explain to patients with overweight and obesity. Nutrition research is somewhat contentious, contradictory, and political. The variety of information about food and exercise hampers the delivery of a clear and focused message to patients. As a result, patients are often confused about what they should do to achieve their health goals in regards to weight.

Food and Digestion

Digestion

The digestive system consists of the gastrointestinal (GI) tract and three solid organs: the liver, pancreas, and gallbladder. The GI tract is divided into different parts that provide different functions and absorb different nutrients. The individual parts of the intestinal system are the mouth, esophagus, stomach, small intestine, and large intestine. The GI tract contains the microbiome that includes millions of microorganisms along with multiple bacteria and other microbes that interact with consumed food. The small intestine is rather specialized and is itself divided into the duodenum, jejunum, and ileum. The GI tract and the three solid organs that support it have their own nervous system, called the enteric nervous system, as well as their their own blood supply. All together, this system is responsible for breaking down food and liquid ingested by a person and converting it into energy.

As food moves through the digestive tract, various digestive juices or fluids are added that break down food to allow the body to absorb the nutrients in food. Although people generally think of taste as being a sensation felt through the taste buds in the mouth, there are "taste" cells, or chemical sensors, all along the GI track. These specialized taste cells have the job of sensing the chemical composition of the digested food at each stage and sending specific signals to the brain. The brain reads the signals and sends specific instructions to the body to do certain things with the chemicals it senses.

Digestion starts in the mouth with chewing, or the mechanical breakdown of food. During this process an enzyme in saliva, salivary amylase, breaks down starches into their component sugars. Once swallowed, the food moves through the esophagus to the stomach. The stomach is a complex organ. It works on the food mechanically by contracting and relaxing. The stomach secretes hydrochloric acid into the food and liquid to further break it down. The stomach can dilate to accommodate large volumes of food. The cells of the stomach produce the hormone ghrelin that influences appetite and satiety. The stomach is a critical place for absorption of calcium and B vitamins and produces a carrier protein that allows the body to absorb iron.

Once food is broken down in the stomach it is released through the pylorus into the first portion of the small intestine, the duodenum. The food is moved through the small and large intestine via peristalsis. The duodenum receives digestive juice enzymes from the pancreas that break down starch, fat, and protein. It also receives bile from the liver that breaks down fat. These enzymes are aided by the action of the microbiome. The digested nutrients of the food and liquid originally consumed are then absorbed through the walls of the intestine into the bloodstream. Most of the nutrients, including most carbohydrates and proteins, are absorbed in the jejunum; a few are absorbed in the ileum. The inside lining of the small intestine is like velvet and is called the brush border. It has multiple nooks and crannies full of transport cells and enzymes that aid the digestive process. Water and waste moves on to the large intestine, which absorbs water and bile salts and then pushes the food into the distal large intestine (sigmoid colon) and anus for storage until it can be eliminated as waste. All along the way, specific parts of the GI track absorb specific nutrients.

The absorptive capacity of the alimentary canal, through which food passes from mouth to anus, is limitless. The GI tract produces per day about 1500 ml of secretions in the stomach and another 400 ml of secretions in the liver (bile), pancreas, and intestine. In addition, an average person typically ingests about 2000 ml of liquid and produces about 750–1500 ml of saliva per day. These massive amounts of secretions are largely absorbed in the distal small intestine so that less than 1000 ml makes it to the large intestine. Feces contain only about 150 ml of water per day.

Recommended Mechanics of Eating

Eat Slowly

Eating slowly allows food to reach the part of the intestine that turns off hunger signals and contributes to satiety. The result is that less food is consumed and therefore fewer calories. The methodology of learning this new food culture is simple. Advise patients to put down the fork or spoon between bites. Chew each bite 20–40 times. This takes practice. Having patients isolate themselves initially from others while eating and advising them to refrain from reading or watching television while eating may help them concentrate on technique. It also helps if they divide food into four portions and spend 5 min eating each portion, taking a full 20 min to finish a meal. In regards to chewing, using a carrot or apple is a great food to help them learn to chew 40 times for each bite, savoring the change in the flavors and textures. These techniques, if adopted for a 6-week period consistently, will generally result in slower, more mindful eating. It takes at least 10 min to get food to the right place in the intestine for chemical feedback to occur, so 20 min total eating time is recommended. Once fairly simple recommended eating mechanics are adopted and mastered, every other effort the patient is making to control his/her weight will be enhanced.

Many patients will say they never feel full and this may be true. The signal, GLP-1, is less potent in patients with overweight and obesity, so in fact they may not feel "full." Somehow feeling "full" is associated with taking in adequate nutrition, but many people who take in very little food actually live the longest. The message to communicate to patients is simple: eating until full increases the likelihood of gaining weight.

Calories and Kilocalories

What is a calorie? The word calorie comes from Latin "calor" meaning "heat". Although we often refer to calories, few know the definition. A calorie is defined at the amount of energy necessary to raise the temperature of 1 g of water by 1 °C. A kilocalorie is the amount of energy needed to raise 1 kg (1000 g) of water by one degree. The kilocalorie is the most common referral for dietary use. Although the word "calorie" is commonly used in nutrition, it is actually a referral to "kilocalories." For example, food labels in the United States list "calories" per serving, but mean "kilocalorie." In Europe they accurately use "kilocalorie."

Macronutrients

Energy is required for the body to operate its complex machinery. The source of energy for the body is from food ingested and the macronutrients absorbed during digestion. Macronutrients for nutrition include protein, carbohydrates, and fats, as well as various chemical elements, vitamins, and minerals. Macronutrients are essential in large amounts for the growth and health of the human body. A discussion of key macronutrients is set forth below.

Protein

Protein is essential to life. It forms the basis of all major structural components in the body including genes, epigenetic material, organs, and muscle as well as almost all hormones and signaling chemicals. The recommended level of protein intake is based on nitrogen balance studies is currently 0.8 g/kg of body weight for a normal, sedentary person. Proteins are made up of basic structural units called amino acids, nine of which are considered essential, five that are dispensable, and six that are conditionally essential.

The defining characteristic of protein from a nutritional standpoint is its amino acid composition. Proteins are polymer chains linked together by peptide bonds. During digestion, proteins are broken down to smaller polypeptide chains by hydrochloric acid and protease actions in the stomach. This allows for the synthesis of essential amino acids that cannot be biosynthesized by the body.

The two major enzymes involved in the digestion of proteins are *endopeptidases* that attack internal bonds and *exopeptidases* that cleave off one amino acid from the end of the protein at a time. Pepsin is the first peptidase to interact with food in the stomach. Gastric or hydrochloric acid (HCL) secreted by the stomach alters the form of pepsin so that it becomes active. Gastric acid also denatures or unfolds the proteins so the enzymes can attack them. Pepsin is particularly good at freeing up amino acids like phenylalanine, tryptophan, and leucine, all essential amino acids. Curiously, although pepsin digests about 10–15 % of the proteins in food, this process is not essential for digestion. People can live without part or all of their stomach, as evidenced by gastric bypass patients and patients who have undergone total gastrectomy. As food passes into the duodenum the pancreas secretes pancreatic proteases and these are complemented by similar peptidases in the brush border of the small intestine. Protein is absorbed primarily in the duodenum and jejunum as amino acids, dipeptides, and tripeptides.

Nine amino acids that are considered necessary for health function are: histidine, lysine, isoleucine, leucine, methionine, phenylalanine, threonine, tryptophan, and valine. These are considered "essential" because the body cannot synthesize them and they must come from the food we eat. Some protein sources contain amino acids in a "complete" sense. Meat, products from milk, eggs, soy, and fish are sources of "complete" protein. Whole grains and cereals are another source of amino acids, but tend to be limited in providing certain amino acids, including lysine. Proteins in plant sources have relatively low concentrations of amino acids by mass in comparison to protein from animal sources. Plant sources, however, are more complete than whole grains and cereals, in that they contain all the amino acids necessary in human nutrition. Eating plant sources in specific combinations may yield higher availability of essential proteins. While certain protein sources are "complete," their digestibility and anti-nutritional factors may render them less desirable as a protein source. *Therefore, in choosing sources of protein to consume, patients should consider digestibility and the source's secondary nutrition profile such as calories, cholesterol, vitamins, and mineral density.* Worldwide, plant protein foods contribute on average over 60 % of the per capita supply of protein. In contrast, North America derives 70 % of its per capita supply of protein from animal sources [1] (Fig. 8.1).

Carbohydrates

Carbohydrates ingested by humans include simple sugars (glucose and fructose), disaccharides (lactose and sucrose), and complex carbohydrates (starch and glycogen). The two key enzymes that break down carbohydrates during digestion are salivary amylase and pancreatic amylase [1] (Fig. 8.2).

New dietary guidelines published by the United States Government (health.gov—2015) recommend that adult diets should be 45–65 % carbohydrates. This recommendation falls within the Institute of Medicine (IOM) Acceptable Macronutrient Distribution Range (AMDR). The IOM further recommends daily intake (RDI) for carbohydrates (i.e., glucose) of 130 g per day for both males and females. If the desired caloric intake is 2000 kcal, 45–65 % carbohydrates would mean 900 to

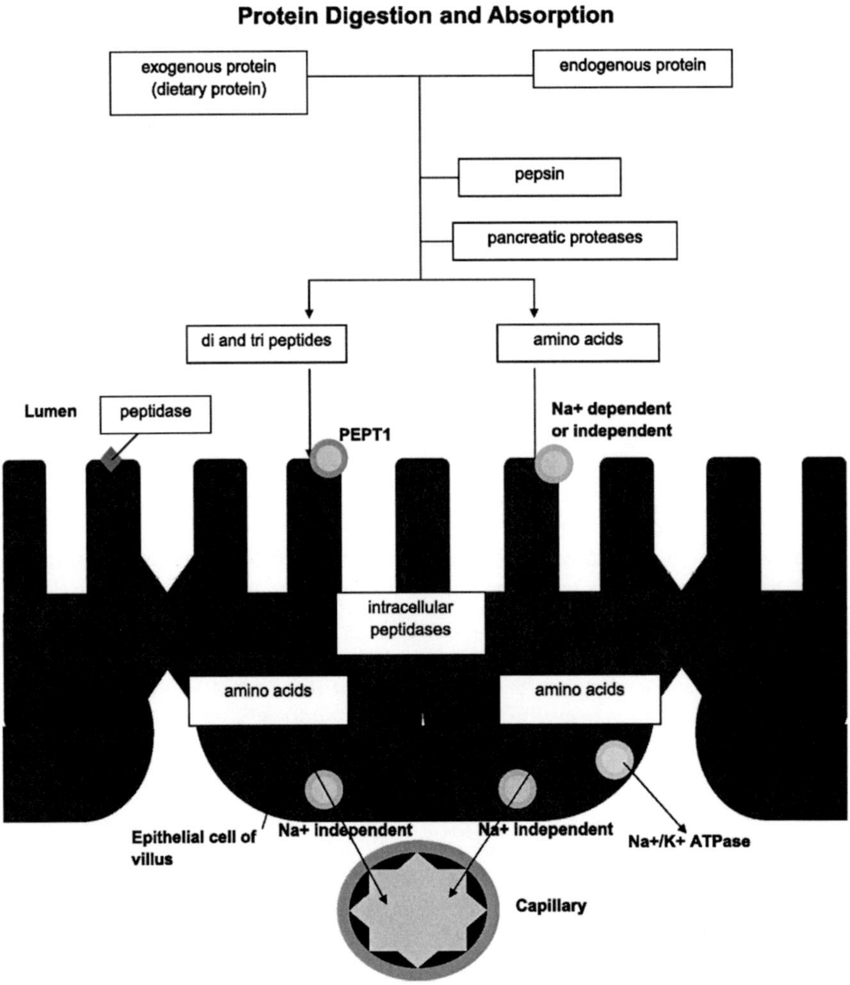

Protein Digestion and Absorption

Fig. 8.1 Protein digestion and absorption (from Goodman [1], with permission)

1300 kcal should come from carbohydrates. The conversion of calories to grams and vice versa is not straightforward. In this example, the 900 to 1300 kcal of carbohydrates converts to 116 to 168 g of carbohydrate per day.

The Food and Nutrition Board of the United States lists an RDI of 175 g/d of carbohydrate in the Dietary References Intakes section of their publication for 2015. The Food and Nutrition Board's RDI is based upon the amount of glucose oxidized daily by the brain (100 g/d) plus an added "margin of safety" to account for use in adult muscle and noncentral nervous system use. It should be noted that the Board also includes the following statement in the same publication, "There is no evidence that establishes the amount of sugar or added sugar that is beneficial in diet." [2]

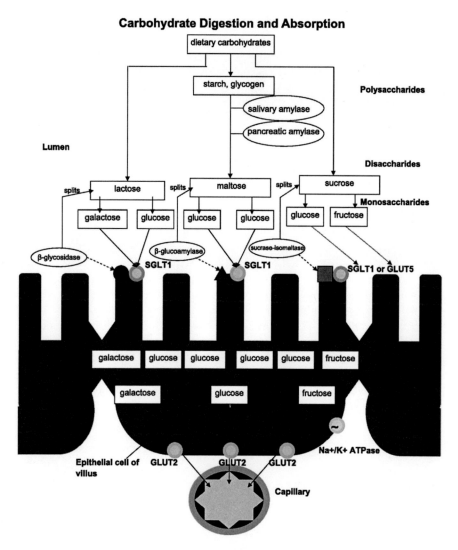

Fig. 8.2 Carbohydrate digestion and absorption (from Goodman [1], with permission)

This confusion begs the question: what amount of carbohydrates is actually required by the body? As shown above, the government recommendation for daily intake of carbohydrates is determined by the amount of glucose required for energy use by the brain, the only glucose dependent organ. The brain requires 100 g of glucose per day. However, in the absence of glucose from carbohydrates, the brain will use glucose from other sources (primarily fat), obtained through a process of ketogenesis and gluconeogenesis. *This means the minimum amount of carbohydrate necessary in the diet is actually zero* [3].

Despite confusion as to what the RDI for carbohydrates should be, *the goal is to maintain a relatively constant level of blood glucose* when carbohydrates are consumed. If blood glucose drops too low, the patient may experience "hunger" or lethargy. If it goes too high, the pancreas secretes excess insulin and converts the excess glucose to fat. The body responds to both the type and the amount of carbohydrate consumed. Carbohydrates are absorbed in the jejunum at a rate of about 120 g/h. However, each patient is different and may have a different response to the particular carbohydrates ingested, especially if the patient is insulin resistant already.

Carbohydrates are sometimes ranked by the rate of conversion to glucose within the body after ingestion. The *glycemic index* (GI) is a scale from 0 to 100, with the higher values representing a more rapid rise in blood sugar. In general, the lower the GI rating, the slower the infusion and absorption of sugars into the bloodstream. Starchy foods like potatoes and white bread are high on the GI scale. Green vegetables, most fruits and bran cereals generally have a low GI. One limitation of GI values, however, is they do not reflect the quantity consumed of a particular food. To address this problem, *glycemic load* (GL) values have been developed which take into consideration both the glycemic index of the food as well as the amount of digestible sugar/starch carbohydrates contained in that quantity of the food item.

Eating a food high on the glycemic index results in an initial elevation in energy, followed by increased storage as fat and increased hunger. When choosing carbohydrates to eat, the lower the GI/GL, the healthier the choice. Caution is necessary, however, when using a low GI/GL diet exclusively as a weight loss tool because GI and GL give no other nutritional information such as calories, fiber, protein, or fat content.

Dietary Fiber

Dietary fiber consists of all parts of plant foods that the body cannot digest or absorb. Fiber is generally classified as soluble or insoluble. Soluble "viscous" fiber dissolves in water to form a gel-like substance and can help lower blood cholesterol and glucose levels. Insoluble fiber promotes the movement of material through the digestive system and increases stool bulk. Some fibers that stay in the stomach may contribute to a feeling of fullness by delaying gastric emptying and reducing blood glucose levels after eating. These same fibers may reduce cholesterol and absorption of dietary fat through the interference with the enterohepatic circulation. The amount of adequate dietary fiber intake decreases with age. The IOM (2012) states the daily recommended amount of fiber is 38 g for adult men 50 and younger, and 30 g for men age 51 and older. For women, the recommended daily amount is 25 g for adult women 50 and younger, and 21 g for women 51 and older.

Fat

Dietary fat is essential for producing energy, for cell growth, to protect the organs and to keep the body warm. Dietary fat also helps the body absorb certain nutrients and produces hormones. About 30–40 % of calories in the typical American diet come from fat, 90 % of which is in the form of triglycerides. Most ingested fat takes the form of long chain fatty acids (C16, C18, and C20). Medium chain fatty acids are rarely found in the diet outside of coconut. The digestion of fat begins in the mouth and stomach with lingual and gastric lipase, but only about 15 % of fat digestion occurs in this part of the GI tract. Chewing and the churning and peristalsis of the stomach all contribute to turn the fat into fine droplets of oil prior to its entering the duodenum. This facilitates digestion of fat in a key way. When fat enters the duodenum the pancreas is stimulated to secrete pancreatic lipase and the gallbladder is stimulated to release bile. These key secretions of pancreatic lipase, colipase, and bile appear in the second portion of the duodenum. The fat/water interface is coated with both bile salts and cholesterol in a constantly changing environment as the pancreatic lipases attack the fat droplet from the outside [1] (Fig. 8.3).

The breakdown products of this hydrolytic processing of dietary fat results in transport across the intestinal epithelial cell lining into the smooth endoplasmic reticulum where they are packaged into chylomicrons that flow through the lymph system [1] (Fig. 8.4). Those chylomicrons provide lipids that are stored within fat cells throughout the body.

The body synthesizes saturated fatty acids, monounsaturated fatty acids, and cholesterol. The majority of dietary lipids/fats (95 %) are absorbed in the small intestine.

Water

It is important to remember that water is a macronutrient. Water makes up more than two-thirds of the weight of the human body. All the cells and organs of the body need water to function. Water serves many purposes: it makes up saliva and the fluid surrounding the joints, it regulates body temperature through perspiration, and it helps move food through the intestines. Water in the body is obtained from liquids, solid food, and through the process of metabolism. The recommended daily intake (RDI) of water is 3.7 L for men and 2.7 L for women, gleaned from both solid food and liquid sources [4].

Alcohol and Sweetened Beverages

In the United States, alcoholic beverages and sugar sweetened beverages (SSB) represent 19 % (>9 billion gallons) and 27 % (>13 billion gallons), respectively, of the total gallons of liquid beverages consumed [5].

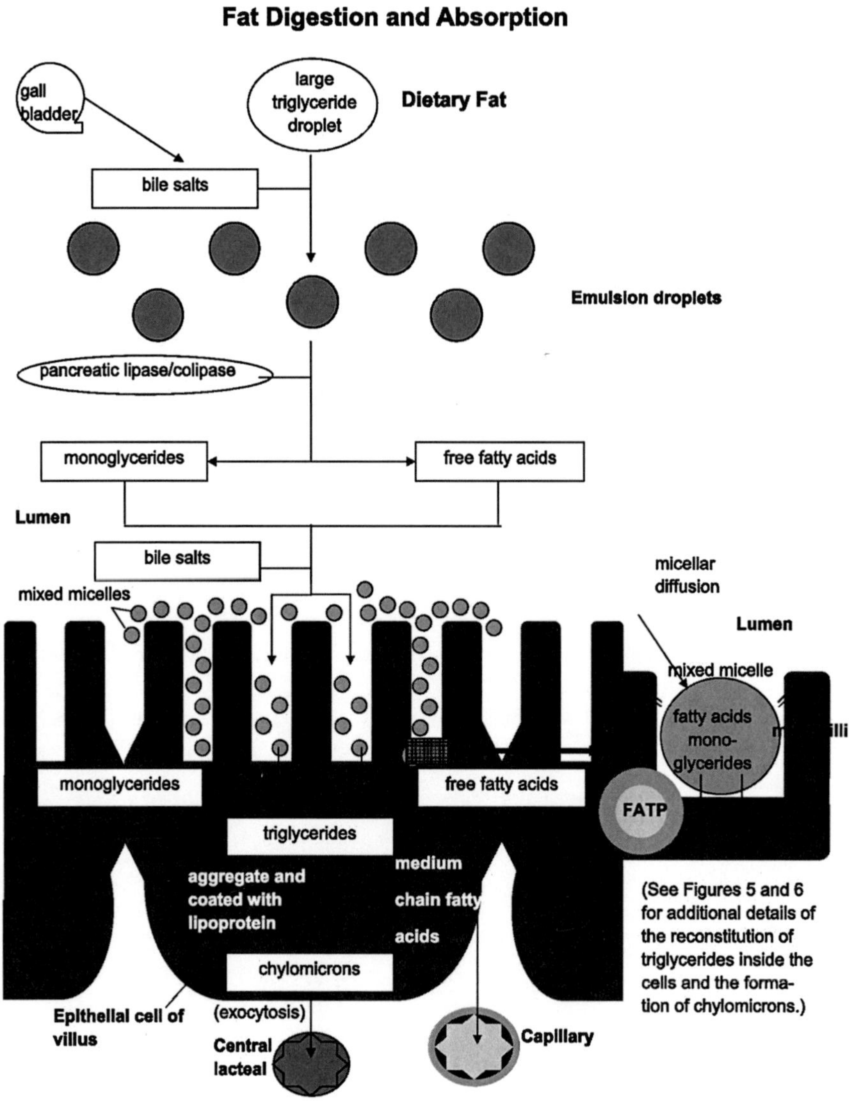

Fat Digestion and Absorption

Fig. 8.3 Fat digestion and absorption (from Goodman [1], with permission)

Alcohol is consumed by many patients and contributes to many chronic health problems. It is absorbed in the small intestine and diffuses into all tissue into which water diffuses, except bone and fat. The major detoxification of alcohol occurs in the liver through a two-step process of oxidation. The first step is oxidation of the alcohol into acetaldehyde. The second step is the oxidation of acetaldehyde into acetate. There is variability in the absorption of alcohol due to physical size and

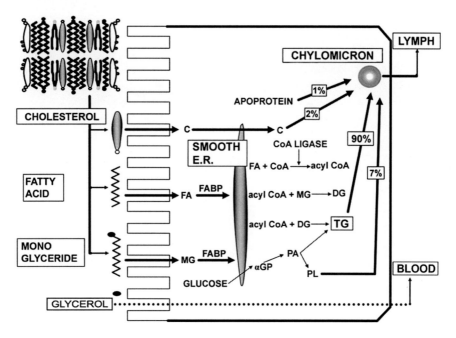

Fig. 8.4 Reconstitution of triglycerides and formation of chylomicrons (from Goodman [1], with permission)

genetic factors as well as medication use. Alcohol use has been shown to cause epigenetic changes through the methylation of DNA.

A causative role of alcohol in contributing to overweight and obesity has not been established [5]. Some types of alcohol used in moderation, like wine, has beneficial health effects. Wine contains polyphenols and resveratrol that can have a positive effect on cardiovascular health [6]. On the other hand, alcohol contributes as a risk factor to breast cancer [7]. While a causative role has not been established, alcohol can affect weight. The caloric content of alcohol can add up quickly and is not its only impact on weight. The body has to metabolize by priority the food and drink consumed. The body prioritizes the metabolism of alcohol and will stop metabolizing food when alcohol is present. Those food calories are put "on hold" and get stored as fat. Alcohol is a simple carbohydrate and blood glucose levels rise during alcohol ingestion. When those glucose levels start to drop, the sensation of hunger materializes. In addition, alcohol use disinhibits the prefrontal cortex where decision-making is located in the brain, thereby contributing to one's lack of ability to be mindful about food choices.

Sugar sweetened beverages (SSB) have been a focus of public policy debate for some years with efforts to limit the access to these beverages by children and adolescents. SSB's are the single largest source of added sugar and energy intake in the United States. Recent data supports the causative role of SSB's in overweight and obesity, as demonstrated in three meta-analyses and two randomized controlled trials (RCT). These studies show that intake of SSB's among children is associated with a 55 % risk of being overweight, and two servings per day of SSB is associated with a risk of 26 % for T2DM. The two RCT's demonstrate that reducing consumption of SSB decreased weight gain and adiposity in children and adolescents [8]. Studies discussed earlier in this book demonstrate the mechanism of epigenetic silencing of the SuVar gene in Drosophila when the Drosophila were fed sugar water. These studies have raised the question of whether this may also be the primary mechanism by which SSB intake causes obesity.

Fatty Acids

Two fatty acids are included in the essential nutrients required for health: linoleic acid (omega-6 essential fatty acid) and alpha-linolenic acid (omega-3 fatty acid). These fatty acids must be derived from sources outside the body because the body does not synthesize them. Americans eat more omega-6 than omega-3 fatty acids.

Linoleic acid is the main polyunsaturated fat found in certain vegetable oils (sunflower, canola), nuts, and seeds. It lowers the risk of coronary artery disease by decreasing total and LDL cholesterol. Concerns have been raised about linoleic acid promoting inflammation but multiple studies show that it may be anti-inflammatory [9]. Unfortunately, in the typical American diet, linoleic acid comes largely from refined carbohydrates and saturated fats, both of which are linked to coronary artery disease.

Alpha-linolenic acid is a component of cell membrane and receptors throughout the body and provides the starting component for making steroid hormones. Alph-linolenic acid is primarily derived from foods like fish, leafy vegetables and vegetable oils including walnut oil and flax seed oil.

Vitamins and Minerals

Vitamins and minerals are essential nutrients because together they perform hundreds of roles in the human body. There is a fine line between getting enough of each nutrient for good health and getting too much. Vitamins are organic and can be broken down by heat, air, or acid. Minerals are inorganic and hold on to their chemical structure.

Table 8.1 Recommendations of macronutrients in adults

Macronutrient	EAR	RDI
Carbohydrate[a]	130 g/d	175 g/d
Protein		0.8 g/d/kg of body weight 56 g for men 46 g for women
Total fat	Not determined to have value	Not determined to have value
Total fiber	AI of 38–30 g/d (male) AI of 25–21 g/d (female)	

Definitions
EAR Estimated average requirements
RDI Recommended daily allowance
AI Adequate intake
[a]Although carbohydrates are marked as recommended, there is no scientific evidence that requires any carbohydrates in the diet
From food and Nutrition Board [2], with permission

The following vitamins are considered essential nutrients: vitamin A, vitamin B, vitamin B-6, ascorbic acid (one form of Vitamin C), vitamin D, vitamin E, vitamin K, thiamine, riboflavin, niacin, pantothenic acid, folic acid, and biotin.

The following minerals are considered essential nutrients: calcium, phosphorus, magnesium, and iron.

The following trace minerals are considered essential nutrients: zinc copper, manganese, iodine, selenium, molybdenum, and chromium.

Dietary References Intakes (DRI) for Macro and Micronutrients

Dietary Reference Intakes (DRIs) are issued by the Food and Nutrition Board of the IOM. The DRIs provide a set of reference values to assess and plan for nutrient intake of healthy people. Often these recommendations have to be adjusted for age, gender, and specific situations like pregnancy. The DRI is broken down into Estimated Average Requirements (EAR), which is the intake needed to meet the nutrient needs of approximately 50 % of the population, as opposed to the RDI, which is the intake that meets the needs of 97–98 % of healthy individuals (Table 8.1).

Reading a Food Label

The Food and Drug Administration (FDA) is responsible for ensuring that foods sold in the United States are safe and properly labeled. The Nutrition Labeling and Education Act (NLEA) require most foods to have nutrition labeling that complies with specific requirements. Food labels are a key source of information for anyone wanting to know the precise contents of the food they are consuming, but labels can be confusing. One major source of confusion on the food label is the serving size.

Many people assume one "package" is one serving size, when in fact it may contain multiple servings.

When evaluating a food label it is helpful to start with the serving size per package and calories per serving. Next consider the amounts per serving for total fat, cholesterol, sodium, and carbohydrates. Again, it is important to know what *one serving* contributes in each of these categories. Finally, the amounts of dietary fiber, protein, and minerals and vitamins per serving should also be taken into account. There is some evidence that keeping an accurate record of foods consumed on a daily basis can have a significant impact on choices made and, ultimately, on weight loss. Patients interested in weight loss should be encouraged to use food labels and to accurately track food intake and associated calories.

Energy Expenditure

The Recommended Dietary Intake (RDI) reference values for adults correspond with energy expenditure of 3067 kcal/d for men and 2403 kcal/d for women [10]. *The majority of daily energy expenditure is from basal metabolism. Physical activity contributes only a small additional proportion of total energy expenditure, unless you exercise 8 or more hours a day.* Total energy expenditure in human beings has three major components: (1) basal metabolic rate (BMR), (2) thermic effect of food (TEF), also called diet-induced thermogenesis (DIT), and (3) thermogenesis (i.e., physical activity). All three components of total energy expenditure are discussed in more detail below.

Energy Expenditure: Basal Metabolic Rate (BMR)

Basal Metabolic Rate (BMR) is the largest component of energy expenditure, accounting for about 60 % of a person's total energy expenditure. BMR is essentially the rate at which the human body uses energy while at rest, to keep vital organs and bodily functions operating. BMR is affected by whether you are lean or obese, as well as by gender, age, and genetic inheritance. When taking all these factors into account, the BMR is variable from one individual to another by approximately 200 kcal/d.

Energy Expenditure: Thermal Effect of Food (TEF)

The thermal effect of food (TEF) is an increase in metabolic rate (i.e., caloric burn) that occurs after ingesting food. When you ingest food, the body must expend extra energy (calories) to digest, absorb, and store nutrients, thereby increasing metabolism. TEF is the difference between energy expenditure after food consumption and BMR, divided by the rate of nutrient energy administration. The TEF of different key nutrients is: Alcohol 10–30 %; Protein 20–30 %; Carbohydrate 5–10 %; and Fat 0–3 %. These assigned values for nutrient energy administration account for the amount of extra energy required to metabolize and store each nutrient [11]. Alcohol is included because it accounts for a significant part of some people's dietary intake although it is not strictly a "nutrient".

Patients with obesity have a significantly lower TEF than lean individuals [12]. Alcohol itself does not always increase body weight, as people who consume alcohol may in fact be more active [13]. TEF was increased by 100 % on a high-protein diet over a high-carbohydrate diet [14]. A high-protein diet is also favored after weight loss [15]. The mechanism by which protein increases TEF is through the induction of satiety [16]. A mixed diet consumed at energy balance showed that TEF accounts for 5–15 % of daily energy expenditure.

Energy Expenditure: Thermogenesis (Exercise and Physical Activity)

Physical activity, or thermogenesis, is an important component of energy expenditure and is beneficial beyond simply the burning of energy. There is both exercise-related thermogenesis and non-exercise thermogenesis. Non-exercise activity thermogenesis (NEAT) in most people is the predominant energy expenditure outside of BMR, as well as the most highly variable type of energy expenditure. NEAT includes the energy expended for everything that is not sleeping, eating or sports-like exercise. For instance, NEAT in a "couch potato" accounts for a very large part of their total energy expenditure whereas a cyclist in the Tour de France will have a very small NEAT expenditure.

When you have a high amount of exercise-related physical activity as opposed to a high amount of NEAT, you compensate for it by not only having an increased appetite, but also by decreasing your amount of NEAT. Both of these compensatory mechanisms are driven centrally in the brain and are largely outside your volitional control. In addition, the efficiency of NEAT is genetically programmed. Some scientists believe that NEAT could be the secret to achieving or maintaining weight loss. It can increase energy expenditure by up to 2000 kcal/d. Implementing ways to increase NEAT expenditure in everyday activities might compensate for the increase in energy intake and mitigate the weight gain of aging [17].

The muscle in your body does more than provide locomotion. The 640 + muscles account for about 30–40 % of total body weight and utilize 25 % of the energy consumed by the body at rest. Muscle has "plasticity" and can adjust its own composition when needed. For instance, an immobilized limb can lose up to 1/3 of its mass in a few weeks. Genes modulate changes in muscle. *Changes in gene expression caused in part by physical activity are good examples of epigenetic modulation* [18]. Lack of physical activity influences your susceptibility for chronic disease. Genes that require physical activity are also disease susceptible genes [19].

Exercise-related thermogenesis, as opposed to NEAT, is highly variable, and should perhaps be viewed as "medicine" designed to stave off chronic disease. Lack of physical activity is a risk factor for all-cause mortality independent of BMI [20]. Physical activity and exercise provide protection against diabetes, cardiovascular disease, cancer, dementia, and depression. In muscle, which is the most abundant tissue in the body, proteins can respond within a few seconds with changes that allow increase in the body's use of glycogen and oxygen [18]. The effect of inactivity is so profound that the Centers for Disease Control and Prevention (CDC) have designated physical *in*activity as a cause of chronic disease, including obesity.

Exercise does not always work as a treatment for patients with obesity primarily because achieving a significant calorie deficit requires exercise of a higher intensity and longer duration/frequency than many obese patients are physically capable of performing. A patient may even gain weight in the early stages of an exercise program as muscle, which is heavier, replaces fat. *Once a patient has lost weight, the amount of energy burned doing the same exercise decreases approximately 20 %. This is one of the reasons that weight regain is so prevalent: even with the same amount of exercise, the patient is no longer burning as much energy* [17].

In addition, there is variability in how people respond to exercise. Just like people respond to a particular medication differently based on their genetics, people respond to exercise differently as well. In a group of people matched for body type, there was wide variability in their response to the same exercise regimen [21]. It appears that high intensity intermittent exercise may be more effective at reducing subcutaneous and abdominal body fat and lowering insulin resistance through muscle adaptation [22].

A person's maximal aerobic capacity (VO2 Max) is determined by maternal mitochondrial DNA. Physical training can increase VO2 Max to one's "genetic ceiling." Other inheritable traits include the type of fibers in muscle and the muscle's response to training. Proteins can respond within a few seconds with changes that allow an increase in the muscle's use of glycogen and oxygen [18].

Skeletal muscle is the biggest endocrine organ in the body. The first myokine (irisin) was the first protein hormone isolated from muscle and is reported to induce the browning of white adipose tissue [23]. The effect of irisin in metabolic disease remains to be defined [24]. Other exercise-derived factors play a role in signaling. For example, the release of nitric oxide (NO) during exercise in small doses helps to decrease insulin resistance in skeletal muscle but in larger doses is harmful [25].

Most adults gain on average 1–2 lb per year as they age. Accordingly, it is estimated that 100 additional calories per day in extra energy expenditure or a combination of increased EE and decreased energy intake totaling 100 kcal/d is necessary each year to prevent weight gain. Preventing weight gain is relatively easy compared to inducing weight loss, which requires large behavior changes with more intense and longer periods of exercise. This becomes an important concept for all providers working with patients, and especially those patients in the "overweight" BMI groups. *In the "overweight" group of patients, as opposed to the clinically obese BMI group, holding the line is relatively inexpensive and can be effective with effort and commitment.*

Patients with established obesity do not simply need to maintain weight, they need to actively lose weight. For this group, achieving weight loss through exercise is very difficult. Nevertheless, making the effort to identify safe options for exercise and helping the patient to establish consistent exercise habits is important because even outside of weight loss, exercise plays a role in keeping a person healthy. The new science indicates that exercise is medicine. See www.Exerciseismedicine.org.

Mental Health in the Bariatric Population

Psychiatric illness and psychological disorders in people with obesity should be taken as seriously as other obesity-related diseases the patient may be experiencing. Just as diabetes and the medications the patient takes to treat it may affect the ability of a patient to lose weight, a psychological disorder and the medications a patient takes, or the limitations a patient may have because of it, may affect the patient's ability to lose weight or maintain weight loss.

There is a high incidence of psychiatric illness and psychological disorders in people with obesity compared to populations that are not obese. The true incidence, however, is difficult to discern. The National Comorbidity Survey–Replication predicted much lower rates of Axis 1 disorders (Table 8.2) in overweight and obesity, however the highest quality data detailing the incidence of psychological illness was reported in the prospective Longitudinal Assessment of Bariatric

Table 8.2 Axis I disorders

Major depressive disorder	Dysthymia
Generalized anxiety disorder	Social phobia
Agoraphobia	Specific phobia (animal, natural environment, blood-injection-injury, situational or other)
Panic disorder	Post-traumatic stress disorder
Anorexia nervosa	Pain disorder
Conduct disorder	Alcohol abuse/dependence
Cannabis abuse/dependence	Hard drugs abuse/dependence (including opiates, sedatives, cocaine, amphetamine, hallucinogens, inhalants and polysubstance)

Data from Roysamb, E, Tambs K, Orstavik RE, Torgersen S, Kendler KS, Neale MC et al. The Joint Structure of DSM-0IV Axis I and Axis II Disorders

Surgery (LABS) NIH funded trial [26]. The LABS cohort was 82.9 % female/Caucasian with a median age of 46 and body mass index (BMI) of 44.8 kg/m^2 and showed the following pathology:

- 38.7 % lifetime history of depressive disorder
- 33.2 % lifetime diagnosis of alcohol abuse or dependence
- 13.1 % lifetime diagnosis of binge eating disorder
- 33.7 % once current Axis I disorder
- 68.8 % at least one lifetime Axis I disorder

Additional high-quality studies support these findings and confirm lifetime rates of psychiatric disorders in patients affected by obesity to be 66.3 % and 72.6 % [26, 27].

Specific Psychiatric Disorders Related to Obesity: Depression and Anxiety

Association between obesity and depression has been repeatedly established yet the nature and underlying mechanisms of the association and the reciprocal link between depression and obesity are still unclear and subject to ongoing research. Studies have shown that people who consider themselves as being overweight or obese often experience weight-related stigma and discrimination and consequently present with symptoms of low self-esteem, low self-worth, and guilt. Obesity is also related to sleep apnea, low socioeconomic status, and reduced physical activity, all of which are additional strong predictors of depression [28].

It has been established that depression and anxiety in patients with obesity varies by gender. Men with Class 3 obesity (BMI $\geq$ 40 kg/m^2) have higher levels of depression and anxiety than normal weight men. Women had increased depression and anxiety if they were either underweight, overweight, or obese compared to normal weight women. These effects were independent of other lifestyle and social factors [28].

Clinicians should consider the possibility of depression and anxiety in patients with excess body weight and comorbidities. Likewise, patients who present with symptoms of common mental disorders such as depression and anxiety should be assessed for obesity and related chronic diseases, particularly given the possible side effect of weight gain with antidepressant medications.

Food Addiction: Science or Silly?

One current model of explaining overeating and obesity attempts to cast obesity in the framework of addiction. The idea of food addiction is an evolving nonlinear science. The model presents people with obesity as being physically dependent on food rather than being personally in charge of their dietary and exercise choices. Presenting obesity in this way shapes the message the public perceives and may influence the way we communicate about this issue [29]. There are compelling arguments to embrace this model, including the biologic effect of food on the brain and related behavior, as well as society's errant belief that obesity is a result of personal flaws or lack of self-control.

Obesity is currently recognized as a disease and is characterized by frequent relapses after dieting. Treatment of obesity, like the treatments for many other addictions, is often ineffective or achieves a less than optimal rate of success. Like addicts of alcohol or drugs, people who suffer from obesity often under-report or deny the true amount of the abused substance, in this case food, that they ingest. Some evidence implies that using the food addiction model results in less bias and stigma [30] while others believe that pairing the "food addict" label with obesity results in more stigma. [31]. The real question is whether the food addiction model is based on facts and science.

The Diagnostic and Statistical Manual of Mental Disorders, Fifth Edition (DSM-V), acknowledges food addiction [32]. Central to the addiction argument is that certain foods, specifically sugar, fat, salt, and processed foods, contain addictive substances that produce behavioral adaptations comparable to the effects of drugs, tobacco, and alcohol on the brain.

Food addiction has also been viewed as a behavioral phenotype. In an effort to quantify the food addiction phenotype, a new evaluation tool has been proposed and validated: the Yale Food Addiction Scale (YFAS) [33, 34]. While there is currently no official diagnosis of "food addiction," the YFAS was developed in 2009 to identify people who exhibited symptoms of dependency toward certain foods. The YFAS is still recognized as an important tool for evaluating whether an addictive process contributes to certain types of problematic eating behaviors.

Another school of thought is that food addiction is the cause of obesity only in special subsets of people, such as people suffering from Binge Eating Disorder. Adding to the debate is the fact that functional neuroimaging, assessing whether external food cues evoke the desire to eat and result in obesity, do not seem to support the addiction model [35, 36].

Another model that attempts to integrate food addiction with diet/nutritional science and psychology is the Stress/Weight Matrix [37] (Fig. 8.5). This matrix

Circle all that apply:

Marital Status: Single Married Divorced Separated Widowed
Have you been hospitalized in the last year? Y N
Have you been hospitalized for more than 7 days in your lifetime? Y N
Do you drink coffee or tea? Y N
Did any of the following happen to you in the last year?
Y N Death of a family member or a very close friend
Y N Separation from spouse or long-time partner
Y N Recent change of job
Y N Moving within the same city
Y N Moving to another city
Y N Financial difficulties
Y N Legal problems
Y N Beginning of a new relationship

How many hours do you work per week? _____
Y N Are you satisfied with your work?
Y N Do you feel under pressure at work?
Y N Do you get along with your colleagues at work?
Y N Do you get along with your spouse or partner?
Y N Do you get along with other relatives?
Y N Has any close relative been seriously ill in the past year?
Y N Do you feel tension at home?
Y N Do you live by yourself?
Y N Do you feel lonely?
Y N Do you have anyone whom you can trust and confide in?
Y N Do you get along well with people?
Y N Do you often feel overwhelmed by the demands of every day life?
Y N Do you often feel you cannot make it?
Y N Do you tend to be influenced by people with strong opinions?
Y N Do you tend to worry about what other people think of you?
Y N Do you have stomach or bowel pains?
Y N Does your heart beat quickly or strongly without a reason?
Y N Do you have feelings of dizziness or fainting?
Y N Do you have feelings of pressure or tightness in your head or body?
Y N Do you have difficulty breathing or feel you cannot get enough air?
Y N Do you feel tired and lack energy?
Y N Are you irritable?
Y N Do you feel sad or depressed?
Y N Do you feel tense or "wound up"?
Y N Have you lost interest in most things?
Y N Do you get "panic" attacks?
Y N Do you believe you have a physical disease but doctors have not diagnosed it correctly?
Y N When you read or hear about an illness, do you get similar symptoms?

How would you rate your level of stress? Low/Medium/High/ Intermittent High
How do you rate the quality of your life? Excellent/Good/Fair/Poor/Awful

Fig. 8.5 Stress/Weight Matrix (adapted from Sonino and Fava [39], with permission)

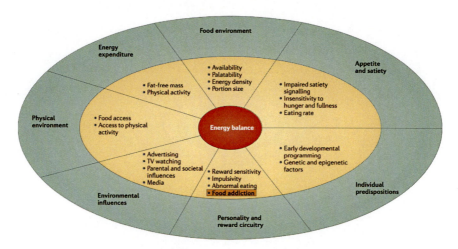

Fig. 8.6 Mediators of energy balance and body weight. The outer ring represents the major classes of mediators, the inner ring some of the individual mediators in each class. We suggest that food addiction is one of many factors in a more complex model of the obesity epidemic that require further exploration and refinement. The data on which the figure is based come from the Obesity Systems Map introduced by the UK Foresight programme 2007, a multidisciplinary effort to plan the UK response to obesity (from Ziauddeen et al. [38], with permission)

demonstrates how food addictions impact obesity by food cueing and food craving. It identifies three drivers of weight: Metabolic (homeostatic), Addictive (hedonic), and Relationship (anthroponic). The Stress/Weight Matrix model helps explain many of the unpredictable, nonlinear reactions that patients have toward food. The vulnerability to relapse is often driven by hedonic or addictive elements [37].

These are complex and difficult issues to sort through. The drivers of overweight and obesity are many [38]. In some people with obesity an addiction to food may be a factor (Fig. 8.6). Using tools like the YFAS (Table 8.3) and the Stress/Weight Matrix, along with the other known drivers of overweight and obesity, to determine whether food addiction is present in any given patient may facilitate referral of the patient to appropriate colleagues and result in more effective therapy for obesity. As research continues, we may see that the neurobiological models that break obesity down into biological and physiological processes against a background of genetic predisposition may supplant the "addiction" model. Nevertheless, food addiction neuroscience research and neuroimaging during fasting and eating is revolutionizing our understanding of how obesity evolves and sustains itself [35–37].

Table 8.3 Yale food addiction scale

In the past 12 months	Never	Once a month	2–4 times a month	2–3 times a week	4 or more times or daily
1. I find that when I start eating certain foods, I end up eating much more than planned	0	1	2	3	4
2. I find myself continuing to consume certain foods even though I am no longer hungry	0	1	2	3	4
3. I eat to the point where I feel physically ill	0	1	2	3	4
4. Not eating certain types of food or cutting down on certain types of food is something I worry about	0	1	2	3	4
5. I spend a lot of time feeling sluggish or fatigued from overeating	0	1	2	3	4
6. I find myself constantly eating certain foods throughout the day	0	1	2	3	4
7. I find that when certain foods are not available, I will go out of my way to obtain them. For example, I will drive to the store to purchase certain foods even though I have other options available to me at home	0	1	2	3	4
8. There have been times when I consumed certain foods so often or in such large quantities that I started to eat food instead of working, spending time with my family or friends, or engaging in other important activities or recreational activities I enjoy	0	1	2	3	4
9. There have been times when I consumed certain foods so often or in such large quantities that I spent time dealing with negative feelings from overeating instead of working, spending time with my family or friends, or engaging in other important activities or recreational activities I enjoy	0	1	2	3	4
10. There have been times when I avoided professional or social situations where certain foods were available, because I was afraid I would overeat	0	1	2	3	4
11. There have been times when I avoided professional or social situations because I was not able to consume certain foods there	0	1	2	3	4
12. I have had withdrawal symptoms such as agitation, anxiety, or other physical symptoms when I cut down or stopped eating certain foods. (Please do NOT include withdrawal symptoms caused by cutting down on caffeinated beverages such as soda pop, coffee, tea, energy drinks, etc.)	0	1	2	3	4
13. I have consumed certain foods to prevent feelings of anxiety, agitation, or other physical symptoms that were developing. (Please do NOT include consumption of caffeinated beverages such as soda pop, coffee, tea, energy drinks, etc.)	0	1	2	3	4

(continued)

Table 8.3 (continued)

In the past 12 months	Never	Once a month	2–4 times a month	2–3 times a week	4 or more times or daily
14. I have found that I have elevated desire for or urges to consume certain foods when I cut down or stop eating them	0	1	2	3	4
15. My behavior with respect to food and eating causes significant distress	0	1	2	3	4
16. I experience significant problems in my ability to function effectively (daily routine, job/school, social activities, family activities, health difficulties) because of food and eating	0	1	2	3	4

In the past 12 months	No			Yes	
17. My food consumption has caused significant psychological problems such as depression, anxiety, self-loathing, or guilt	0			1	
18. My food consumption has caused significant physical problems or made a physical problem worse	0			1	
19. I kept consuming the same types of food or the same amount of food even though I was having emotional and/or physical problems	0			1	
20. Over time, I have found that I need to eat more and more to get the feeling I want, such as reduced negative emotions or increased pleasure	0			1	
21. I have found that eating the same amount of food does not reduce my negative emotions or increase pleasurable feelings the way it used to	0			1	
22. I want to cut down or stop eating certain kinds of food	0			1	
23. I have tried to cut down or stop eating certain kinds of food	0			1	
24. I have been successful at cutting down or not eating these kinds of food	0			1	

	1 or fewer times	2 times	3 times	4 times	5 or more times
25. How many times in the past year did you try to cut down or stop eating certain foods altogether?		2 times	3 times	4 times	5 or more times

This survey asks about your eating habits in the past year. People sometimes have difficulty controlling their intake of certain foods such as: sweets like ice cream, chocolate, doughnuts, cookies, cake, candy, and ice cream; starches like white bread, rolls, pasta, and rice; salty snacks like chips, pretzels, and crackers

Fatty foods like steak, bacon, hamburgers, cheeseburgers, pizza, and French fries

Sugary drinks like soda pop. When the following questions ask about "CERTAIN FOODS" please think of ANY food similar to those listed in the food group or ANY OTHER foods you have had a problem with in the past year

From Gearhardt et al. [33], with permission

Conclusion

These fundamental components of healthy food, exercise, and behavior modification are the building blocks of any sound program for body weight maintenance or weight loss. Patients and providers are often confused about these fundamentals in part due to the plethora of books and articles in the popular press giving advice of various kinds that is often directly contradictory. Also, some of the recommendations from the scientific community create confusion in recommended daily allowances of nutrients, as we see in the case of carbohydrates. It is important to separate the facts from fiction for the patient but also to educate them on this topic. The essential next step is to identify the patient at risk (Overweight BMI of 27 kg/m^2 and above), assess the patient, and determine how to intervene specifically in a way that helps the patient maintain or lose weight and restore health. These topics are all addressed in detail in the next chapter.

References

1. Goodman BE. Insights into digestion and absorption of major nutrients in humans. Adv Physiol Educ. 2010;34(2):44–53.
2. Food and Nutrition Board. Dietary reference intakes for energy, carbohydrate, fiber, fat, fatty acids, cholesterol, protein and amino acids. Washington, DC: National Academies of Sciences, Engineering and Medicine, The National Academies Press; 2015.
3. Westman EC. Is dietary carbohydrate essential for human nutrition? Am J Clin Nutr. 2002;75(5):951–3.
4. Popkin BM, D'Anci KE, Rosenberg IH. Water, hydration and health. Nutr Rev. 2010;68(8):439–58.
5. Poppitt SD. Beverage consumption: are alcoholic and sugar sweetened beverages tipping the balance towards overweight and obesity? Nutrients. 2015;7:6700–18.
6. Biagi M, Bertelli AA. Wine, alcohol and pills: what future for the French paradox? Life Sci. 2015;131:19–22.
7. Ferrini K, Ghelfi F, Mannucci R, Titta L. eCancer. 2015;9:557. doi:10.3332/ecancer.2015.557.
8. Hu FB. Resolved: there is sufficient scientific evidence that decreasing sugar-sweetened beverage consumption will reduce the prevalence of obesity and obesity-related diseases. Obes Rev. 2013;14(8):606–19.
9. Farvid MS, Ding M, Pan A, Sun Q, Chiuve SE, Steffen LM, Willett WC, Hu FB. Dietary linoleic acid and risk of coronary heart disease: a systematic review and meta-analysis of prospective cohort studies. Circulation. 2014;130(18):1568–78.
10. National Academies of Sciences, Institute of Medicine. Dietary references intakes for energy, carbohydrate, fiber, fat, fatty acids, cholesterol, protein and amino acids; 2002.
11. Acheson KJ. Influence of autonomic nervous system on nutrient-induced thermogenesis in humans. Nutrition. 1993;9(4):373–80.
12. De Jonge L, Bray GA. The thermic effect of food and obesity: a critical review. Obes Res. 1997;5(6):622–31.
13. Westerterp KR, et al. Alcohol energy intake and habitual physical activity in older adults. Br J Nutr. 2004;91(1):149–52.
14. Johnston CS, Day CS, Swan PD. Postprandial thermogenesis is increased 100 % on a high-protein, low-fat diet versus a high-carbohydrate, low-fat diet in health, young women. J Am Coll Nutr. 2002;21(1):55–61.

References

15. Westerterp KR, Plantenga MS. The significant of protein in food and body weight regulation. Curr Opin Lin Nutr Metabl Care. 2003;6(6):635–8.
16. Westerterp KR. Diet induced thermogenesis. Nutr Metabol. 2004. doi:10.1186/1743-7075-1-5.
17. Villablanca PA, Alegria JR, Mookadam F, Holmes DR, Weight RS, Levine JA. Nonexercise activity thermogenesis in obesity management. Mayo Clin Proc. 2015;90(4):509–19.
18. Neufer PD, Booth F. Exercise controls gene expression. Am Sci. 2005;93:1–5.
19. Ntanasis-Stathopoulos J, Tzanninis JG, Philippou A, Koutsilieris M. Epigenetic regulation on gene expression induced by physician exercise. J Musculoskeletal Neuronal Interact. 2013;13(2):133–46.
20. Pedersen BK. Muscles and their myokines. J Exp Bio. 2011;214:337–46.
21. King NA, Hopkins M, Caudwell P, Stubbs RJ, Blundell JE. Individual variability following 12 weeks of supervised exercise: identification and characterization of compensation for exercise-induced weight loss. Int J Obesity. 2008;32:177–84.
22. Boutcher SH. High–intensity intermittent exercise and fat loss. J Obes. 2011;868305.
23. Bostrum P, Wu J, Jedrychowski MP, Korde A, Ye L, Lo JC, et al. A PGC1α-dependent myokine that drives browning of white fat and thermogenesis. Nature. 2012;481(7382):463–8.
24. Chen J, Huang Y, Gusdon AM, Qu S. Irisin: a new molecular marker and target in metabolic disorder. Lipids Health Dis. 2015; 14(2).
25. McConell GK, Rattigan S, Lee-Young RS, Wadley GD, Merry TL. Skeletal muscle nitric oxide signaling and exercise: a focus on glucose metabolism. Am J Physiol Endocrinol Metab. 2012;303:E301–7.
26. Mitchell JE, et al. Psychopathology prior to surgery in the longitudinal assessment of bariatric surgery-3 (LABS-3) psychosocial study. Surg Obes Relat Dis. 2012;8(5):533–41.
27. Kalarchian MA, et al. Psychiatric disorder among bariatric surgery candidates: relationship to obesity and functional health systems. Am J Psychiatry. 2007;164:328–34.
28. Zhao G, Ford ES, Shingra S, Li C, Strine TW, Mokdad AH. Depression and anxiety among US adults: associations with body mass index. Int J Obes. 2009;33(2):257–66.
29. Chong D, Druckman JN. Framing theory. Annu Rev Polit Sci. 2007;10:103–26.
30. Latner JD, Puhl RM, Murakami JM, O'Brien KS. Food addiction as a causal model of obesity. Effects on stigma, blame, and perceived psychopathology. Appetite. 2014;77C:77–82.
31. DePierre JA, Puhl RM, Luedicke J. A new stigmatized identity? Comparisons of a "food addict" label with other stigmatized health conditions. Basic Appl Soc Psychol. 2013;35:10–21.
32. American Psychiatric Association. Diagnostic and statistical manual of mental disorders. 5th ed. Arlington: American Psychiatric Association. p. 350–2.
33. Gearhardt AN, Corbin WR, Brownell KD. Preliminary validation of the Yale food addiction scale. Appetite. 2009;52:430–6.
34. Gearhardt AN, Corbin WR, Brownell KD. Yale Food Addiction Scale (YFAS). Measurement instrument database for the social science. Retrieved from www.midss.ie (2012).
35. Passamonti L, Rowe JB, Schwarzbauer C, Ewbank MP, von dem Hagen E, Calder AJ. Personality predicts the brain's response to viewing appetizing foods: the neural basis of a risk factor for overeating. J Neurosci. 2009;7(29):43–51.
36. Kullman S, Henri M, Veit R, Ketterer C, Schick F, Haring HU, Fritsche A, Preissi H. The obese brain: association of body mass index and insulin sensitivity with resting state network functional connectivity. Hum Brain Mapp. 2012;33(5):1052–61.
37. Shriner R, Gold M. Food addiction: an evolving nonlinear science. Nutrients. 2014;6(11):5370–91.
38. Ziauddeen H, Farooqi IS, Fletcher PC. Obesity and the brain: how convincing is the addiction model? Nat Rev Neurosci. 2012;13:279–86.
39. Sonino N, Fava GA. A simple instrument for assessing stress in clinical practice. Postgrad Med J. 1998;74:408–10.

Chapter 9
The Assessment of the Adult Patient with Overweight and Obesity

Key Message

Every person who is overweight or obese needs guidance and support from their physician to get back to better health. To facilitate this, a thorough medical assessment of the overweight/obese patient is crucial, as the factors contributing to obesity in this particular patient must be ascertained. Many obese patients have an inherited predisposition to obesity. The question is: can these patients modulate the epigenetics that are impacting their weight? Can these patients do this by modifying their diet, their exercise, their sleep, their stress levels, their cultural and family influences and any other impactful components of their daily environment?

A thorough and comprehensive intake history followed by a complete physical examination unique to the patient with obesity will allow the practitioner to identify and quantify the weight issues of the patient and design an appropriate treatment plan. The goal is to educate and encourage the patient to embrace specific methods that will effectively modulate or "reset" their epigenetics. Frequent and consistent follow up by the practitioner is required.

The specific format for taking a history in a patient with obesity is laid out in this chapter. It then goes on to outline the mechanics and unique challenges of performing a complete physical assessment and the various tools that can be used, including necessary or recommended diagnostic tests. Information regarding additional assessments on patients with non-alcoholic fatty liver disease (NAFLD) and type 2 diabetes (T2DM) is also provided in this chapter, along with a discussion about disordered sleep. Finally, this chapter explains the importance of doing a summary assessment in which patient goals are established and a treatment plan is created. Treatment often starts with realistic and more easily attainable goals before bigger goals are set because asking a patient to do everything at once will likely result in failure and frustration.

Learning Objectives

1. Understand how to take a comprehensive health history in a patient with obesity. Understand the mechanics and challenges of performing a proper and

thorough physical assessment of a patient with obesity, including the necessity of specific diagnostic tests that should be ordered. Understand the importance of using the history and physical assessment to design an effective treatment program for the patient that also encompasses meaningful follow up care.
2. Outline the evaluation of a patient with non-alcoholic fatty liver disease (NAFLD) for liver biopsy.
3. Summarize the assessment of disordered sleep and the role it plays in obesity management.
4. Understand the need for and most effective use of the Weight Related Health Indicators (WRHI) obtained through the health history and physical assessment of the patient.
5. Summarize the EKG changes in a patient with obesity and discuss which ones indicate an abnormal EKG that requires further evaluation.

Obesity affects almost all body systems (Fig. 9.1). Performing a thorough and accurate patient assessment on the patient who is overweight or obese is critical. An astute assessment will allow the medical practitioner to identify potential obesity-related issues (see summary of complications in Fig. 9.1) that may have gone unrecognized, or to detect insulin resistance and inflammation or other early signs of adipose tissue dysfunction that can lead to obesity-related diseases. Even the patient with simple obesity, uncomplicated by obesity-related disease, has an increased risk of early mortality and requires a thorough assessment [1] (Fig. 9.2).

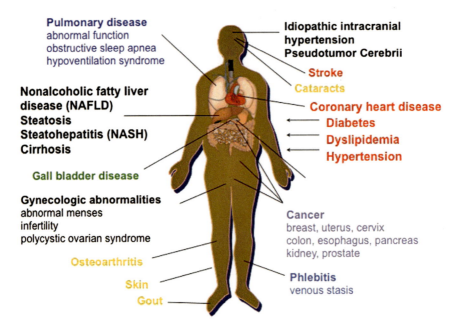

Fig. 9.1 Adult obesity-related disease

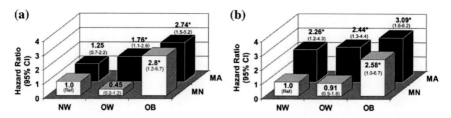

Fig. 9.2 Relative risk of all-cause mortality by RMO category and metabolism status as defined by METSyn factors **a** and insulin resistance **b** criteria. *Asterisk* HR significantly different from MNNW referent ($P < 0.05$). Data are adjusted for age, sex, income, ethnicity, smoking status, and alcohol consumption. Metabolically normal (*MN*) was defined as one of less MetSyn risk factor or HOMA <2.5 *MA* metabolically abnormal; *NW* normal weight; *OB* obese; *OW* overweight. From Kuk and Ardern [1] with permission

The Health History

The history serves to document factors that may be influencing obesity. *It is important to carefully note the patient's responses to the history as they relate to eating habits and diet, physical activity, stress, sleep, circadian patterns, family culture, and medications. Some of these factors are potentially reversible or modifiable and may provide ways to impact the patient's weight almost immediately.* Taking a thorough history consists of the following 14 areas of inquiry, each of which is discussed in more detail below.

> **Historical Survey of Weight Gain and Loss**
> **Family History of Obesity and Related Disease**
> **Medications**
> **Dietary History**
> **Stress Factors**
> **Circadian Patterns**
> **Disordered Sleep Analysis**
> **Lifestyle, Cultural and Occupational Factors**
> **Physical Activity**
> **Obesity-Related Disease**
> **Psychosocial and Psychiatric Disorders**
> **Previous Surgical History**
> **Allergies**
> **Review of Systems**

Historical Survey of Weight Gain and Loss

This section allows the provider to gain insight into the patient's personal burden of obesity over his/her lifetime. The historical survey chart in Table 9.1 below is a useful tool as it provides a visual timeline of the patient's personal journey to obesity and may highlight the patient's "triggers" for weight gain and weight loss.

It is important for the medical practitioner to solicit from and make notes of additional comments or pertinent explanations offered by the patient that will render the historical survey even more helpful in the treatment of the patient. There are usually specific triggers to eating high calorie, high sugar, and fat foods that need to be elicited during this part of the history.

Family History of Obesity and Related Disease

Key insights are gained from the patient's family history. It allows the medical practitioner to understand how many generations of family members have been affected by obesity and what obesity-related diseases they may have suffered. It also provides insight into possible motivations the patient may have to change his/her lifestyle. For example, one profound risk factor is whether the patient's mother experienced gestational diabetes. This should be discussed with the patient because the presence of gestational diabetes means the patient may be genetically predisposed to early chronic disease, and particularly diabetes. It should also be determined whether the patient's father had diabetes at time of conception, as that may be a risk factor, as well. The family history of obesity and related disease charts in Tables 9.2 and 9.3 are helpful tools to make sure all areas are covered.

Medications

Obtaining a complete history of medication/vitamin/supplement use is essential to the assessment of the overweight or obese patient. Every practitioner should be

Table 9.1 Individual historical survey of weight gain and loss

	Age	Weight	Trigger
Birth weight			
After undergoing puberty			
High school graduation			
Marriage			
Divorce			
Lowest weight in past 5 years			
Highest weight in past 5 years			

Adapted from RP Blackstone patient intake questionnaire

The Health History

Table 9.2 Family histories of obesity and related disease

	Living (circle one)		Current age (if living)	Deceased at age	Illness/cause of death		
Overweight/obese							
Mother	Yes	No				Yes	No
Father	Yes	No				Yes	No
Maternal grandmother	Yes	No				Yes	No
Maternal grandfather	Yes	No				Yes	No
Paternal grandmother	Yes	No				Yes	No
Paternal grandfather	Yes	No				Yes	No
Sibling	Yes	No				Yes	No
Sibling	Yes	No				Yes	No
Sibling	Yes	No				Yes	No
Sibling	Yes	No				Yes	No

Adapted from RP Blackstone patient intake questionnaire

Table 9.3 Medical conditions in close family members

Did your mother or father have type 2 diabetes? Y N		
Did your mother have gestational or type 2 diabetes during her pregnancy? Y N		
Was your father already diabetic when you were conceived? Y N		
Please circle medical conditions that have affected a close family member including your father, mother, grandparent, or siblings		
High blood pressure	Obesity	Colon cancer
High blood cholesterol	Diabetes	Breast cancer
Bleeding tendency	Heart disease	Kidney disease

Adapted from RP Blackstone patient intake questionnaire

aware of the possibility that a patient may be on medications for obesity-related disease that actually *cause* weight gain or hinder the patient's ability to lose weight. A change in medication to one that does not promote weight gain, made in consultation with the primary care physician (PCP), can beneficially impact both the education of the PCP as well as the weight of the patient. As patients experience weight loss or gain their need for certain medications may change and/or the doses of those medications may need to be adjusted. Thus, it is crucial to maintain an accurate list of current medications for each patient. *Encourage or require that patients bring a current written list of medications with them to every appointment to ensure that an accurate record is maintained.*

In addition, it is critical to know whether a patient has used specific weight loss medication and the result of that usage. Different weight loss medications have different mechanisms of action. Knowing what worked or did not work may give the provider information about how the individual patient's physiology responds to different mechanisms of medications (Table 9.4).

Table 9.4 Weight loss medication histories

	Date(s)	Check if medically supervised	Total duration (months)	Maximum weight loss
Phentermine (Adipex, Ionamin) Phendimetrizine, Diethylpropion (Tepanil)				
Zonisamide				
Topamax/Topiramate				
Bontril/Phendimetrazine				
Tenuate (Amfepramone)				
Orlistat (Alli/Xenical)				
Bupropion (Amfebutamone)				
Metformin				
Exenatide (Byetta, Bydureon) Liraglutide (Victoza)				
Lorcaserin (Belviq)				
Naltrexone				
Phentermine + Topiramate				
Bupropion + Naltrexone (Contrave/NB32)				
Empatic				
HcG *Circle one: shots or oral*				
B12 Injections				
Over-the-counter *Such as SlimShots, Stacker, Cortislim, Xenadrine, Hydroxycut*				

Adapted from RP Blackstone patient intake questionnaire

Patients often decide on their own to supplement their normal diet with vitamins or take other over-the-counter medications/supplements to augment weight loss. Many of the vitamins or supplements commonly taken have not been scientifically proven to be beneficial. In fact, they may trigger drug interactions that are harmful or may in some other way be unhealthy or dangerous.

Diet pills, weight loss supplements, and workout supplements from both foreign and domestic sources are readily available over-the-counter or online. These untested supplements can contain potentially dangerous and unexpected substances, including phenolphthalein, amphetamines, steroids, the compound DNP, antianxiety medication, antidepressants, and stimulants. Two popular supplements are human chorionic gonadotropin (HCG) and human growth hormone (HGH). Both are available on line and through physician offices. One example of the risk of using these types of products that derive from the tissue of human beings arises out of the time when HGH was used historically in medicine to treat short stature. HGH was obtained at that time from cadavers infected with prions. The infection was transmitted to the patients treated with HGH thereby increasing the patient's risk of Creutzfeldt-Jakob Disease (CJD), a fatal neurological disease. There is evidence that the use of HGH is still creating problems years after the practice of obtaining HGH from cadavers was discontinued [2].

Asking questions of patients about vitamin and supplement use not only establishes the patient's reasons for taking the supplements and the source of the supplements, but it also increases the opportunity for the provider to direct the patient to evidence-based vitamins and supplements that have been proven to be scientifically effective.

Dietary History

One patient behavior that may be open to change is the patient's dietary habits. Often a person who is gaining weight has little idea of the value of their food choices not only from the standpoint of how many calories the food contains or the nutrient makeup of that food, but also how the body breaks that food down and uses it to send messages to the brain about whether to burn or store what has been eaten. Asking questions and understanding a patient's level of knowledge about food is necessary in order to achieve meaningful change. Having a patient complete the personal eating habits survey can help start the conversation. Patients should also be asked about any commercial diet programs they have tried and whether/how they track calories consumed and energy expended (Table 9.5).

Many patients have participated in commercial weight loss programs or are using electronic devices to keep track of food and exercise. A survey of these programs will help the provider understand the level of concern the patient has had about his/her about weight as the patient has invested time and money in participating in these programs (Tables 9.6 and 9.7).

Stress Factors

Stress is a trigger for the release of the stress hormones norepinephrine and dopamine. Chronic stress causes these hormones to stimulate the release of cortisol as well as mobilize fat stores for additional energy. Chronic stress is now counted as a risk factor for obesity and contributes to the development of insulin resistance and obesity-related disease. A stress assessment can be made in clinical practice by having the patient fill out a screening questionnaire that provides a basis for engaging the patient in a discussion of his/her significant stressors and helps guide a strategy around stress. That strategy may include a referral for further testing and assessment by a trained psychologist [3] (Table 9.8).

Table 9.5 Personal eating habits survey

Who is responsible for grocery shopping?
What grocery items are regularly purchased?
Who does the majority of the cooking?
How many times per week do you eat out?
Is your home cooked food of a particular ethnic influence? (Please circle)
Latino Middle Eastern East Indian Kosher Asian African Other_____
Do you get food through WICK or food assistance? Y N
Do you eat breakfast every day? Y N
When do you eat most of your food? Breakfast Lunch Dinner
Do you snack during the day? Y N
If you do snack what is your favorite treat? _____
Are you a "fast" eater or a "slow" eater? (Please circle)
What feelings or events trigger episodes of overeating? (Circle all that apply)
Depression, feeling down Celebration/happiness Feeling very hungry Boredom
Sports/social events Loss of control Social/habit Family culture
How to you feel about eating genetically modified foods?
How often do you eat processed food? Everyday Seldom Rarely Never (Please circle)
Do you buy your fruits and vegetables at a farmers market? Y N
Do you eat "organic" foods? Y N
How many times per week do you eat away from home? _____
What meals do you typically eat away from home? _____
When you eat out, where do you usually go/what do you order? _____
Do you generally have "seconds"? Y N
Do you generally have dessert? Y N
Do you smoke cigarettes? Y N How many a day? _____ Are you willing to quit? Y N
Do you drink alcohol? Y N How many times per week? _____
How many glasses per day (wine) or beers? _____
Do you drink "hard" alcohol? Y N How many drinks per day? _____
Do you get fancy coffee drinks in the morning? Y N What is your favorite? _____
Do you drink sugar-sweetened beverages like soda or sport drinks? Y N
What type? _____ How many servings a day? _____ Size? _____
Do you drink diet drinks? How often?

Table 9.6 Use of commercial weight loss programs and outcomes

			Date(s)	Check if medically supervised	Duration in months	Maximum weight loss	Do you have records of this effort?
Jenny Craig	Yes	No					
Nutri-systems	Yes	No					
Weight watchers	Yes	No					
Opti/medi fast	Yes	No					
Very low calorie diet	Yes	No					
Meal replacements	Yes	No					
Other	Yes	No					

Adapted from RP Blackstone patient intake questionnaire

Table 9.7 Use of a personal fitness tracking device

			When did you get it?	Do you enter food you eat?	Do you enter exercise?	Have you lost weight?	Would you like to join a group?
Fitbit	Yes	No					
Apple watch (or other smart watch)	Yes	No					
Jawbone	Yes	No					
Garmin	Yes	No					
Other_____	Yes	No					

Adapted from RP Blackstone patient intake questionnaire

Table 9.8 Stress screening survey

Circle all that apply
Marital status: Single_____Married_____Divorced_____Separated_____Widowed_____ Have you been hospitalized in the last year? Y N Have you been hospitalized for more than 7 days in your lifetime? Y N Do you drink coffee or tea? Y N Did any of the following happen to you in the last year? Y N Death of a family member or a very close friend Y N Separation from spouse or long-time partner Y N Recent change of job Y N Moving within the same city Y N Moving to another city Y N Financial difficulties Y N Legal problems Y N Beginning of a new relationship
How many hours do you work per week? _____ Y N Are you satisfied with your work? Y N Do you feel under pressure at work? Y N Do you get along with your colleagues at work? Y N Do you get along with your spouse or partner? Y N Do you get along with other relatives? Y N Has any close relative been seriously ill in the past year? Y N Do you feel tension at home? Y N Do you live by yourself? Y N Do you feel lonely? Y N Do you have anyone whom you can trust and confide in? Y N Do you get along well with people? Y N Do you often feel overwhelmed by the demands of every day life? Y N Do you often feel you cannot make it? Y N Do you tend to be influenced by people with strong opinions? Y N Do you tend to worry about what other people think of you? Y N Do you have stomach or bowel pains? Y N Does your heart beat quickly or strongly without a reason? Y N Do you have feelings of dizziness or fainting? Y N Do you have feelings of pressure or tightness in your head or body? Y N Do you have difficulty breathing or feel you cannot get enough air? Y N Do you feel tired and lack energy?

(continued)

Table 9.8 (continued)

Y N	Are you irritable?
Y N	Do you feel sad or depressed?
Y N	Do you feel tense or "wound up"?
Y N	Have you lost interest in most things?
Y N	Do you get "panic" attacks?
Y N	Do you believe you have a physical disease but doctors have not diagnosed it correctly?
Y N	When you read or hear about an illness, do you get similar symptoms?
How do you rate the quality of your life? Excellent/Good/Fair/Poor/Awful	

Circadian Patterns

Circadian rhythms are based upon 24-h intervals and are affected by light and darkness. These rhythms send essential signals that tell our bodies when to sleep and they regulate many body systems including those that control metabolism and eating behavior. Disruption of the circadian rhythm can cause disorders as diverse as dementia, cardiovascular disease, obesity, and cancer. Researchers have identified certain genes that direct circadian rhythms in people, as well as fruit flies, mice, fungi, and other organisms used for genetic studies. Medical practitioners should survey their patients' habits relating to circadian rhythms to determine if a disruption may be contributing to obesity.

The International Classification of Diseases (ICD-10-CM, 2014) lists six subtypes of circadian rhythm sleep disorder, each of which have certain characteristics: (1) delayed sleep phase type; (2) free-running type; (3) advanced sleep phase type; (4) irregular sleep–wake type; (5) shift work type; and (6) jet lag type.

The diagnosis of circadian rhythm disorder is challenging and often requires the assistance of a sleep specialist. It is also important to exclude other sleep disorders that often mimic circadian rhythm disorder. There are tests that can be used to help determine if a circadian rhythm order exists and what type it is. Patients can also be encouraged to keep sleep logs or diaries, undergo sleep studies, complete the Epworth Sleepiness Scale Questionnaire or the Stop Bang Questionnaire, and use a wrist monitor to measure sleep–wake cycles. Treatment options may include behavior therapy to advance or delay sleep, medications such as melatonin or short term sleep aids, bright light therapy done in a controlled environment, or chronotherapy to shift the sleep cycle over time. The energy level survey in Table 9.9 along with the questionnaire contained in the following section on disordered sleep may provide additional patient information for the medical practitioner.

Disordered Sleep Analysis

Patients with obesity often have disordered sleep. This covers a range of problems that include insomnia, obstructive sleep apnea, restless leg syndrome, and others.

Table 9.9 Energy level and circadian rhythm survey

Energy level survey
What is your energy level in the morning: very low, low, moderate, high, very high
What is your energy level in the evening: very low, low, moderate, high, very high
What hours of the day do you usually: go to bed____fall asleep_____wake up_____
Do you work the afternoon or evening shift at work?
Does your job require you to shift from days to nights?
Do you consider yourself a "morning person" or a "night owl?"
What hours of the day/night do you feel most alert and most productive?
Adapted from RP Blackstone patient intake questionnaire

Obstructive Sleep Apnea

Patients with obesity should always be screened for obstructive sleep apnea (OSA) as it has implications for the development of heart failure. Often these same patients have low oxygen tension during the night that affects their level of hypoxia and contributes to the tissue hypoxia that contributes to inflammation of white adipose tissue.

The questions outlined below help the medical provider to determine if the patient should be referred for a portable home monitoring test (no evidence of heart failure and the provider only suspects OSA) or to a formal polysomnogram test performed in a sleep lab. The diagnosis of OSA is an Apnea Hypopnea Index (AHI) ≥ 15 without signs of arousal or ≥ 5 with signs of arousal.

The etiology of obstructive sleep apnea in patients who are obese is due to partial or complete obstruction of the upper airway. OSA is an independent risk factor for systemic hypertension, coronary artery disease, stroke and hyperglycemia and may lead to endothelial dysfunction [4]. Clinical features of OSA are not sufficient for diagnosis and require a sleep study.

Sleep plays a major role in overweight and obesity. The questions found in Table 9.10 should be asked of every patient who is overweight or obese. The Epworth Sleepiness Scale Questionnaire and the Stop Bang Sleep Apnea Questionnaire should also be administered. These questionnaires can be found online.

Lifestyle, Cultural, and Occupational Factors

Lifestyle, family culture, and occupation influence when and how the patient uses food or participates in exercise. Understanding a patient's family food culture may help the provider and patient to discuss family expectations relating to food and how to change those expectations, if necessary. Network theory has shown that obesity tends to cluster in groups and no group has a stronger influence than the family.

Most people develop a culture around food that governs their timing of meals, speed of eating and their food choices. In some ethnic groups there are very strong

Table 9.10 Disordered sleep survey

How much sleep do you get each night on average?
4–5 h   6–8 h   More than 8 h
Do you have restless sleep? Y N
Does it take a long time to fall asleep? Y N How long on average? _____
Do you wake up early and have trouble falling back asleep? Y N
Do you feel tired when you wake up in the morning? Y N
What is your sleep environment like?
Dark room: Y N   Sleep with dogs: Y N   Sleep with a disruptive partner: Y N   Quiet room: Y N
Do you have insomnia? Y N
Do you take any sleep aid medications? Y N Type_____
Do you snore at night? Y N If yes: Always   Intermittently   Never
Has your sleep partner ever told you that you stop breathing while you are sleeping? Y N

Adapted from RP Blackstone patient intake questionnaire

tendencies to enforce eating or overeating as a sign of affluence or love. The well-meaning wife, husband or mother often sabotages the individual's efforts by trying to feed their loved ones, even when they state they are trying to lose weight or are no longer hungry. The rituals of family and societal culture often revolve around food. Common societal events involving food include football games or other sporting events, holidays, birthdays, weddings, funerals, vacations, parties, and other celebrations. It is important to obtain a patient's history with respect to cultural/societal events in order to understand the influence they have on the patient's weight.

Occupational factors can also affect a patient's weight. Many office work environments, including doctors' and nurses' lounges, are notorious for having significant amounts of unhealthy food available on a regular basis, and much of the food is sugar, fat and carbohydrate based. Shift work can also contribute to overweight through disruption of regular eating habits. The culture of routinely "eating out" with coworkers or eating snacks at one's desk or while on break all influence the amount of calories blindly consumed.

Use of alcohol, tobacco, and drugs may also be part of the patient's culture around food and exercise. Discussing and discovering patterns of a patient's use of alcohol is important, especially if the patient intends to undergo bariatric surgery. Bariatric surgery alters alcohol metabolism and can lead to alcohol overuse and physical addiction. Additional inquiries should be made about the use of tobacco and other drugs including those used for enhancing athletic performance (Table 9.11).

Physical Activity

Every patient should undergo a physical activity assessment. Lack of physical activity has been linked to higher mortality from chronic disease, including obesity. The options for exercise for patients with obesity are more limited than the options for a normal weight person. The patient who is obese is less mobile, less tolerant of physical exertion, and less healthy overall. Before starting any exercise program the

The Health History

Table 9.11 Culture and social history

Family culture
Describe the culture of your family around food: _____
What kind of food is part of your family culture and regularly consumed:
How does your family celebrate holidays or important occasions: _____
Do you ever feel pressure to eat more food than you want/should eat? Y N
Do you ever feel pressure to eat fattening or unhealthy food? Y N
Use of alcohol
Do you use alcohol? Y N How many days per week?
How many drinks per day?
Do you ever feel the need to cut down on drinking alcohol? Y N
Do you ever feel annoyed by criticism of your drinking alcohol? Y N
Do you ever have guilty feelings with regard to drinking alcohol? Y N
Do you ever take/have a "morning eye opener"? Y N
Use of tobacco
Do you use tobacco? Y N Number of cigarettes/packs per day? _____
Are you willing to quit?
Use of supplements for athletic performance enhancement?
Have you ever taken substances to enhance athletic performance?
What kinds of supplements did you take?
Have you ever used or are currently using the following substances? Marijuana Cocaine
Crack methamphetamines inhalants stimulants hallucinogens heroin

Adapted from RP Blackstone patient intake questionnaire
The questions with bold shading are part of the CAGE questionnaire [6], reprinted with permission

patient who is overweight or obese should be medically screened to determine if exercise is even advisable, and to what degree. An evaluation by physical therapy and/or physical medicine and rehabilitation can be valuable in ensuring the patient begins to engage in safe exercise practices. The physical assessment should focus not on the patient's weight but rather on the patient's function and ability to be mobile. Objective strength, balance and flexibility are the focus, not weight loss. Low impact exercise options are ideal for patients who have significant musculoskeletal stress such as those patients with extreme obesity. Low impact options include swimming, walking, or riding a stationary bicycle. A survey of the patient's past and current exercise habits are helpful to establish the view the patient has of themselves and their capabilities and commitment in regards to exercise. Often the vision the patient has of himself is more historical than current. Knowledge of this allows the medical practitioner to gently orient the patient to their current situation (Table 9.12).

Obesity-Related Disease

Correctly assessing a patient who is overweight or obese for obesity-related disease is essential. Patients often do not realize they are at risk for obesity-related disease until it is too late. The medical practitioner should assess the patient for

Table 9.12 Physical activity and exercise survey

Were you an athlete in high school or college? Yes No
What was your sport? _____

How many minutes of exercise do you get every week?
30 min   60 min   120 min   180 min   Other: _____

What level of exercise do you do? Circle one:
Mild (i.e., walking on flat surface)
Moderate (i.e., house work/gardening)
Intense (i.e., running/cycling/swimming)

When you walk, what is your usual pace of walking? Circle one:
Casual (<2 mph)   Normal (2, 3 mph)   Fairly brisk (3–4 mph)   Brisk or striding (>4 mph)

Is there any opportunity to increase physical activity at work?
How does your work impact your ability to exercise?

How many flights of stairs do you climb each day?
Do you lift weight? Y N   How many times per week?

What form of exercise do you most enjoy?
Walking   Spinning   Yoga   Running   Swimming   Hiking   Cycling   Dancing   Other _____

What is the best time of day for you to exercise? _____
What are the barriers you have to doing exercise?
Do you have physical limitations that prevent exercising? Y N
Explain: _____

How many times per week are you willing to commit to exercise?
Explain how you think exercise impacts your weight: _____

Adapted from: RP Blackstone patient intake questionnaire

musculoskeletal disease, high cholesterol, hypertension, heart disease, non-alcoholic fatty liver disease (NAFLD), insulin resistance, prediabetes and diabetes, polycystic ovarian syndrome, pulmonary disease, gastrointestinal disease, urinary stress incontinence, endocrine disorders and cancer, all of which are described in more detail below.

Musculoskeletal Disease

Patients who are overweight or obese will often present with joint pain and overall body aches. These are often the first physical symptoms they notice. It affects their ability to exercise and contributes to further weight gain. Obtaining a history of orthopedic disease/symptoms can help assess the patient's risk for musculoskeletal disease (Table 9.13).

It is helpful to educate patients at the same time you are taking their history. This can be accomplished by grouping together all the risk factors that impact certain diseases and discussing those factors with the patient. For example, discussing with the overweight or obese patient the risk for cardiovascular disease will include a discussion of several risk factors, including high cholesterol, hypertension, heart disease, NAFLD, insulin resistance and diabetes.

High Cholesterol

Often the first sign of high cholesterol is picked up in routine testing. The current guidelines for testing, finalized by the US Preventive Services Task Force, indicate

Table 9.13 History of musculoskeletal disease

Do you have pain in your joints or back? Y N Back pain: Neck   Thoracic spine   Lower back
Please indicate what joints are affected: Elbows R L   Shoulders R L   Hip R L   Knees R L   Ankles R L
Plantar Fasciitis? Y N Neuropathy of your feet? Y N How were you diagnosed? X-rays   MRI   Other: _____
Have you been treated for any these problems? Y N If yes, mark all that apply: Over the counter medication? Y N Type: _____ Prescription medication? Y N Type: _____ Physical therapy? Y N Joint replacement? Y N Specify which joint(s)_____ R L
Can you walk unassisted? Y N If not, do you use assistance? Cane: Y N   Walker: Y N   Wheelchair: Y N
Have you had any weight-related injuries? Y N Please describe: _____ Do you have any swelling in your legs? Y N

Adapted from RP Blackstone patient intake questionnaire

Table 9.14 History of high cholesterol and triglycerides

Specific questions for patients about cholesterol
Have you been diagnosed with high cholesterol? Y N
If so, what year were you diagnosed? _____
Do you have high triglycerides? Y N
If so, what year were you diagnosed? _____
When was the last time you were tested for high cholesterol?
Are you currently undergoing treatment?
If so, what type of treatment?

Adapted from RP Blackstone patient intake questionnaire

screening of men age 25–35 if they are at increased risk for coronary heart disease, and all men at 35 years and older. The Task Force recommends screening for women 20 years and older only if they are at increased risk for coronary heart disease (CHD).

Increased risk is defined as the presence of any ONE of the following risk factors: diabetes, previous personal history of CHD or non-coronary atherosclerosis, a family history of cardiovascular disease before age 50 in male relatives or age 60 in female relatives, tobacco use, or hypertension of obesity (BMI ≥ 30 kg/m^2).

(http://www.uspreventiveservicestaskforce.org/Page/Document/RecommendationStatementFinal/lipid-disorders-in-adults-cholesterol-dyslipidemia-screening#consider)

The primary assessment for the patient is to determine what risk they have for atherosclerotic cardiovascular disease (ASCVD) and to direct testing according to the guidelines. The preferred screening test is a fasting lipid panel. The 2013 recommendations are somewhat complex, including implementing statin therapy with LDL-C levels >190 mg/dl in specific populations.

Prevention recommendations include maintaining a healthy body weight, cessation of smoking, and control of hypertension and diabetes when present [6] (Table 9.14).

Hypertension

High blood pressure most often is asymptomatic and detected only by measurement. Generally, physical symptoms like facial flushing, dizziness, blood spots in the eyes and nosebleeds are not indicative of high blood pressure unless the patient is in hypertensive crisis, i.e., systolic blood pressure of 180 or higher and diastolic blood pressure of 110 or higher. In the case of hypertensive crisis, severe anxiety, shortness of breath, nosebleed, and severe headache may be experienced.

If a patient has already been diagnosed with hypertension the relevant issue is whether the condition is under adequate control on the medications they are taking. It is important to determine if they are on rate control medications as it may have implications for exercise regimens and for the timing of a bariatric surgery procedure.

Heart Disease

Cardiovascular disease is an indication of end stage disease. The primary types include atherosclerosis of carotid arteries or coronary arteries, peripheral vascular disease, cardiomyopathy, arrhythmias and heart failure. The presence of metabolic syndrome (MetS) is also linked to the development of CVD. A leptin level reading may give you an indication of the risk the patient has for heart disease. Leptin levels have recently been suggested as a component to be used to improve the specificity of a metabolic syndrome (MetS) diagnosis.

Non-alcoholic Fatty Liver Disease (NAFLD), Insulin Resistance (IR), Intermediate Diabetes (ID) and Type 2 Diabetes Mellitus (T2DM)

Every medical practitioner treating patients who are overweight or obese needs to be aware of the risk of liver disease in patients with obesity. The incidence of NAFLD in patients with BMI 30–39 kg/m^2 is 65 % versus 15 % in the non-obese. This incidence increases to 85 % in patients with a BMI of 40 kg/m^2 and above. With respect to non-alcoholic steatohepatitis (NASH), which is a more severe form of NAFLD, research shows the incidence is 3 % in the non-obese, 20 % in BMI 30–39 kg/m^2, and 40 % in BMI 40 kg/m^2 and above [8]. The tipping point into cirrhosis seems to be marked by the development of fibrosis and is associated with intestinal dysbiosis with translocation of bacteria to the liver. *Significantly, weight loss generally reverses the ongoing liver damage if fibrosis is not advanced.* Suspicion and confirmation of NAFLD can be based on BMI, signs of insulin resistance, liver function/liver enzyme tests, imaging procedures including ultrasound CT scan, MRI, and/or liver biopsy.

Suspicion of insulin resistance (IR) should be based on body mass index and signs of insulin resistance like acanthosis nigricans. Confirmation with liver function testing and fasting insulin levels should also be used if suspicion is high. The overweight/obese patient should be educated and informed that a 20–30 lb weight gain plus the development of insulin resistance presents a significant risk factor for developing chronic obesity-related diseases (Table 9.15).

The staging and management of NAFLD is a complex topic best summarized by Rinella in Table 9.16 below [9].

Polycystic Ovarian Syndrome

The diagnosis of polycystic ovarian syndrome (PCOS) is based on the Rotterdam criteria, meaning the presence of two of three criteria: androgen excess (noted by hirsutism/acne unresponsive to topical agents), ovulatory dysfunction indicated by menstrual irregularities indicating anovulation, and polycystic ovaries. PCOS is often first noticed due to the effect on fertility, however we increasingly think of it as a cardio metabolic problem that indicates IR, dysregulation of the sympathetic

Table 9.15 Personal history of non-alcoholic fatty liver disease (NAFLD), insulin resistance (IR), intermediate diabetes (ID), and type 2 diabetes mellitus (T2DM)

Have you ever been told you have any of the following?
An elevation of liver function? Y N
An elevated insulin level? Y N
Have you ever been told that you had "prediabetes"? Y N
Have you been diagnosed with type 2 diabetes? Y N or type 1 diabetes? Y N
How was the diagnosis of diabetes confirmed?
Fasting blood glucose?
Hemoglobin A1c?
Glucose tolerance test?
Did you have gestational diabetes during pregnancy?
Do you have complications of diabetes? Neuropathy   Kidney disease   Vascular disease

Adapted from RP Blackstone patient intake questionnaire

Table 9.16 Diagnosis, monitoring and management considerations for non-alcoholic fatty liver disease (NAFLD)

	NAFLD disease stage		
	Non-alcoholic Steatohepatitis with fibrosis		
	Stages 0–1[a]	Stages 2–3[b]	Isolated hepatic steatosis
Evaluate clinical evidence	Development of worsening of metabolic diseases	For features of cirrhosis: development or worsening of metabolic diseases	Development or worsening of metabolic diseases
Monitor laboratory evidence of disease progression	Monitor liver chemistry test results; screen for dyslipidemia and diabetes	Monitor liver chemistry test results; screen for dyslipidemia and diabetes; laboratory features of advanced disease: ratio of AST to ALT >1; low platelet count; increased INR and bilirubin or lower albumin	Monitor liver chemistry test results; screen for dyslipidemia and diabetes
Management considerations			
Liver-directed therapy	Consider treatment with pioglitazone or vitamin E; consider eligibility for a clinical trial	Consider treatment with pioglitazone or vitamin E; consider eligibility for a clinical trial	No proven benefit
Other	Manage comorbidities; including behavioral and weight loss therapy; consider bariatric surgery if appropriate	Manage comorbidities; including behavioral and weight loss therapy; consider bariatric surgery if appropriate	Manage comorbidities; including behavioral and weight loss therapy; consider bariatric surgery if appropriate

[a]Indicates early or no fibrosis
[b]Indicates moderate to severe fibrosis (precirrhosis)
ALT alanine aminotransferase; *AST* aspartate aminotransferase; *INR* international normalized ratio
Adapted from Rinella [9] with permission

nervous system and a state of chronic inflammation. PCOS may also be the early warning signal of a person at risk for MetS in later life.

When other causes are excluded and PCOS is suspected, the patient should be screened with an 8 am free testosterone level. If testosterone levels are increased, then other etiologies for androgen excess should be explored prior to diagnosing PCOS, if normal PCOS is unlikely. There are several baseline screenings to evaluate women suspected of having PCOS, including: thyroid function tests, serum prolactin levels, total and free testosterone levels, free androgen index, serum hCG level, cosyntropin stimulation test, serum 17-OHPG level, urinary free cortisol and creatine levels, low dose dexamethasone suppression test and serum insulin like growth factor level. In addition, ovarian ultrasound using the transvaginal approach and a pelvic CT scan or MRI may be useful [10].

Pulmonary Disease

Asthma and reactive airways disease often complicate recommendations for exercise and other aspects of health. The questions outlined below can help establish a patient's history of breathing issues and/or asthma (Table 9.17).

Pulmonary hypertension is a disease that is often extremely difficult to diagnose until late stages because the initial signs and symptoms are not distinguishable from many complaints for other reasons. Women are usually more symptomatic than men. The most common presentation is dyspnea (60 %), weakness (19 %), and recurrent syncope (13 %). In addition, patients may complain of fatigue and lethargy, anorexia, chest pain and right upper quadrant pain. Awareness that pulmonary hypertension could be present, especially in the patient with untreated sleep apnea, may prompt a more comprehensive evaluation by a specialist.

Gastrointestinal Disease

Patients who are overweight or obese often have associated gastrointestinal disease. Obesity is associated with 1.5-to 2-fold increase in the risk of gastroesophageal

Table 9.17 History of pulmonary disease

Do you ever have trouble breathing? Y N
Do you find yourself out of breath as a result of regular daily activities? Y N
Have you been diagnosed with asthma or reactive airways disease? Y N
How old were you when you were diagnosed? _____
Are you on daily medications for asthma? Y N If yes, what medication? _____
Are you on inhalers for asthma? Y N
How many emergency room or hospital admissions have you had for asthma over the last five years? _____
Have you ever been given steroids for a cold, bronchitis, or asthma attack? Y N
Adapted from RP Blackstone patient intake questionnaire

reflux disease (GERD and erosive esophagitis) and a 2–2.5-fold increase in the risk of esophageal adenocarcinoma [11] (Tables 9.18 and 9.19).

Urinary Stress Incontinence

Urinary stress incontinence (UI) is a problem affecting over 50 % of middle-aged and older women. In women with obesity there is a 20–70 % increase in incontinence with every 5-unit increase in BMI, documented with an incidence of 11 % per year [13]. The theoretical cause of UI is increased abdominal pressure causing an increase in bladder pressure and overactive bladder. Many women with incontinence also have a history of pregnancy that may be an initial cause of weakening

Table 9.18 The GERD questionnaire

Total score 0–2 point = 0 % likelihood of GERD 3–7 points = 50 % likelihood of GERD 8–10 points = 79 % likelihood of GERD 11–18 points = 89 % likelihood	How many times does this occur this week			
Symptom	0 days	1 day	2 or 3 days	4–7 days
Burning feeling behind the breastbone (heartburn)	0	1	2	3
Stomach contents moving up to the throat or mouth (regurgitation)	0	1	2	3
Pain in the middle of the upper stomach area	3	2	1	0
Nausea	3	2	1	0
Trouble getting a good night's sleep because of heartburn or regurgitation	0	1	2	3
Need for over-the-counter medicine for heartburn or regurgitation (such as Tums, Rolaids, Maalox, or other antacids), in addition to the medicine your doctor prescribed	0	1	2	3

Adapted from Jones et al. [12] with permission

Table 9.19 Supplemental questions to GERD questionnaire

Additional questions
Have you had an EGD (esophagogastroduodenoscopy)?
Have you been tested for Helicobacter pylori?
Have you been treated for H. pylori?
Have you been told you have a hiatal hernia?
Have you ever been told you had Barrett's esophagitis?
Have you ever been diagnosed with hepatitis?
What type of hepatitis did you have? A B C D E

Adapted from RP Blackstone patient intake questionnaire

Table 9.20 The questionnaire for female urinary incontinence diagnosis (QUID)

	None of the time	Rarely	Once in awhile	Most of the time	All of the time
Do you leak urine (even small drops), wet yourself, or wet your pads or undergarments					
1. When you cough or sneeze?	☐	☐	☐	☐	☐
2. When you bend down or lift something up?	☐	☐	☐	☐	☐
3. When you walk quickly, jog, or exercise?	☐	☐	☐	☐	☐
4. While you are undressing in order to use the toilet?	☐	☐	☐	☐	☐
5. Do you get such a strong and uncomfortable need to urinate that you leak urine (even small drops) or wet yourself before reaching the toilet?	☐	☐	☐	☐	☐
6. Do you have to rush to the bathroom because you get a sudden, strong need to urinate?	☐	☐	☐	☐	☐

Scoring each item scores *0* none of the time, *1* rarely, *2* once in awhile, *3* often, *4* most of the time or *5* all of the time. Responses to items *1*, *2* and *3* are summed for the stress score; and responses to items *4*, *5*, and *6* are summed for the urge score

Adapted from Bradley et al. [14], with permission

of pelvic floor structures. Obesity exacerbates all these mechanical factors. Women with visceral adiposity may be more affected.

Table 9.20 validated questionnaire helps distinguish stress urinary incontinence from urge urinary incontinence or a mixed disorder [14].

Endocrine Disorders

Thyroid disorders and Vitamin D deficiency is common in patients with a BMI >30 kg/m^2.

Vitamin D deficiency is usually asymptomatic but may also present with fatigue, bone pain and muscle weakness. The screening test is a 25 hydroxy-vitamin D blood level. Many patients believe that a dysfunctional thyroid is the cause of their weight gain but that explanation is not always a factor. On the other hand, if the patient does have hypothyroidism it can contribute to weight gain or difficulty losing weight. The signs of hypothyroidism can be elicited by asking specific questions (Table 9.21).

Cancer

Most people do not think of obesity and cancer as being related. However, obesity is among the top two related risk factors for cancer. The publication of a survey of

Table 9.21 Endocrine disorder survey

Please circle any of the following symptoms if they apply to you
Fatigue
Increased sensitivity to cold
Constipation
Dry skin
Unexplained weight gain
Puffy face
Hoarseness
Muscle weakness
Muscle aches, tenderness and stiffness
Pain, stiffness or swelling in your joints
Heavier than normal or irregular menstrual cycles
Thinning hair
Slowed heart rate
Impaired memory

Adapted from RP Blackstone patient intake questionnaire

mortality from obesity-related cancers ranging from prostate cancer to liver cancer was published in 2003, prompting an increased interest in this relationship.

The primary driver of cancer recurrence is obesity. Multiple intra and extra cellular signaling events have been documented and the crown structures noted in fatty liver tissue are also seen in cancer recurrence. The challenge of cancer in the patient with obesity is threefold. First, cancer is more likely to be diagnosed later in a person with obesity due to the fact that symptoms or signs are often discounted as being related to obesity rather than raising the suspicion of cancer as it might in people who are lean. In addition, people who are obese often suffer physical discomfort and anxiety in having to undergo preventative testing and consequently postpone testing or choose not to go. Second, the same treatments for cancer may not be practical or even attainable due to the physical size of the patient. Third, dosing of chemotherapeutic medications has to be carefully matched to body size and body fat percent in order to achieve therapeutic doses. Even in patients dosed correctly the endothelial dysfunction results in less blood flow to the affected area, meaning the chemotherapy cannot reach its target as easily as it does in a person who is lean. Body fat is now being taken into account in dosing chemotherapy of lipophilic agents.

The three cancers that correlate most strongly with obesity in women are breast cancer, endometrial cancer and colon cancer. In men who are obese the highest correlation is with colon cancer, malignant melanoma and pancreatic cancer. Questions concerning basic preventative testing should be asked of all patients who are overweight or obese (Table 9.22). Practioners should ensure that basic screening tests are conducted.

Table 9.22 Survey of health maintenance

Women
When was your last mammogram? Was it normal?
When was your last Pap Smear? Was it normal?
Have you ever had a colonoscopy?
Men
Have you had a prostate exam?
Have you ever had a colonoscopy?

Adapted from RP Blackstone patient intake questionnaire

Idiopathic Intracranial Hypertension

The most common presentation of idiopathic intracranial hypertension (IIH) (formerly Pseudotumor Cerebri) is headache, transient visual disturbances, and sixth nerve palsy. Patients presenting with a BMI >25 kg/m^2 and headache should undergo a screening optic fundus examination.

Pregnancy, Infertility and Low Testosterone

Many women of reproductive age experience infertility. With even modest weight loss they often recover ovulatory function and normal menstrual cycles. Men with obesity often have low testosterone attributed to inflammatory cytokines. Testing and repletion of testosterone helps facilitate weight loss. Weight loss itself often improves the testosterone level (Table 9.23).

Table 9.23 Pregnancy, infertility and low testosterone

Infertility
Do you consider yourself infertile? Y N
Have you undergone any treatment for infertility? Y N
Age at first menstrual period? Date of last period:
Pregnancy
Total # of pregnancies? _____ # of live births? _____ # of miscarriages/abortions? _____
Did you have type 2 diabetes before you became pregnant? Did the father of the baby have type 2 diabetes before you became pregnant?
While you were pregnant did you have:
Gestational Diabetes? Y N
Preeclampsia? Y N
Hypertension? Y N
Did your doctor put you at bed rest during your pregnancy? Y N
Did you have other obstetric complications? Y N What were they?
What were the birth weights of your children?
Hormone replacement therapy
Do you presently use birth control pills? Y N
Are you on hormonal replacement therapy? Y N
Have you ever been told you have a low testosterone level? Y N
Have you ever been tested for testosterone? Y N

Adapted from RP Blackstone patient intake questionnaire

Table 9.24 Most commonly used surveys in assessing patients with obesity

Beck depression inventory
Beck anxiety inventory
Questionnaire on eating and weight patterns—revised
Eating disorder examination questionnaire
Yale food addiction scale
Minnesota multiphasic personality inventory-2
Millon behavioral medicine diagnostic

Adapted from RP Blackstone patient intake questionnaire

Psychosocial and Psychiatric History

Behavioral aspects of a person's life may be affecting the ability of that person to lose weight or to understand why they have gained weight. These behavioral aspects include mood and anxiety disorders, including depression. They may also reflect frustration with self-efficacy in work or personal life. A variety of personal questions along with an assessment of the patient's use of alcohol, tobacco, and other drug use may provide deeper understanding of how behavioral aspects play a role in the patient's weight. In order to assess these aspects of behavioral health the use of surveys or inventories such as those listed below may be useful. The structured interview even without the use of the surveys and inventories may be invaluable (Table 9.24).

Patients may need to be referred to a psychologist for evaluation and testing for personality disorder, depression, anxiety, or food addiction, which may then allow a more targeted approach to the management of obesity. It is essential that the treating psychologist have credentials in treating patients with overweight and obesity [15–22] (Table 9.25).

Surgical History

Patients often experience multiple surgical procedures during their lifetime. A survey of those procedures, the kind of approaches used in the surgeries, and any complications may help explain some of the patient's current medical complaints (Table 9.26).

Allergies

It is important to document any known allergies the patient has to items commonly used for treatment. Patients with obesity are either on many medications or may need them, making allergic interactions important to identify (Table 9.27).

Table 9.25 Screening questions for pertinent psychosocial history

Screening questions psychosocial history—please circle all that apply	
Have you ever had?	
Y N	Suicide attempt
Y N	Family history of suicide
Y N	History of depression
Y N	History of bipolar disorder
Y N	History of anxiety or panic disorder
Y N	Obsessive compulsive disorder
Y N	A phobia or avoidance of specific things or situations?
Y N	Post traumatic stress disorder
Over the last two weeks have you experienced any of the following?	
Y N	Loss of interest in activities that you formerly enjoyed
Y N	Guilt worthlessness/helplessness/hopelessness
Y N	Reduced energy
Y N	Lack of concentration
Y N	Appetite disturbance increased or decreased
Y N	Agitation
Y N	Depressed mood
Y N	Death of close family member or friend
Abuse assessment:	
Y N	In the past year have you been hit, kicked, or physically hurt by another person?
Y N	Are you ever been in a relationship with someone who threatens or physically harms you?
Y N	Have you ever been forced to have sexual contact that you were not comfortable with?
Y N	Have you ever been abused? If yes, describe by whom, when, and how

Adapted from RP Blackstone patient intake questionnaire

Table 9.26 History of surgery in patient with obesity

Type of procedure	Date	Reason for surgery	Approach
Shunt for pseudotumor cerebri			
Thyroid surgery			
Parathyroid surgery			
Cardiac surgery			
Coronary artery bypass graft (CABG)			
Coronary artery stent			
Carotid artery surgery (carotid endarterectomy)			
Peripheral artery shunt			
Shunt for access for kidney dialysis			
Mastectomy or bilateral mastectomy			
Axillary lymph node dissection			
Liver biopsy			
Removal of the gallbladder			
Surgery on the stomach or intestines			

(continued)

Table 9.26 (continued)

Type of procedure	Date	Reason for surgery	Approach
Removal of a part of the colon (large intestine)			
Appendectomy			
Hysterectomy			
Oophorectomy			
Prostatectomy			
Carpal tunnel surgery			
Shoulder surgery			
Hip replacement R L			
Knee replacement R L			
Foot surgery R L			
Major car accident with intra-abdominal injuries			
Previous bariatric surgery procedure Adjustable gastric band Sleeve gastrectomy Gastric bypass Roux-en Y Vertical banded gastroplasty Other			

Adapted from RP Blackstone patient intake questionnaire

Table 9.27 History of allergic reactions

Allergy to	Name of medication (if known)	Reaction
PCN/sulfa		
Narcotic		
Latex		
Surgical tape		
Dye used in radiology procedures		

Adapted from RP Blackstone patient intake questionnaire

Review of Systems

A comprehensive review of systems (ROS) should be documented in each office visit. Use of a standard electronic health record (EHR) is sufficient to document ongoing problems the patient is experiencing.

Physical Assessment of Patients with Obesity and Related Diseases

Anthropometrics

Anthropometric measurements, taken at every office visit, should include *measured* height and weight, body fat percentile using a standing scale, and *measured* waist circumference. Do not rely on the patient's self-reporting for these measurements as it is somewhat unreliable. These measured health indicators should be used to complete a weight-related report card. A copy of the weight-related report card should be given to every patient at every visit (Table 9.28).

Pattern of Body Fat Distribution

The most dangerous location to carry fat is in the belly. This is called visceral adiposity. Subcutaneous fat distribution is a pattern associated with less risk of chronic disease, where the weight is carried in the buttocks and legs. It should be noted that when the subcutaneous fat depot in a patient is maximally utilized, the patient will begin to accumulate fat in the abdomen. Men and people of Asian and Indian descent usually carry much of their weight in their abdomen and very little in subcutaneous depots. Women generally store much of their fat in the subcutaneous depot.

Table 9.28 Weight-related health indicators™

		RANGE	POINTS	SCORE
BMI (Measured height and weight)		18.5 - 24.9	0	
		25.0 - 29.9	1	
		30.0 - 39.9	2	
		> 40	3	
Waist Circumference	Male	</=40 in	0	
		>/=40 in	1	
	Female	</=35 in	0	
		>/=35 in	1	
Body Fat %	Male	</=25	0	
		>/=25	1	
	Female	</=35	0	
		>/=35	1	
Health Report Card			Total Points	

Total Points	Health Report Card
0	Green
1	Green
2	Yellow
3	Orange
4	Red
5	Red +

The patient should be visibly assessed for the presence of Cushing's disease. Although fairly rare, the physical signs are recognizable and indicate further testing. Physical signs of Cushing's disease include: moon facies, dorsal adiposity, and central adiposity with peripheral wasting, proximal muscle weakness, and purple striae over the abdomen and shoulders. They can present with hypertension and laboratory testing will indicate glucose. The diagnosis is made definite by screening tests, including a 24-h urine free cortisol, low dose dexamethasone suppression test or a late night salivary cortisol test. Positive screening should be made on two occasions to verify a diagnosis.

A neck circumference greater than 17 inches for men and 16 inches for women increases the risk of obstructive sleep apnea (OSA) prompting the administration of the Epworth Sleepiness Score Questionnaire or the Stop Bang Questionnaire and other indicators of OSA to determine if formal sleep testing is required.

Vital Signs

It is important to note if the patient has tachycardia or bradycardia as these are not common findings in patients with obesity. Bradycardia may be a sign the patient is on a beta blocker or other heart rate control medication. Hypertension must be confirmed by taking the blood pressure with an *appropriate sized cuff*. Be sure to allow the patient with obesity to relax and rest before taking blood pressure readings as the physical effort of just getting all the way into the exam room can be stressful. You can create a set of vital signs that reflect the effort of movement. Patients with BMI 35 kg/m^2 may benefit from a pulse oximetry in addition to the standard set of vital signs in order to detect and document abnormalities in oxygenation.

General Observation

Observation of the patient often gives important clues as to the patient's self-regard via their dress and demeanor. In addition, visual observation may immediately reveal problems that affect the patient's health, such as breathlessness or edema of the lower extremities. It should also be noted whether the patient looks older or younger than their stated age. Visual observation can also be suggestive of more significant nutritional deficiencies or syndromic obesity syndrome.

Head, Eyes, Ears, Nose and Throat

Signs of various syndromes may be present on physical examination of the head, eyes, ears, nose and throat (HEENT). The signs of Prader Willi include a round face with narrow bitemporal diameter and almond shaped eyes. Prader Willi can go unrecognized until adulthood. Retinitis pigmentosa can be a sign of Laurence-Moon syndromic obesity. A large tongue can indicate Beckwidth-Weiderman.

Examination of the bilateral neck for lymphadenopathy and examination of the skin on the back of the neck for acanthosis nigricans may reveal either cancer or insulin resistance. The veins of the neck are examined for distension that may provide a sign of right heart or advanced left heart failure. Examination of the thyroid gland should be done to look for masses or asymmetry and to ensure the thyroid moves appropriately with swallowing. Carotid pulses should be exculpated and bruits ruled out. Neck range of motion should also be noted.

Chest and Breast Exam

The examination of the thorax gives an idea of the patient's size and whether there may be mechanical issues with breathing or reflux.

In listening to the heart the practitioner should rule out any murmur, rubs or gallops and ensure there is a regular rhythm and rate.

Auscultation of the chest may detect wheezing, rales, or rhonchi suggestive of asthma, reactive airways disease or lack of air movement in the lower lungs, which in turn can be suggestive of irregular heartbeat, murmurs, tachyarrhythmia, or bradycardia. Signs of pulmonary hypertension are subtle but may include an increase in the pulmonic component of the second heart sound, or a palpable second heart sound in advanced cases of pulmonary hypertension, tricuspid regurgitation, pulmonic regurgitation (Graham Steell murmur) and a right-sided S3 gallop. In pulmonary hypertension the lung examination is usually normal.

Breast and axillary examination should be done on women patients and allows for a good opportunity to confirm that women are doing a breast self-exam. It is an opportunity to discuss preventive screening as well. Breast cancer occurs more frequently in women who are affected by obesity. Implementation and follow up of screening recommendations is essential.

Abdomen

The abdomen of an obese patient can be very difficult to examine. Upon physical inspection, it should be generally determined whether the patient has symmetry from one side to the other and whether there are any obvious hernias, scars, rashes, or swelling that may be caused by fluid accumulation. Fluid accumulation may be associated with heart failure or cirrhosis. Auscultation will check for healthy bowel sounds and provides a good opportunity to discuss bowel habits in general with the patient. A bruit may be a sign of aortic aneurysm. The extent of the pannus should be documented and the possibilities of disability or intertriginous infections resulting from the pannus should be discussed with the patient. This documentation can assist the patient after massive weight loss in getting an abdominoplasty that may have a positive effect on body image. If a patient with obesity loses a significant amount of weight, he/she may be able to have a panniculectomy to remove the excess skin and fat.

Extremities

Disability due to size is often an issue for patients with obesity. Observation of the extremities as well as observations of the patient's ease of movement and ease of sitting/standing will help the provider understand the extent of any disability the patient may be experiencing. Inspection of the extremities may also point out lipomas, edema of the lower legs and skin tags. Obese patients may have forms of lipomatosis and associated syndromes (Table 9.29).

The extremities often reflect changes of malnutrition and other pathology. For instance, iron deficiency can present with pallor and brittle nails. Unsteady stance and gait can indicate thiamine deficiency. Clubbing of the nails can reflect lung, heart, and gastrointestinal or thyroid disease and chiefly tips off the provider to look more deeply into sources of the clubbing.

Ankle swelling in a patient with obesity is often a sign of right heart failure or sleep apnea. Oftentimes there can be signs of "brawny edema" where deposits of melena pigment are deposited on the lower legs. The skin becomes shiny and thin and there is a tightness in the tissue of the lower leg almost like a cicatrices. The pigmentation is usually permanent. With weight loss and a decrease of intra-abdominal pressure the swelling recedes and the skin become thicker. At times there may be both swelling and redness of the lower legs which is not normally infectious but more likely inflammatory in nature.

Table 9.29 Forms of lipomatosis and associated syndromes in patients with obesity

Name	Description
Proteus syndrome	Congenital overgrowth of skin, adipose, and lymphatic tissue and muscle
Adiposis dolorosa (Dercum's disease)	Multiple painful lipomas primary on the trunk and associated with obesity. Women more affected than men with onset at 35–45 years of age
Cowden syndrome	Rare; presents with multiple hamartomas that are at an increased risk of cancer due to a mutation in a tumor suppressor gene (PTEN)
Benign symmetric lipomatosis (Madelung's disease or cephalothoracic lipodystrophy)	Fatty deposits in soft tissue of the neck, shoulder girdle, and head associated with alcohol abuse and more common in men than women

Adapted from RP Blackstone patient intake questionnaire

Swelling, tenderness, and loss of motion commonly affect the musculoskeletal system of patients who are overweight or obese. The musculoskeletal system can be graded by scoring each muscle group's range of motion: 1 (Trace), 2 (Poor), 3 (Fair), 4 (Good), and 5 (Normal). The muscle groups that should be graded are: deltoid, triceps, biceps, wrist flexion, wrist extension, quadriceps, plantar flexion, and dorsiflexion. Determining the range of motion of joints is helpful in understanding and documenting the mobility of each patient.

Neurologic

Patients with obesity should be evaluated for neurological disorders related to or exacerbated by obesity, including stroke, Alzheimer's Disease, sleep disorders, headache, and diabetic neuropathy. In addition, given the high rate of thiamine deficiency in obese individuals, the patient who is obese should be evaluated for weakness, polyneuropathies, beriberi, Wernicke's encephalopathy (WE), nystagmus, and hearing loss. Thiamine deficiency in the most extreme form, WE, presents with changes in mental status, including confusion, apathy, and difficulty concentrating. A patient may be at heightened risk for WE after bariatric surgery especially if there is persistent vomiting and intravenous administration of glucose without thiamine. When the syndrome bumps up to Korsakoff's Syndrome, symptoms can include retrograde amnesia and aphasia, apraxia, anosmia, and a deficiency in executive functioning.

Pelvic and Anorectal Exam

Pelvic exams and anorectum exams are often difficult to perform in patients who are obese, however, it is important that these preventive exams are performed, including pap smears for women and prostate exams for men. The anorectum exam is also important for detecting masses in the rectum. If the history indicates the patient has unusually heavy menses or post menstrual bleeding there is an indication for a workup for endometrial cancer.

Skin, Trunk, and Extremities

Evaluating the patient for symptoms of insulin resistance like acanthosis nigricans may provide the basis for further laboratory testing with HOMA-IR and insulin levels. In addition, any swelling in the lower extremities may indicate the development of right heart failure from untreated sleep apnea. Documenting range of motion of joints and overall movement status of the patient may assist you in evaluating whether the patient will be at risk for falls. Lipomatosis is also an important finding. Physical examination of the trunk and extremities can detect many of the manifestations of the genetically inherited syndromes of obesity.

The skin can also provide clues to vitamin deficiencies through rashes. Any rash present under the pannus should be documented. The resection after massive weight loss of this excess skin (to prevent infection) may be paid for by insurance if the rash is repeatedly documented.

Determination of Metabolic Factors

Resting Metabolic Rate

There are many tests that are done in isolation for specific obesity-related diseases. There are also certain tests that are required in order to accurately "stage" obesity. Staging helps guide the proper strategy for weight loss. Determining the resting metabolic rate (RMR) is one of the key tests for staging obesity. This test allows the provider to counsel the patient about how many calories they will burn as a baseline and allows the planning of calorie intake.

The most accurate method of evaluating RMR is a "metabolic cart". This is not a tool that can be utilized for most patients as the cost is prohibitive, it takes many hours to complete, and it is rarely available outside of a research setting. The most often used tool to measure RMR is a handheld calorimeter. The patient prepares by fasting for at least four hours prior to the test, with no consumption of caffeine, no exercise for four hours prior to the test, and no nicotine consumption for one hour before the test. The calorimeter will give the patient and provider a reasonably accurate idea of how many calories the patient can eat before his/her body begins to store the excess food as fat. Some of the current body composition analysis scales can now roughly estimate RMR for patients . Patients will understand their specific calorie intake and expenditure based on a determination of their RMR and can also use a wrist watch type tool to calculate their daily activity and food intake.

Body Composition Analysis

Body composition, or the ratio of fat mass to lean tissue (including bone, muscle, ligaments, tendons, and organs), can be measured by a variety of methods ranging from the quick and painless to more complicated and detailed methods. Variation in method also results in fluctuations in accuracy. Range of error is greater in some methods than in others.

The most accurate approach to measuring body composition is by chemical analysis of cadavers. This approach is obviously of limited value in ongoing clinical evaluation of the living obese patient.

Hydrostatic Weighing: The most accurate modern assessment of body composition in living persons is hydrostatic weighing. The underwater weight method coupled with labeling of water with radioactive deuterium and tritium remains the gold standard for measuring volumes and body composition but is only used in specialized research settings. It has been widely replaced by newer methods proved to be nearly as accurate. Methods that are newer and nearly as accurate and that can be utilized in large patient populations are used in clinical settings.

Magnetic resonance imaging (MRI): MRI allows for the specific evaluation of adipose tissue around organs but its use is time consuming, expensive, and difficult for large patients to endure due to table size and patient immobility. In addition, MRI cannot be used with metal implants. Quantitative MRI underestimates fat mass. MRI is rarely used for standard obesity evaluation.

Dual Energy X-ray Absorptiometry (DEXA): DEXA is a non-invasive test that can be applied to people of all ages. It can accurately estimate the three main components of the body: water, fat, and the remaining fat-free dry mass. The DEXA test has good accuracy and reproducibility and can give an assessment in disease states, growth disorders and in various states of nutrition. There is a small amount of radiation with DEXA testing and there may be an upper weight restriction limit due to the size of the tables that are used during testing. The DEXA loses some accuracy when used with patients who have a "thick" body style.

Bioelectrical Impedance Scale: *To date, the best tool to use on a daily basis to assess body composition is a simple scale that measures bioelectrical impedance.* The tradeoff in accuracy is made up in "trending" the evaluation of body composition (for each component) and the ease of use. *Single frequency* bioelectrical impedance analysis (BIA) can determine total body water and fat-free mass. If the BIA is *multifrequency* the instrument will also provide information on intracellular water and extracellular water components. *Note: Bioelectrical impedance scales are not recommended for use in patients with a pacemaker* [23, 24].

Diagnostic Tests for Obesity-Related Disease

One of the key diagnoses that needs to be ruled out in a patient who is overweight or obese is NAFLD. The following algorithm demonstrates the approach to the evaluation of NAFLD and lays out the steps for deciding whether a liver biopsy should be recommended [9] (Fig. 9.3).

Laboratory Test Recommendations

The primary lab tests that can be performed as a baseline screening for specific obesity-related diseases within the patient are the following:

HbA1c: HbA1c is the primary tool to use to diagnosis intermediate diabetes and type 2 diabetes. This replaces fasting blood glucose, which is often difficult for the

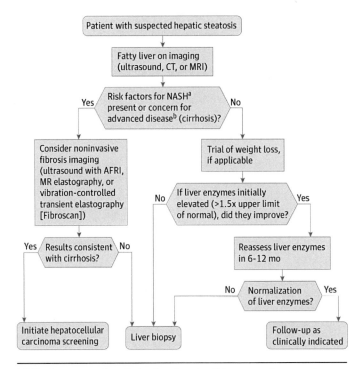

Fig. 9.3 Algorithm for the decision to perform liver biopsy in patients with presumed non-alcoholic fatty liver disease after negative serological evaluation and exclusion of alcohol as a contributing factor. From Rinella [9] with permission

patient to do and requires two different episodes of testing. The level of hyperglycemia is the level that causes retinopathy. A normal HbA1c is <5.7 %, intermediate diabetes is 5.7–6.4 % and diabetes: ≥ 6.5 %.

Lipid Panel: This blood test measures fats and fatty substances and identifies lipid abnormalities.

TSH: The thyroid-stimulating hormone test evaluates thyroid function and/or symptoms of a thyroid disorder.

Liver Function Tests: Liver function tests (including Alt, AST, Alkaline phosphatase, and total bilirubin) often yield normal results in obese patients, but elevated transaminase levels may indicate fatty infiltration of the liver.

Renal Function Tests: Comprehensive Metabolic Profile.

Uric Acid: The uric acid blood test is used to detect high levels of uric acid which may suggest diabetes and/or a kidney disorder, among other things.

EKG: Electrocardiograms (EKG) are routinely ordered to check for problems with the electrical activity of a patient's heart, particularly in overweight or obese patients. *It is important to note that multiple changes that can occur in an EKG associated with obesity.* There is usually an elevation in heart rate of approximately 7 beats per minute. When both bradycardia and tachycardia are abnormal further workup is required. In addition, adipose tissue builds up around the heart causing it to assume a more horizontal position than usual. This is often seen in the EKG as a left axis deviation. The P wave morphology is similar to what is seen with left atrial enlargement. The PR interval can be normal, but can also become prolonged with increased levels of obesity. The QRS complex may show low voltage due to a thick chest wall and can exhibit changes consistent with left ventricular hypertrophy from an increased blood volume. Cardiac hypertrophy occurs relatively early in obesity and is found in 87 % of patients with obesity. The EKG may underestimate it. The duration of the QRS may be prolonged. Although there may be a nonspecific T wave flattening and inversion there is usually no ST segment changes. If ST segment change occurs that should be interpreted the same as it would be interpreted in a lean patient. Finally the QT segment is longer than normal because of a delay in repolarization of the ventricle, which increases the patient's risk for tachyarrhythmia. These changes are generally reversed with weight loss [25].

Vitamin D Level: Vitamin D deficiency is very common in patients with BMI >30. It may be asymptomatic, although patients may complain of symptoms like fatigue, bone pain, and muscle weakness. A screening test with a serum 25 hydroxy-vitamin D level is generally obtained during the workup of the patient with obesity. When necessary, repletion with high doses is done until normal levels are obtained.

Conclusion: The Summary Assessment Based on History, Physical Exam and Diagnostic Testing

In the patient's first appointment, information is gathered, tests may be ordered, and initial actions, like changing medications, can be done. In the second appointment the results of the practitioner's comprehensive review of information should be communicated to the patient and engagement in specific goals should be achieved. Subsequent appointments should focus on the execution, barriers and progress toward those goals.

In addition, the final assessment of the patient should include the following:

1. Identification and communication of the patient's Weight-Related Health Indicator Score (body mass index, waist circumference and body fat percentile).
2. Determination of whether the patient is exhibiting signs of metabolic syndrome. If MetS is suspected, determine how that translates into a risk of future disease.
3. Determination of the patient's Edmonton Obesity Stage.
4. Communication to the patient about the level of risk based on this assessment.

The final assessment should allow a determination to be made as to what individualized program the patient needs to maximize his/her success with traditional therapy. The final assessment may determine that a more intensive strategy is necessary, including medications and multidisciplinary management. Chapter 10 will provide a thorough discussion of the types of medications that are available for weight loss and suggest specific strategies for a multidisciplinary approach.

References

1. Kuk JL, Ardern CI. Are metabolically normal but obese individuals at lower risk for all-cause mortality? Diab Care. 2009;32(12):2297–9.
2. Jaunmuktane Z, Mead S, Ellis M, Wadsworth JD, Nicoll AJ, Kenny J, et al. Evidence for human transmission of amyloid-B pathology and cerebral amyloid angiopathy. Nature. 2015;525(7568):247–50.
3. Sonino N, Fava GA. A simple instrument for assessing stress in clinical practice. Postgrad Med J. 1998;74:408–10.
4. Budhiraja R. J Clin Sleep Med. 2007;3:407–15.
5. Johns MW. A new method for measuring daytime sleepiness: the epworth sleepiness scale. Sleep. 1991;14(6):540–5.
6. Steinweg DL, Worth H. The keys to the CAGE. Am J Med. 1993;94:520–3.
7. Stone NJ, Robinson JG, Lichtenstein AH, Goff DC, Lloyd-Jones DM, Smith SC, et al. Treatment of blood cholesterol to reduce atherosclerotic cardiovascular disease risk in adults: synopsis of the 2013 American College of Cardiology/American Heart Association cholesterol guideline. Ann Intern Med. 2014;160:339–43.
8. Fabbrini E, Sullivan S, Klein S. Obesity and nonalcoholic fatty liver disease: biochemical, metabolic and clinical implications. Hepatology. 2010;51(20):679–89.
9. Rinella ME. Nonalcoholic fatty liver disease: a systematic review. JAMA. 2015;313 (22):2263–73.
10. Legro RS, Arslanian SA, Ehrmann DA, Hoeger KM, Murad H, Pasquali R, Welt CK. Diagnosis and treatment of polycystic ovary syndrome: an endocrine society clinical practice guideline. JCEM. 2013; doi:10.1210/jc.2013-2350.
11. El-Serag H. The association between obesity and GERD: a review of the epidemiological evidence. Dig Dis Sci. 2008;53(9):2307–12.
12. Jones R, Junghard O, Dent J, et al. Development of the GerdQ, a tool for the diagnosis and management of gastroesophageal reflux disease in primary care. Aliment Pharmacol Ther. 2009;30(10):1034.
13. Subak LL, Richter HE, Hunskaar S. Obesity and urinary incontinence. J Urol. 2009;182(6): S2–7.
14. Bradley CS, Rahn DD, Nygaard IE, Barbar MD, Nager CW, Kenton KS, Siddiqui NY, Abel RB, Spino C, Richter HE. The questionnaire for urinary incontinence diagnosis (QUID):

validity and responsiveness to change in women undergoing non-surgical therapies for treatment of stress predominant urinary incontinence. Neuroural Urodyn. 2010;29(5):727–34.
15. American Psychiatric Association. Diagnostic and statistical manual of mental disorders. 4th ed. Washington, D.C: American Psychiatric Association; 2000.
16. Benazzi F. Bipolar disorder—focus on bipolar II disorder and mixed depression. Lancet. 2007;369:935.
17. Center for Disease Control. Suicide: risk and protective factors. 2012. http://www.cdc.gov/violenceprevention/suicide/riskprotectivefactors.html.
18. Center for Disease Control. Mental health basics. 2011. http://www.cdc.gov/mentalhealth/basics.htm.
19. Hilty DM, Brady KT, Hales RE. A review of bipolar disorder among adults. Psychiatr Serv. 1999;50(2):201–13.
20. Hirschfeld RM, Cass AR, Holt DC, Carlson CA. Screening for bipolar disorder in patients treated for depression in a family medicine clinic. J Am Board Fam Pract. 2005;18(4):233–9.
21. World Health Organization. Mental health: a state of well being. 2011.
22. Lengel RA. Psychosocial assessment: a nursing perspective. CEUFAST, Inc.; 2015.
23. Heymsfield SB, Ebbeling CB, Zheng J, Petrobelli A, Strauss BJ, Silva AM, Ludwig DS. Multi-component molecular-level body composition reference methods: evolving concepts and future directions. Obes Rev. 2015;16(4):282–94.
24. Lee SY, Gallagher D. Assessment methods in human body composition. Curr Opin Clin Nutr Metab Care. 2008;11(5):566.
25. Fraley M, Birchem JA, Senkottaiyan N, Alpert MA. Obesity and the electrocardiogram. Obes Rev. 2005;6(4):275–81.

Chapter 10
Beyond Traditional Management: The Use of Medications in the Treatment of Obesity

Key Message

Traditional management of obesity focuses mainly on diet and exercise and results in a target weight loss of 5-10 %. In a person with obesity, however, most weight loss is regained as the body system ferociously asserts metabolic adaptation (genetic resetting^{TM}) in an attempt to return the person to his/her previous level of obesity. Unfortunately this means that weight loss through traditional methods of diet and exercise is generally unsustainable in the person with obesity. Nonetheless traditional management is important, particularly in patients who are merely "overweight" rather than obese. Early intervention at lower BMI (i.e. when BMI begins to edge up into the 27Kg/m^2 range) is when traditional management may be most effective. Medications along with traditional management techniques have been used to treat overweight and obesity for years with mixed results and many side effects. It is crucial that providers of care for persons with overweight and obesity understand the role of pharmaceuticals, their mechanisms of action, their potential interactions with other drugs, and their side effects.

This chapter lists and classifies all the medications prescribed for weight loss, for treating obesity-related diseases, for use in connection with bariatric surgery, and for treating other medical problems in patients with obesity. It details the unique challenges of using prescription medications in patients with obesity and defines the criteria for using pharmacotherapy in the management of weight loss. Finally, this chapter explains the mechanism of action of FDA-approved medications for weight loss. As our understanding of obesity improves and the efficacy of prescription medications evolves our management strategies will improve as well, resulting in a positive and lasting impact on patients with obesity and on the disease itself.

Learning Objectives

1. Outline the traditional approach to the management of obesity and how medications can add to that treatment.
2. Recognize and classify the medications used in patients with overweight and obesity for weight loss, for obesity-related diseases, for use in bariatric

surgery, and for treatment of other medical problems, including medications that *promote* weight gain.
3. Explain the challenges in using medications in patients with obesity.
4. Define the criteria for use of pharmacotherapy in the management of weight loss.
5. Explain the mechanism of action of FDA-approved medications for weight loss.

Any attempt to treat obesity must embrace diet, exercise, and epigenetic modulation through lifestyle management as a means to achieving good health. Unfortunately for many people, this approach alone does not result in sufficient weight loss, or the weight loss is merely temporary. For these reasons nontraditional management options including the use of prescription medications for weight loss may need to be considered.

The use of prescription medications in patients with obesity, however, is not without its drawbacks. Medications are often prescribed to patients with obesity not to treat the obesity per se, but to treat obesity-related diseases or other medical problems. In addition, the patient with obesity often receives a prescription drug in which the dosage does not take into account the patient's level of body fat, which can alter absorption or elimination rates. Moreover, the drugs themselves may contribute to weight gain or worsening of adipose tissue dysfunction. Weight gain as a result of prescribed medication is a common *unintended* consequence. Despite all these pitfalls, medication plays a major role in managing the health of the patient with obesity and facilitating weight loss. Medical practitioners must understand both the upsides and the pitfalls.

The Use of Medications for the Treatment of *Other* Medical Problems in Patients with Obesity

Morbid obesity is associated with several pathophysiological changes that can profoundly affect drug distribution and clearance. Most data on the use of drugs in human beings are based upon "ideal" patient populations; few have been studied rigorously in patients with obesity. For example, most medications being used in the treatment of children in the emergency department have been studied only in lean children [1]. Other categories of medications that have not been tested/addressed for use specifically in patients with obesity are perioperative pain medications, antibiotics and other medications for treating infections, and VTE prophylaxis [2]. The physiology of adipose tissue can have important implications for dosing and effectiveness depending on the mechanism by which the medication works. Drug dosing for CVD risk factors is another area that is untested/unaddressed in patients with obesity [3].

The distribution of a drug between fat and lean tissue will influence the kinetics and metabolism of the drug. People of obesity have a larger absolute amount of lean tissue as well as a larger fat mass. The behavior of a drug with weak or moderate lipophilicity, like lithium or vecuronium, is generally predictable because they are primarily distributed in lean tissue. Dosage in these cases should be based on lean body weight. Some medications, like antibiotics and anticancer drugs, are partly distributed in adipose tissue and the dosage must be based on ideal body weight plus a percent of excess body weight or body fat, thereby making it dose specific to the patient [4]. There are no drug dosing recommendations for antibiotics in obese patients. Dosing is based on pharmacokinetic characteristics and dosing recommendations in other disease states [5].

In medications that are fat loving (i.e., have high lipophilicity), like beta blockers and some opioids, there is no consistent systematic relationship with distribution. The loading dose is adjusted to total body weight or ideal body weight and the adjustment of the maintenance dosage will depend on clearance.

Some drugs have a very small therapeutic index and should be administered very carefully using drug plasma concentrations for making adjustments. This category of drugs includes narcotics and VTE prophylaxis. The risk of overdose in these situations compounds the baseline complexity. The unique physiology of a patient with obesity can lead to mortality or severe morbidity in situations where an ideal weight patient might otherwise recover. In addition, sometimes monitoring does not give early warning and patients with obesity may have a higher rate of failure to rescue due to unique physiological concerns.

Failure to rescue means death in a patient with one or more defined complications. Failure to rescue is usually considered to be independent of patient factors and dependent on hospital factors. In the population of the obese, however, the elements that contribute to failure to rescue become more complicated and profound. The use and dosage of medication in a patient with obesity can be a contributing element in the failure to rescue.

Physicians rely upon monitoring to help determine when a medication is having an undesirable effect on the patient. Patients in hospitals often get a "cocktail" of multiple medications they are not accustomed to receiving. Dosing of medication in patients with obesity is already particularly problematic. It becomes even more problematic because standard monitoring may fail to tell us when a patient with obesity is in trouble. This is because medication monitoring is based on a "fire alarm" model. Specific parameters are set and when they are breached we are alerted to a potential problem. This is problematic in the patient with obesity for two reasons. First, the breach notifications do not detect clinical instability early enough to allow effective intervention. Second, there is a false sense of security because, despite reliance upon machine monitoring, sometimes signs and symptoms of instability are present but ignored because the monitoring machine indicates everything is "OK" [6].

An evaluation of deaths between 1956 and 2010 by Lynn and Curry found that there are three distinct patterns of unexplained hospital deaths (PUHD). Type I occurs with hyperventilation compensated by respiratory distress as the result of sepsis, pulmonary embolus, and congestive heart failure (Fig. 10.1); Type II is progressive unidirectional hypoventilation as the result of CO_2 narcosis. What is observed in Type II is a progressive rise in $PaCO_2$ and fall in SPO_2 usually due to

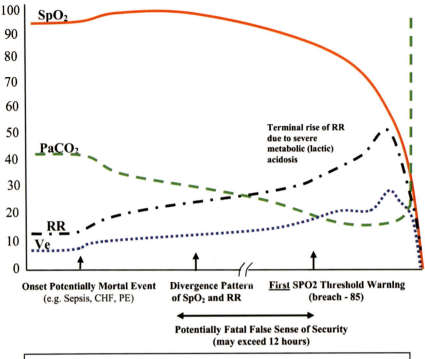

Fig. 10.1 Type 1 pattern of unexpected hospital death (e.g., sepsis, CHF, PE). Values on Y-axis are for reference; actual values for each parameter will vary significantly (from Lynn and Curry [6], with permission)

an overdose of narcotics or sedatives or a combination (Fig. 10.2). Type III exhibits arousal failure allowing a precipitous hypoxemia during apnea that causes terminal arousal arrest (Fig. 10.3).

The second pattern, Type II, is caused by progressive unidirectional hypoventilation from narcotic overdose and has specifically higher risk of occurrence in a patient with obesity who may also be a chronic pain patient. Due to the lipophilicity of many narcotics the basal rate dosing of a patient-centered analgesia machine is not utilized. Patients with obesity may have a PHO2XB mutation (Congenital Central Hypoventilation Syndrome) which means they are at even higher risk of narcotic sensitivity. Other common findings in patients with obesity that may contribute to higher risk are hypothyroidism, COPD, chest wall deformities, and garden-variety obesity hypoventilation. While the patient may be asymptomatic while awake, the genetic mutation the patient carries causes CO2 narcosis under sedative/narcotic effects.

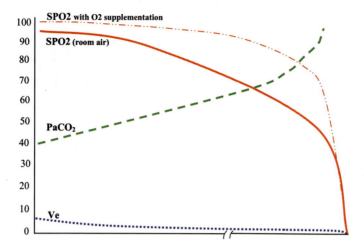

Fig. 10.2 Type II pattern of unexpected hospital death (CO2 narcosis) (from Lynn and Curry [6], with permission)

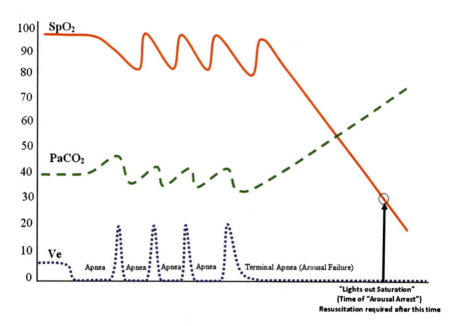

Fig. 10.3 Type III pattern of unexpected hospital death (sleep apnea with arousal failure) (from Lynn and Curry [6], with permission)

In short, the failure of medical practitioners to recognize obesity as a factor in dosing medications may contribute to the inability to rescue a patient from an adverse event when it occurs.

Medications that Cause Weight Gain

Medications that cause weight gain fall into three categories: (1) drugs given for manipulation of the central nervous system, (2) endocrine agents, and (3) all other medications without a common cause of action. The practitioner should be aware of all three categories of medicine and their potential repercussions when prescribing medications for patients with obesity [7]. During initial consultation with a patient with obesity, an evaluation and substitution to medications that do not cause weight gain but are equally effective, in collaboration with the patient's primary physician, may be an easy first step to prevent the patient from gaining additional weight.

The choice of medications for treatment of obesity-related disease in patients with obesity can also have a major impact on a system of healthcare in terms of cost and prevention of disease. Antipsychotic medication is one example. Investigators using the electronic medical record data in two health care systems examined the records of 18–79 year-old patients put on antipsychotic medications, looking for weight gain ≥ 7 % body weight. While not all patients on antipsychotic medications gained weight, the incidence was 7–17 % in 1 year in those who did gain weight, and the average weight gain was 10 kg. The antipsychotic medication most associated with weight gain was olanzapine (17/100 users; 95 % CI: 14.2–20.5) versus ziprasidone (7.7/100; 95 %CI: 4.6–13.0). Although antipsychotic medications provide just one example, it is clear that prescribing other types of medications with similar efficacy *that do not promote weight gain* is advisable in patients with obesity.

Tables 10.1, 10.2, 10.3, 10.4, 10.5, 10.6, 10.7, 10.8, and 10.9 contain most of the drugs commonly prescribed for various medical conditions. These tables also indicate at-a-glance the medication's effect on body weight. The direction of the blue arrow denotes whether a medication tends to increase or decrease body weight, or has no discernible effect.

It should be noted that some of the medications prescribed to treat insulin resistance and diabetes often have the effect of causing weight gain, even though weight loss is the primary treatment for diabetes. The best approach is Weight-Centered Management of Hyperglycemia. As practitioners begin to treat hyperglycemia in a patient with obesity, the choice of medications becomes paramount to preventing further weight gain (11).

Table 10.1 Antipsychotic drugs

Effect on body weight	Generic and proprietary examples
⇈	Clozapine (Clozaril, FazaClo), olanzapine (Zyprexa), zotepine
↑	Asenapine (Saphris), chlorpromazine, iloperidone (Fanapt), paliperidone (Invega), quetiapine (Seroquel), risperidone (Risperdal), sertindole, lithium
⇔	Amisulpride, aripiprazole, haloperidol, lurasidone, ziprasidone

Data from Manu et al. [8]

Table 10.2 Antiseizure drugs

Effect on body weight	Generic and proprietary examples
↑	*Carbamazepine* (Tegretol, Carbatrol, Equetro, Epitol), *gabapentin* (Gralise, Neurontin, Horizant, Fanatrex), *valproate* (Depakene, Depacon, Depakote, Stavzor, Valproic)
↓	*Lamotrigine* (Lamictal), *topiramate* (Topamax), *zoniasamide* (Zonegran)

Table 10.3 Antidepressant drugs

Effect on body weight	Generic and proprietary examples
↑	*Amitriptyline, doxepin* (Silenor, Zonalon, Prudoxin), *imipramine* (Tofranil-pm, Tofranil), *isocarboxazid* (Marplan), *phenelzine* (Nardil), *paroxetine* (Pexeva, Paxil), mirtazapine (Remeron, Remeronsoltab)
↔	*Desipramine* (Norpramin), *nortriptyline* (Pamelor), *protriptyline* (Vivactil), *tranylcypromine* (Parnate), *citalopram* (Celexa), *escitalopram* (Lexapro), *fluoxetine* (Sarafem, Prozac), *sertraline* (Zoloft), *desvenlafaxine, duloxetine* (Cymbalta), *venlafaxine* (Effexor)
↓	*Bupropion* (Buproban, Aplenzin, Wellbutrin, Budeprion, Zyban)

Data from Reekie et al. [9]

Table 10.4 Hypnotic drugs

Effect on body weight	Generic and proprietary examples
↑	*Diphenhydramine* (Benadryl, Sominex, Diphenhist, Wal-Dryl, Banophen, Hydramine, Silphen, Dicopanol)—an antihistamine (hypnotic) used to treat allergic reactions, motion sickness, symptoms of Parkinson's disease
↔	*Benzodiazepines* (Diazepam, Alprazolam, Clonazepam, Lorazepam), nonbenzodiazepine hypnotics, melatonergic hypnotics, trazodone (Oleptro)

Table 10.5 Migraine drugs

Effect on body weight	Generic and proprietary examples
↑	*Amitriptyline, gabapentin* (Gralise, Neurontin, Horizant, Fanatrex), *paroxetine* (Pexeva, Paxil), *valproic acid* (Depakene, Depacon, Depakote, Stavzor, Valproic)
↓	*Topiramate* (Topamax)
↑	Serotonin Antagonists—*pizotifen* (Sandomigran)—used to treat recurrent migraines

Table 10.6 Anti-diabetes drugs

Effect on body weight	Generic and proprietary examples
↑	Insulin in any formulation, sulfonylureas, meglitinides, thiazolidinediones
↓	*Metformin* (Glumetza, Glucophage, Fortamet, Fiomet), glucagon-like peptide-1 agonists like *exenatide* (Byetta) and *liraglutide* (Victoza), sodium glucose cotransporter 2 inhibitor like *canagliflozin*, alpha glucosidase inhibitors like *acarbose* (Precose)
⇔	*Dipeptidyl peptidase-4 inhibitors like sitagliptin* (Januvia), *vildagliptin and saxagliptin* (Onglyza)

Data from Cheng and Kashyap [10]

Table 10.7 Cardiovascular drugs

Effect on body weight	Generic name
↑	Beta blockers: *propranolol, atenolol* (Tenormin), and *metoprolol* (Lopressor), calcium channel blockers like *dihydropyridine, nifedipine* (Procardia), *amlodipine* (Norvasc), *felodipine* (Plendil)
↓	Diuretic use in patient with peripheral edema
⇔	Angiotensin converting enzyme inhibitors and angiotensin II receptor blockers

Table 10.8 Steroid medications

Effect on body weight	Generic name
↑	Glucocorticoids, estrogens, diphenhydramine
⇔	Progestins

Table 10.9 Antiviral and chemotherapy drugs

Effect on body weight	Generic name
↑	HAART protease inhibitors without HIV lipodystrophy
↓	HAART protease inhibitors with HIV lipodystrophy
↑	Tamoxifen, cyclophosphamide, methotrexate, 5-fluorouracil, aromatase inhibitors

HAART Highly active antiretroviral therapy

Medications for Use as Weight Loss Medications

The use of medications specifically for weight loss is not the first line of defense, but it may become a necessary treatment strategy. Preparation and education of the patient through traditional treatment strategies involving diet, exercise, and educating the patient about the risk and consequences of obesity-related diseases should be undertaken first.

Historical Perspective of Weight Loss Medications

Medications for weight loss include both FDA-approved medications and over-the-counter (OTC) medications. OTC medications are widely used with unknown or poorly documented effectiveness and side effects, yet people spend billions of dollars each year on OTC supplements. Over history, the use of medications to induce weight loss has resulted in a number of serious and fatal unintended consequences [12] (Table 10.10). This history of serious adverse side effects and mortality has profoundly inhibited the use of prescribed drugs for weight loss therapy by physicians.

Table 10.10 Unintended consequences of weight loss medications

Year	Medication	Consequence
1892 [13]	Sheep thyroid extract	Hyperthyroidism, cardiac arrhythmias, and cardiac arrest
1932 [14]	Dinitrophenol (DNP)	Cataracts/neuropathy, fatal hyperthermia, agranulocytosis
1937 [15]	Amphetamine and the "rainbow pill" regimens: amphetamines, digitalis, thyroid hormone, diuretics and laxatives with barbiturates used to calm people down	Addiction, myocardial toxicity, and sudden death
1968 [16]	Aminorex	Pulmonary hypertension with a mortality rate of >50 % in those who developed this side effect
1997 [17]	Phen/fenfluramine (phen-fen)	Pulmonary hypertension and heart valve dysfunction
1998 [18]	Phenylpropanolamine (PPA)	Intracranial bleeding and hemorrhagic stroke
2003 [19]	Ephedra alkaloids combined with caffeine and/or guarana (Ma Huang)	Heart palpitations, hypertension, heart attack, stroke, sudden death

(continued)

Table 10.10 (continued)

Year	Medication	Consequence
2008 [20]	Rimonabant (CB-1 endocannabinoid receptor antagonist)	Psychiatric side effects including depression and suicide
2010 [21]	Sibutramine	People with preexisting cardiovascular conditions may have an increased risk of nonfatal heart attack and stroke
Over-the-counter (OTC) medications [22]	1. Modulation of carbohydrate metabolism (chromium, ginseng) 2 Increase satiety (fiber containing supplements like guar gum, glucomannan and psyllium) 3. Enhance fat oxidation (hydroxycitric acid, conjugated linoleic acid, green tea, licorice, pyruvate, vitamin B6, L-carnitine) or 4. Block lipid absorption (chitosan)	Appear to be tolerated but no evidence exists regarding their long-term safety and no clinical trials document their efficacy People spend billions of dollars on OTC supplements

Data from Bray [12]

This history of complications has likely curtailed the use of medications in treating obesity. This is partly due to strong obesity bias that implies that any risk is unacceptable when obesity is so easily fixed without medication if the person with obesity would simply employ self-control when it comes to diet and exercise. It is only in recent years, as the impact of epigenetic inheritance and gene expression of phenotype have become more widely known, that the risk/benefit ratio of prescribing medicine for weight loss has become more acceptable.

Of perhaps greater concern is the wide variety of unregulated OTC medications and supplements that are frequently used for weight loss. Perhaps the best example currently is the hCG (Human Chorionic Gonadotropin) diet, which promotes the use of the hCG hormone (normally produced during pregnancy) paired with a very low calorie diet (VLCD), between 500 and 800 calories/day. As a prescription medicine, hCG is used mainly to treat infertility. It is not approved for OTC use, nor has it been proven effective for weight loss, yet it is purchased OTC and on the internet in staggering amounts. The minimal calorie diet, not the hCG, is what generally results in some initial weight loss at least short term. The risks of following a low-calorie unsupervised diet can include gallstone formation, irregular heartbeat, and an imbalance of electrolytes. Taking hCG for weight loss also presents a serious risk of blood clot formation in the legs or lungs [23]. The current literature contains multiple case studies, some of which also document pregnancies in conjunction with the thromboembolic compilation. Perhaps even more concerning is the continuing report of transmission of human prion proteins with injectable hCG. Over 300,000 women annually receive urine-derived hCG for infertility (not just for weight loss). These proteins have a very long incubation time, and are associated with Creutzfeldt–Jakob disease. The incidence of this disease is rising [24].

Although hCG may be one of the most widely misused weight loss medications at the current time, the medication with arguably the most long-term negative impact was the drug combination fenfluramine/phentermine (usually referred to as fen-phen, also known as Redux). Fen-phen was heavily marketed in the mid-1990s as an antiobesity treatment. Studies in 1996–1997 showed that fen-phen was linked with potentially fatal pulmonary hypertension and heart valve damage, and the FDA requested its withdrawal from the market in 1997. Fen-phen users filed more than 50,000 product liability lawsuits against the manufacturer, who set aside over $21 billion to cover the cost of the lawsuits.

The rapidly increasing number of patients affected by obesity means that safe and effective medications for treatment are sorely needed. Research for the development of new obesity medications is ongoing. Research concerning brain circuitry, the microbiome, and metabolism are allowing medications to be developed with specific targets in mind. Safe and effective obesity medications have the potential to deliver less expensive and more widely applicable options for treatment.

Indications for the Use of Prescription Medications in a Patient with Obesity

Once a physician has assessed a patient as being overweight or obese, the patient should be counseled appropriately about the use of traditional methods for weight loss and the importance of epigenetic modulaton via the implementation of a lifestyle modification program. That foundation of behavioral modification is considered essential and is recommended for a 6-month period prior to implementing any medications to assist in the weight loss. After 6 months of behavioral work, medications designed to promote additional weight loss or sustain the weight loss already achieved may need to be considered. Such medications may be able to help correct the adipose tissue dysfunction of obesity [25].

The goal of weight loss therapy, including the use of pharmaceuticals, is to achieve a 5–10 % reduction in weight and fat mass. *The indication for use of pharmaceuticals in the treatment of obesity via monotherapy or combination drug therapy, is as follows*:

> Patient with a BMI of ≥ 30 kg/m^2
> Patient with a BMI of ≥ 27 kg/m^2 plus the presence of obesity-related disease*

(*T2DM, Hypertension, Dyslipidemia)
If no clinical improvement after 12 weeks, increase the dosage or change to an alternative

For each medication prescribed, the medical practitioner should first:

1. Know and understand the primary mechanism of the medication's action in the body and the mechanism of action for weight loss (if known).
2. Know and understand the indications, contraindications, benefits, specific risks, and side effects of the medicine.
3. Determine if the medication has any special categories of use that require satisfaction of additional requirements;
4. Establish a plan for monitoring and follow up.
5. Discuss all of the above with the patient and obtain consent and agreement.

Note: *Many practitioners of obesity medicine will have a standard consent form that the patient is required to sign prior to beginning use of pharmaceuticals for weight loss.*

Some patients with obesity may be girls and women who are within childbearing age. The practitioner needs to understand the Pregnancy Risk Categories and provide written information to the patient regarding this risk if a weight loss medication is prescribed.

The Pregnancy Risk Categories include the following:

Category A: Human studies demonstrate no risk
Category B: Animal studies demonstrate no risk, no study in pregnant women
Category C: Animal studies demonstrate adverse effect, no study in humans. The potential benefit may warrant use in pregnant women
Category D: Evidence of risk to fetus
Category X: Studies in animals or humans demonstrate fetal abnormalities. The risks outweigh any potential benefit
Category N: Not an FDA-classified drug

For all medications with Pregnancy Category X designations, a negative pregnancy test is required prior to initiating the medication and contraceptive use should be confirmed with the patient and included in the informed consent document.

Mechanism of Action

Any attempt to understand the value of using weight loss medications should start with mechanism of action. In prescribing weight loss medication for a patient with obesity the practitioner should understand, in general terms, the biochemical interaction through which a drug produces its pharmacological effect. Some of the pertinent mechanisms of action can be found in the individual drug summaries set forth below. Additional information on other drugs not listed below can be obtained via research and/or the drug facts sheet pertaining to each pharmaceutical.

Understanding the mechanism of action is helping researchers develop new and promising drugs for the treatment of obesity. Current research indicates that it may be possible to modulate the activity of exogenous hormones with pharmaceuticals to make them more effective at weight control. As discussed in previous chapters, the physiology of energy metabolism is controlled in the hypothalamus. Two sets of neurons in the hypothalamus control hunger and satiety. These neurons send signals to the rest of the body that cause other downstream body systems to react. Receptors in these systems provide targets for manipulation by pharmaceuticals. For example, receptors that create satiety when activated, like Y2 and Y4, are targets for the exogenous hormones pancreatic polypeptide and PYY. Similarly, blocking receptors that stimulate hunger are another target for manipulation by pharmaceuticals [26] (Figs. 10.4 and 10.5).

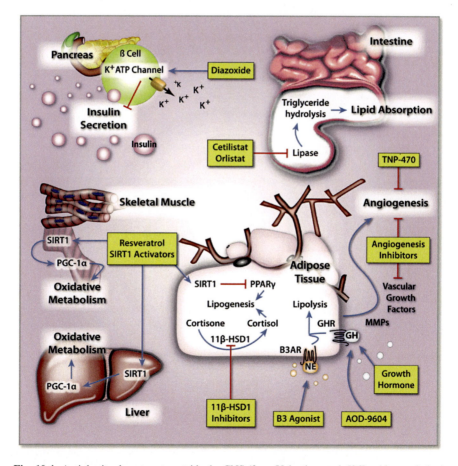

Fig. 10.4 Antiobesity drug targets outside the CNS (from Valentino et al. [26], with permission)

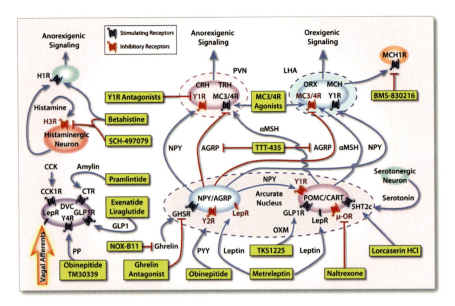

Fig. 10.5 Endogenous signaling of appetite-regulating hormones, neuropeptides, and neurotransmitters and the drugs targeting these pathways (from Valentino et al. [26], with permission)

When the hormone leptin was first used to treat obesity it failed because people with high body fat percent are generally leptin-resistant. New approaches have emerged that may bring leptin back as a target for manipulation by pharmaceuticals. One approach is to administer medications that sensitize the body to leptin, like tauroursodeoxycholic acid (TUDCA). Another approach is to administer a drug like 4-phenyl butyric acid (PCA) that decreases the endoreticular stress of leptin resistance. Other medications like Pramlintide, which is a synthetic analogue of the hormone pancreatic amylin, may be able to provide essential sensitivity to leptin that might allow exogenous leptin to create weight loss. The combination drug Pramlintide/Metreleptin is currently in human trials.

Medications Currently Approved for the Treatment of Obesity

Below is a list of current medications that are approved by the FDA for the treatment of obesity, and a brief summary of pertinent drug facts. *Practitioners should consult the package inserts for detailed and accurate pharmaceutical information and not rely upon the summaries provided below.*

Note: *For all medications with Pregnancy Category X designations, a negative pregnancy test is required prior to initiating the medication and contraceptive use should be confirmed with the patient and included in the informed consent document.*

Phentermine

The group of adrenergic medications are designed to reduce appetite and may increase energy expenditure. Phentermine is the prototype drug in this category and one of the most widely used medications for weight loss in the United States. Phentermine is also currently the least expensive and best selling obesity treatment medication in the United States [27].

Description

This group includes phentermine (Adipex, Ionamin), phendimetrazine, and diethylpropion (Tepanil), all of which act through the inhibition of norepinephrine (NE); as well as bupropion (Wellbutrin), which is a weaker NE and a dopamine reuptake inhibitor. Phentermine and diethylpropion are Drug Enforcement Administration (DEA) schedule IV medications. Phendimetrazine and benzphetamine are DEA schedule III drugs. *All of these drugs are Pregnancy Category X.*

Dosage

This drug requires a hard copy prescription with a DEA number. A verbal order can be given but must be followed up with a faxed or hard copy prescription. It can be dispensed for 1 month with a 5-month refill. Phentermine is administered once per day, usually in the morning, and comes in both long-acting and more immediate formats. Phentermine HCL dose ranges from 8 to 37.5 mg versus 6.4 to 30 mg for long-acting phentermine resins.

Contraindications

Patients with uncontrolled hypertension (HTN), seizures, known coronary artery disease (CAD), cardiac arrhythmias, anxiety disorders, hyperthyroidism, glaucoma, and history of drug abuse, pregnancy and nursing mothers are all excluded from use of Phentermine.

Safety Warning for Phentermine

- *Phentermine cannot be used in people within 14 days before starting or following a Monoamine Oxidase (MAO) inhibitor due to the risk of hypertensive crisis.*

- *Use of alcohol while on Phentermine may precipitate an adverse drug reaction.*
- *If the patient is taking insulin or other medications to treat hyperglycemia the doses may need to be adjusted.*
- *Addition of Phentermine may decrease the effect of adrenergic neuron blocking medications for hypertension.*

Metabolism

Phentermine is metabolized by the liver. The kidneys excrete 70–80 %.

Side Effects

The list of potential side effects includes: cardiac problems including palpitations, tachycardia, hypertension, and ischemia; overstimulation of the central nervous system including restlessness, dizziness, insomnia, euphoria or dysphoria, tremor, headache and psychosis; gastrointestinal complaints including dry mouth, diarrhea, and bad taste in the mouth; allergic reactions including urticaria; changes in libido; impotence; primary pulmonary hypertension and valvular heart disease—although the latter two side effects are rare unless combined with Fenfluramine.

Lorcaserin (Belviq)

Serotonin levels play a role in both energy balance and feeding. Fluoxetine (Prozac, Sarafem) and Sertraline (Zoloft), all of which are selective serotonin inhibitors, induce some weight loss with use. The proposed mechanism is through stimulation of central 5-HT_{2c} receptors. Lorcaserin is an FDA-approved example of this type of drug.

Description

Lorcaserin is a 5-hydroxytryptamine-**2c**-receptor agonist that stimulates α-MSH production from POMC neurons that activates the Melanocortin 4 Receptor (MC4R), thereby increasing satiety. Lorcaserin was approved by the FDA in 2012. It is a DEA schedule IV drug.

Dosage

10 mg twice daily. Discontinue if the person does not achieve 5 % weight loss in the first 12 weeks (nonresponder).

Clinical Evidence

Initially, Lorcaserin was denied FDA approval due to three concerns: the risk of developing tumors, the risk of valvulopathy, and the risk of developing psychiatric disorders. The European Union still has not approved the drug for use. In the United States, the risk for adenocarcinoma in female rats was reviewed by the FDA and it was found that the dose at which it occurs is 87 times the dose in humans. An analysis of three trials found that the 1-year rate of echocardiographic FDA-defined valvulopathy was 2.04 % in the placebo group and 2.37 % in the Lorcaserin group with missing values imputed, which is an insignificant difference [28].

In the BLOOM, BLOSSUM, and BLOOM-DM Trials, a total of 6897 patients aged 18–65 years with BMI ranging from 30 to 45 or 27 to 29.9 kg/m^2 plus one or more obesity-related diseases were randomized to placebo or Lorcaserin 10 mg twice daily. The Lorcaserin treated group achieved a mean weight loss of 10.6 kg (if they did not have diabetes) versus 9.3 kg (if they had diabetes).

In these trials the people who lost more than 4.5 % total body weight by week 12 were responders at week 52, losing 10.22 % of their weight versus 2.46 % if there was no response in 12 weeks. Lorcaserin also showed significantly decreased waist circumference, diastolic blood pressure, total cholesterol, and triglycerides [29] (Fig. 10.6).

Safety Warnings

- Use caution if the person is on any of the following medications:
  - Selective serotonin reuptake inhibitors
  - Serotonin–norepinephrine reuptake inhibitors
  - Monoamine oxidase inhibitors
  - Triptans
  - Bupropion
  - Dextromethorphan
  - *St. John's Wort*
- Signs or Symptoms of heart valve disease
- There is potential for cognitive impairment—this may not be the best drug for someone who operates heavy machinery as both attention and memory may be affected.
- Psychiatric disorders, especially if predisposed to depression or suicidal thoughts

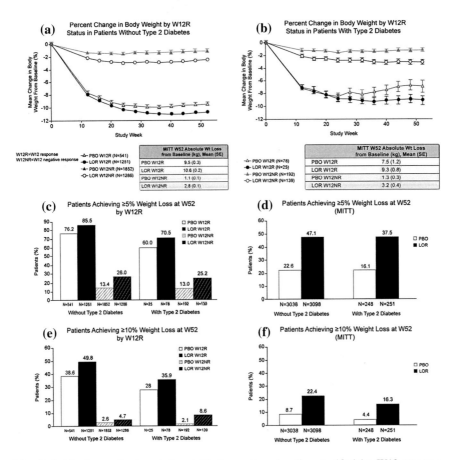

Fig. 10.6 Absolute and categorical weight change from baseline stratified by W12 response. LOR, lorcaserin; PBO, placebo; R, responders; W12NR, nonresponders (<5 % weight loss) at week 12; W12R, responders (>5 % weight loss) at week 12 (from Smith et al. [29], with permission)

- May produce hypoglycemia if the patient is diabetic
- Men with a history of priapism or a predisposition to it
- Pregnancy or Nursing Mothers (Pregnancy Category X)

Metabolism of Drug

Lorcaserin is metabolized in the liver and its metabolites are excreted in the urine.

Side Effects

The side effects can include headache, dizziness, fatigue, nausea, dry mouth, constipation, cough, reduced heart rate, and hyperprolactinemia.

Liraglutide (Saxenda)

Endogenous glucagon-like peptide-1 (GLP-1) that has an effect on the brain of creating satiety.

Description

The FDA-approved GLP-1 analogues Exenatide and Liraglutide are approved for treatment of Type 2 Diabetes Mellitus (T2DM) and have been observed to cause weight loss. Based on this observed effect on obesity and the safety profile, Liraglutide underwent large-scale clinical trials in nondiabetic patients to determine the effectiveness of the drug on weight loss. The mechanism of weight loss appears to be through reduced appetite and energy intake similar to endogenous GLP-1. Liraglutide has 97 % homology to human GLP-1.

Liraglutide comes in two different formulations with different names: Victoza, which is utilized for the treatment of diabetic patients at a dose of 1.2–1.8 mg injections daily; and Saxenda, which is used in nondiabetic patients at a dose of 3.0 mg injected daily.

Clinical Evidence

A trial to establish dosing was conducted in 564 adults with a BMI from 30 to 40 kg/m^2. Patients established a 500 kcal energy deficit and were asked to increase physical activity. Mean weight loss with different dosing regimens showed Liraglutide at 3.0 mg daily has the highest weight loss (7.2 kg) compared to a placebo and Orlistat. Patients who lost more than 5 % of their weight with 3.0 mg daily of Liraglutide were 76 %, versus 30 % with placebo and 44 % with Orlistat [30]. Additional follow up of 2 years showed the patients on 3.0 mg of Liraglutide maintained their weight and lost about 3 kg more weight than those on Orlistat [31].

The SCALE trial was a 56-week double blind trial involving 3731 overweight or obese patients who did not have T2DM and who met criteria for treatment with a medication. Liraglutide at a dose of 3 mg daily by injection was administered to 2487 patients once daily versus administration of a placebo to 1244 patients against a background of lifestyle modification. A total of 61.2 % of patients had intermediate diabetes (also referred to as prediabetes). A total of 63.2 % of patients in the Liraglutide group versus 27.1 % of patients in the placebo group lost at least

5 % of their weight, and 33.1 % and 10.6 %, respectively, lost more than 10 % of their body weight. Both groups were significantly different $p < 0.0001$. The most frequent side effect was mild or moderate nausea and diarrhea. In addition there is a concern about having a higher number of breast cancers diagnosed in the Liraglutide group versus placebo. No cases of C-cell carcinomas of the thyroid or elevated calcitonin levels were observed [32] (Fig. 10.7).

Contraindications

Saxenda is contraindicated in patients who are pregnant or who experienced previous serious hypersensitivity to Liraglutide or related products. Saxenda is contraindicated in a patient with a personal or family history of medullary thyroid cancer, or Multiple Endocrine Neoplasia Syndrome type 2 (MEN 2). Patients need to be counseled to check for neck mass, dysphagia, dyspnea, or persistent hoarseness.

Safety Warnings for Saxenda

- Saxenda should not be used to treat diabetes.
- Saxenda should not be used with insulin.
- Liraglutide causes dose-dependent and treatment duration-dependent thyroid C-cell tumors in rats and mice. The relevance of this to Saxenda is unknown.
- Two medications Saxenda and Victoza share the same key ingredient, liraglutide, and should not be used together.
- Saxenda has not been studied with other products used for weight loss including OTC, herbal preparations, or other prescription medication.
- Saxenda has not been studied in patients with a history of pancreatitis.
- The effects of Saxenda on cardiovascular mortality and morbidity have not been established.
- Patients on Saxenda have a higher risk of having gallstones.
- A Saxenda cause delayed gastric emptying and has potential to impact absorption of other oral medications.

Metabolism

Slowly metabolized by dipeptidyl peptidase-4 [33].

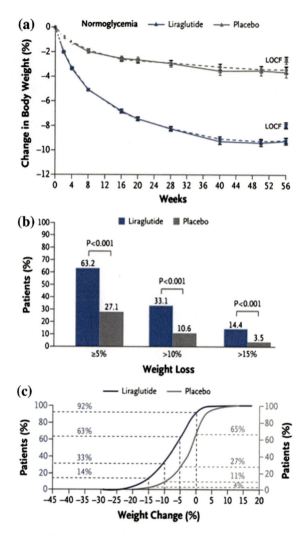

Fig. 10.7 Liraglutide and body weight. **Panel a** shows the mean body weight for patients in the full-analysis set who completed each scheduled visit, according to presence or absence of prediabetes at screening. I bars indicate standard error, and the separate symbols above the curves represent the 56-week weight change using last-observation-carried-forward (LOCF) imputation. The full-analysis set comprised patients who underwent randomization, were exposed to at least one treatment dose, and had at least one assessment after baseline (69 patients were excluded from the full-analysis set: 61 owing to lack of an assessment and 8 owing to no exposure). **Panel b** shows the proportions of patients who lost at least 5 %, more than 10 %, and more than 15 % of their baseline body weight. Data shown are the observed means for the full-analysis set (with LOCF). Findings from logistic regression analysis showed an odds ratio of 4.8 (95 % confidence interval [CI], 4.1–5.6) for at least 5 % weight loss and an odds ratio of 4.3 (95 % CI, 3.5–5.3) for more than 10 % weight loss; the analysis of more than 15 % weight loss was performed post hoc (odds ratio, 4.9 [95 % CI, 3.5–6.7]). **Panel c** shows the cumulative percentage of patients with those changes in body weight after 56 weeks of treatment (from Pi-Sunyer et al. [32], with permission)

Side Effects

Increased heart rate of 2–3 beats per minute, renal insufficiency or failure, hypersensitivity reactions, suicidal behavior and ideation, severe hypoglycemia.

The 2015 approval of Liraglutide for weight loss seems to offer new hope that medications may be helpful in combating obesity, although pharmaceutical treatment of any kind is not without side effects and potential complications. The use of Liraglutide requires a patient to face daily injections at high expense not offset by insurance. In addition, patients who were already obese in the trial remained obese (BMI ≥ 30 kg/m^2) but less so. There was no quantification of the effect on metabolic syndrome. Longer follow up will be required to determine the effect on breast cancer and rule out any side effects that were not apparent at 56 weeks of follow up [34].

Orlistat (Xenical, Alli)

Orlistat (Xenical) is a pancreatic lipase inhibitor that impairs about 30 % of gastrointestinal absorption of fat at a dosage of 60 or 120 mg three times per day. It is approved by the FDA for long-term use as a monotherapy with approximately 3 % weight loss over placebo. *It is Pregnancy Category X*. Most of the side effects include problems with impaired absorption, including flatus with discharge, increased number of defecations, fecal incontinence, and risk of urinary and cholelithiasis and malabsorption of fat soluble vitamins, resulting in potential deficiencies. *The most significant serious side effect is rare reports of severe liver injury.* Nevertheless, a recent report established the long-term evidence for safety of the medication [35]. The limitations of use have been concerns over the question of liver injury and the side effects that can have an effect on lifestyle. The OTC variation is Alli and is available for purchase through the internet. Orlistat is the only agent approved in the European Union for weight loss [36].

Combination medications, as opposed to monotherapies, are designed to use a combination of lower dose medications to create synergistic actions and to reduce side effects.

Phentermine/Topiramate (Qnexa, Qsymia)

Description

The phentermine component acts as a sympathomimetic amine that releases norepinephrine and blunts appetite, while the topiramate increases GABA and prolongs satiety.

This combination medication was initially studied under the name Qnexa, but was not approved by the FDA in 2010 because of concerns about cardiac problems, birth defects, and cognitive effects. In 2012, the FDA approved the medication provided a Risk Evaluation and Mitigation Strategy (REMS) was in place and the company changed the name to Qsymia. Phentermine/Topiramate (Qsymia) is currently FDA approved, is a level IV drug *and is a Pregnancy Category X drug.*

Dosage

Dosing begins with a low dose of phentermine 3.75 mg/topiramate ER 23 mg daily for 2 weeks. Advance is to the treatment dose of phentermine 7.5 mg/topiramate ER 46 mg daily. After 12 weeks, if the patient fails to lose >3 % weight, then the patient is either advanced to the higher dose if being tolerated. If not tolerated it is discontinued and another medication may be considered. The maximum dose is phentermine 15 mg and topiramate ER 92 mg daily. *This medication requires a Risk Evaluation and Mitigation Strategy (REMS) in order to address the concerns about fetal malformations caused by topiramate.* In order to prescribe Qsymia, the provider must use a certified pharmacy and be trained in the use of the drug. The training includes counseling of women of childbearing age regarding the potential for fetal oral and cleft malformations as well as counseling on the use of birth control and pregnancy testing prior to starting the mediation and monthly thereafter.

Clinical Evidence

In a trial comparing Phentermine/Topiramate ER 7.5/46 mg to either placebo or phentermine alone at a dose of 7.5 or 15 mg daily, the combination drug resulted in significantly higher weight loss: 8.46 kg at 28 weeks [37].

Three trials of the combination drug phentermine/topiramate have been done. These include the CONQUER, SEQUEL, and EQUIP studies. SEQUEL was an extension of the CONQUER trial that extended study to 2 years. The CONQUER trial was a 56 week trial of 2487 adults aged 18–70 years with a BMI of 27–45 kg/m^2 and two or more obesity-related diseases. The three arms of the trial compared placebo to phentermine 7.5/topiramate 46 mg or phentermine 15/topiramate 92 mg. The patients were randomly assigned and all parties were blinded to the treatment. Weight loss was achieved by 21 % of patients in the placebo group versus 62 % in the phentermine 7.5/topiramate 46 mg dose and 70 % (10.2 kg weight loss) with phentermine 7.5/topiramate 92 mg dose.

SEQUEL demonstrated long-term weight control out to 108 weeks with weight loss maintenance of −10.5 % for the phentermine 15/topiramate controlled release 92 mg daily dose regimen. There were fewer adverse events between weeks 56 and 108 [38].

The EQUIP trial demonstrated that PHEN/TPM DR compared at either 15 mg/92 mg or 3.75 mg/23 mg showed significantly greater weight loss than the placebo: 10.9 %, 5.1 % and 1.6 %, respectively, with 48 % losing more than 15 % body weight at 15 mg/92 mg. Adverse events caused discontinuation of the medication in less than 1 % of patients. The study had a drop out rate of 40 %, which is consistent with drop out rates of other obesity medications and traditional treatment trials [39].

Contraindications

Phentermine/Topiramate has the following contraindications: glaucoma, hyperthyroidism, during or within 14 days of taking a MOA inhibitor, pregnancy or nursing. In additional trials there were no serious adverse events related to depression, cognition, or anxiety and this medication can be used in patients with stable depression and on selective serotonin reuptake inhibitors.

Safety Warnings

> Fetal toxicity
> Discontinue the medication for unacceptable increases in adrenergic responses, such as an increase in heart rate, especially in patients with a history of cerebrovascular or cardiac disease.
> An increase in suicidal behavior and ideation may occur
> Acute myopia and secondary angle closure glaucoma
> Cognitive Impairment
> Pregnancy or nursing
> Metabolic acidosis
> Hypoglycemia with diabetes medications
> Elevation in Creatine

Side Effects

Side effects include paresthesias, dizziness, change in taste of food, insomnia, constipation, and dry mouth.

Naltrexone SR/Bupropion SR (NB) (CONTRAVE)

Description

Naltrexone is an opioid antagonist used clinically to treat alcohol and opioid addiction. Naltrexone blocks the POMC receptor system. Bupropion is a dopamine and norepinephrine reuptake inhibitor used to treat nicotine dependence, depression, and seasonal affective disorder. Bupropion had been trialed as a monotherapy and was revealed to stimulate opioid mediated pathways that limited its weight loss effect. The combination of Bupropion with Naltrexone, however, was revealed to act on the opioid pathway targeting both the MC4R pathway to create satiety but also affecting the reward pathway in order to change food cravings and control food intake. The two drugs in combination have a synergistic effect on the reward system. The FDA approval of the drug is contingent on postmarketing evaluation of cardiovascular outcomes. *It is a Pregnancy Category X combination drug.*

Dosage

The formulation is 8 mg of Naltrexone and 90 mg Bupropion. In the first week, the patient takes only one tablet in the morning. Beginning in week two, the patient takes one tablet in the morning and one at night. The subsequent dosing in week three is two tablets in the morning and one in the evening. Final dosing in week four and beyond is two tablets in the morning and two tablets in the evening.

Clinical Evidence

NB has been extensively studied. A summary of the major papers and weight loss result is set forth in Table 10.11.

Contraindications

Do not use in patients with uncontrolled hypertension, who have a known allergy or who are using any other bupropion-containing products. Do not use in patients with

Table 10.11 Summary of phase III clinical trial data on sustained-release naltrexone/bupropion (NB)

Trial	Number of patients/time	Effect on weight loss in completers (mean vs. placebo)
COR-I [40]	$N = 1742$ 56 weeks	8.1 versus 1.8 %
COR-II [41]	$N = 1496$ 56 weeks	8.2 versus 1.4 %
COR-BMOD [42]	$N = 793$ 56 weeks Both groups intensive lifestyle modification	11.55 versus 7.3 %
COR-DM [43]	$N = 505$ 56 weeks Type 2 diabetics	5.9 versus 2.2 %

COR Contrave obesity research; *BMOD* Behavioral modification; *DM* Diabetes mellitus seizure disorders, anorexia nervosa or bulimia or who are about to abruptly discontinue alcohol, benzodiazepines, barbiturates, and antiepileptic drugs. Patients cannot take this medication within 14 days after or during treatment with an MAO inhibitor. Patients with chronic opioid use should also be excluded from taking this particular medication.

Safety Warnings

- There is an increased risk of hypertension with MOA inhibitors.
- Dose with caution in drugs that lower seizure threshold
- CNS toxicity can result when used with levodopa and amantadine (dopaminergic drugs)
- Can cause false positive urine tests for amphetamines
- CYP286 interactions
  - CYP286 inhibitors like carbamazepine, phenobarbital, and phenytoin may reduce effectiveness of weight loss by reducing bupropion exposure and these drugs should be avoided.
  - Since bupropion inhibits CYP286, medications that depend on CYP286 for metabolism may have increased concentrations: specifically SSRI's and tricyclic's; antipsychotics, e.g., haloperidol, risperidone and thioridazine; and cardiovascular drugs, e.g., Beta blockers and Type 1C antiarrhythmics.

Metabolism

Both primary drugs and metabolites of naltrexone are active ingredients and cytochrome P450 enzymes metabolize neither. The kidney excretes these metabolites. Bupropion and its metabolites inhibit CYP286 isoenzymes which is the primary pathway of metabolism of many antidepressants. Bupropion is excreted in the urine (87 %) and feces (10 %).

Side Effects

Side effects include nausea, vomiting, dizziness, insomnia, diarrhea, dry mouth, constipation, and headache.

Nutraceuticals

Manipulation of the intestinal microflora has been attempted in medicine for many years and for many reasons. It has become the subject of increasing focus in obesity research as the importance of the microbiome to health has become more fully appreciated. Prebiotics, probiotics, and synbiotics all may play a role in improving health.

A **prebiotic** is a nondigestible food ingredient that promotes the growth of beneficial microorganisms in the intestines. Prebiotics occur naturally in foods such as leeks, asparagus, chicory, Jerusalem artichokes, garlic, onions, wheat, oats, and soybeans. Typical US and European diets include about 2 g of prebiotics/day [44].

Probiotics are beneficial live microorganisms (and in most cases bacteria) that are similar to microorganisms that live in the intestine. They are taken as dietary supplements by consumers and may contain a mixed variety of microorganisms.

Synbiotics combine prebiotics and probiotics in dietary supplements that create a form of synergism. The combination requires constant surveillance to ensure effectiveness because the probiotics can change, due to a natural tendency of bacteria to mutate based on changes in food source and pH [45].

In a meta-analysis of randomized controlled trials, prebiotic supplementation resulted in a reduction of total cholesterol, LDL-c, and triglycerides and increased HDL-c in overweight or obese individuals with diabetes. Synbiotic supplements can reduce fasting insulin and triglyceride levels [46].

There is limited safety data or general data on how prebiotics, probiotics, and synbiotics may affect other medical problems. Moreover, due to the diversity and variability of the microbiome within individuals, the effects may vary. To date, the FDA has not approved any health claims related to prebiotics, probiotics, or synbiotics [47].

Medications as Related to Bariatric Surgery

Patients who are candidates for bariatric surgery are often taking obesity-related medications for management of their health. Part of the initial assessment and strategy for bariatric surgery is to evaluate what medications the patient is already taking, and whether those medications need to be changed in any way in light of the surgery.

Bariatric surgery results in profound and rapid changes in the microbiome of the gut, which in turn leads to alternations that change the absorption of medications and can affect the efficacy of established dosing regimens and formulations of medications (long acting vs. short acting). In addition, the radical change in a patient's food intake after bariatric surgery is both immediate and profound, introducing an urgency in the management of medications that affect blood sugar and anticoagulation. Many medications may need to be rapidly discontinued, changed to shorter acting variations, or changed to a different medication. A recommendation has been made that a therapeutic drug monitoring process be put into place for certain classes of drugs until stable doses are established after bariatric/gastric bypass surgery (RYGB) [48]. In any event, any changes in medication or dosing should be done in consultation with the patient, the primary care physician and the surgeon.

Conclusion

Medications for weight loss offer patients with moderate weight gain (BMI ≥ 27 kg/m^2) an opportunity to reverse weight gain and obesity-related disease. Effectiveness ranges to 11 % in combination with traditional therapy. Therapies that have the ability to reverse or interrupt epigenetic changes or genetic propensities for obesity have yet to be realized. The three most significant limitations of pharmaceuticals are the drop out rate of 40 % in most trials, the serious side effects, and the patient's inability to lose enough weight to meet his/her expectations. Even when medications have been approved, there is very slow adoption of pharmaceutical therapy among patients in the United States.

References

1. Rowe S, Siegel D, Benjamin DK. Best pharmaceuticals for children act-pediatric trials network administrative core committee. Gaps in drug dosing for obese children: a systematic review of commonly prescribed emergency care medications. Clin Ther. 2015;37(1):1924–32.
2. Quidley AM, Bland CM, Bookstaver PB, Kuper K, et al. Am J Health Syst Pharm. 2014;71(15):1253–64.
3. Sankaralingam S, Kim RB, Padwal RS. The impact of obesity on the pharmacology of medications used for cardiovascular risk factor control. Can J Cardiol. 2015;31(2):167–76.
4. Cheymol G. Effects of obesity on pharmacokinetics implications for drug therapy. Clin Pharmacokinet. 2000;39(3):215–31.
5. Tucker CE, Lockwood AM, Nguyen NH. Antibiotic dosing in obesity: the search for optimum dosing strategies. Clin Obes. 2014;4(6):287–95.
6. Lynn LA, Curry JP. Patterns of unexpected in-hospital deaths: a root cause analysis. Patient Saf Surg. 2011;5(1):3. http://www.pssjournal.com/content/5/1/3.
7. Leslie WS, Hankey CR, Lean ME. Weight gain as an adverse effect of some commonly prescribed drugs: a systematic review. QJM. 2007;100(7):395–404.
8. Manu P, Dima L, Shulman M, VanCampfort D, De Hert M, Correll CU. Weight gain and obesity in schizophrenia: epidemiology, pathobiology and management. Acta Psychiatr Scand. 2015;132(2):97–108.
9. Reekie J, Hosking SP, Prakash C, Kao KT, Juonala M, Sabin MA. The effect of antidepressants and antipsychotics on weight gain in children and adolescents. Obes Rev. 2015;16(7):566–80.
10. Cheng V, Kashyap SR. Weight considerations in pharmacotherapy for type 2 diabetes. J Obes. 2011. doi:10.1155/2011/984245.

11. Inzucchi SE, Bergenstal RM, Buse JB, Diamant M, Ferrannini E, Nauck M, Peters AL, Tsapas A, Wender R, Matthews DR. Management of hyperglycemia in type 2 diabetes, 2015: a patient-centered approach: update to a position statement of the American diabetes association and the European association for the study of diabetes. Diabetes Care. 2015;38:140–9.
12. Bray GA. Medical therapy for obesity-current status and future hopes. Med Clin North Am. 2007;91(6):1225–53.
13. Bhasin S, Wallace W, Lawrence JB, Lesch M. Sudden death associated with thyroid hormone abuse. Am J Med. 1981;71:887–90.
14. AMA Council on Pharmacy and Chemistry. Dinitrophenol not acceptable for N.N.R. JAMA. 1935;105:31–3.
15. Asher WL. Mortality rate in patients receiving "diet pills". Curr Ther Res. 1972;14:525–39.
16. Gurtner HP. Aminorex and pulmonary hypertension. A review. Cor Vasa. 1985;27:160–71.
17. Connolly HM, Crary JL, McGoon MD, Hensrud DD, Edwards BS, Edwards WD, Schaff HV. Valvular heart disease associated with fenfluramine phentermine. N Engl J Med. 1997;337:581–8.
18. Kernan WN, Viscoli CM, Brass LM, Broderick JP, Brott T, Feldmann E, Morgenstern LB, Wilterdink JL, Horwitz RI. Phenylpropanolamine and the risk of hemorrhagic stroke. N Engl J Med. 2000;343:1826–32.
19. Haller CA, Benowitz NL. Adverse cardiovascular and central nervous system events associated with dietary supplements containing ephedra alkaloids. N Engl J Med. 2000;343:1833–8.
20. Heal DJ, Gosden J, Smith SL. Regulatory challenges for new drugs to treat obesity and comorbid metabolic disorders. Br J Clin Pharmacol. 2009;68:861–74.
21. James WPT, Caterson ID, Coutinho W, Finer N, Van Gaal LF, Maggioni AP, et al. Effect of sibutramine on cardiovascular outcomes in overweight and obese subjects. N Engl J Med. 2010;363:905–17.
22. Saper RB, Eisenberg DM, Phillips RS. Common dietary supplements for weight loss. Am Fam Physician. 2004;70:1731–8.
23. Pektezel MY, Bas DF, Topcuoglu MA, Arsava EM. Paradoxical consequence of human chorionic gonadotropin misuse. J Stroke Cerebrovasc Dis. 2015;24(1):e17–9.
24. Van Dorsselaer A, Carapito C, Delalande F, Schaeffer-Reiss C, Theirse D, Diemer H, et al. Detection of prion protein in urine-derived injectable fertility products by a targeted proteomic approach. PLoS One. 2011;6(3):e17815.
25. Bays HE. Current and investigational antiobesity agents and obesity therapeutic treatment targets. Obes Res. 2004;12:1197–211.
26. Valentino MA, Colon-Gonzalez F, Lin JE, Waldman SA. Current trends in targeting the hormonal regulation of appetite and energy balance to treat obesity. Expert Rev Endocrinol Metab. 2010;5(5):765–83.
27. Thomas K. Top-selling diet drug phentermine is cheap and easy to get. NYT, Business Day Section. 4 July 2015.
28. Manning S, Pucci A, Finer N. Pharmacotherapy for obesity: novel agents and paradigms. Ther Adv Chronic Dis. 2014;5(3):135–48.
29. Smith SR, O'Neil PM, Astrup A, Finer N, Sanchez-Kam M, Fraher K, et al. Early weight loss while on lorcaserin, diet and exercise as a predictor of week 52 weight-loss outcomes. Obesity. 2014;22:2137–46.
30. Astrup A, Rossner S, Van Gaal L, Rissanen A, Niskanen L, Al Hakim M, et al. Effects of liraglutide in the treatment of obesity: a randomized, double-blind, placebo-controlled study. Lancet. 2009;374:1606–16.
31. Astrup A, Carraro R, Finer N, Harper A, Kunesova M, Lean M, et al. Safety, tolerability and sustained weight loss over 2 years with the once 0-daily human GLP-1 analog, liraglutide. Int J Obes (Lond). 2012;36:843–54.

32. Xavier Pi-Sunyer, Astrup A, Fujioka K, Greenway F, Halpern A, Krempf M, et al. A randomized, controlled trial of 3.0 mg of liraglutide in weight management. N Eng J Med. 2015;373(1):11–22.
33. Malm-Erjefalt M, Bjornsdottir I, Vanggaard J, Helleberg H, Larsen U, Oosterhuis B, et al. Metabolism and excretion of the once-daily human glucagon-like peptide-1 analog liraglutide in healthy male subjects and its in vitro degradation by dipeptidyl peptidase IV and neutral endopeptidase. Drug Metab Dispos. 2010;38(11):1944–53.
34. Siraj ES, Williams KJ. Another agent for obesity-will this time be different? N Engl J Med. 2015;3(73):82–3.
35. Halpern B, Halpern A. Safety assessment of FDA-approved (Orlistat and Lorcaserin) anti-obesity medications. Expert Opin Drug Saf. 2015;14(2):305–15.
36. Torgerson JS, Hauptman J, Boldrin MN, Sjöström L. Xenical in the prevention of diabetes in obese subjects (XENDOS) study. Diabetes Care. 2004;27:155–61.
37. Arrone LJ, Wadden TA, Peterson C, Winslow D, Odeh S, Gadde KM. Evaluation of phentermine and topiramate versus phentermine/topiramate extended-release in obese adults. Obesity. 2013;21(11):2163–71.
38. Garvey WT. New tools for weight-loss therapy enable a ore robust medical model for obesity treatment: rationale for a complications-centric approach. Endocr Pract. 2013;19(5):864–74.
39. Allison DB, Gadde KM, Garvey WT, Peterson CA, Schwiers ML, Najarian T, et al. Controlled-release phentermine/topiramate in severely obese adults: a randomized controlled trial (EQUIP). Obesity (Silver Spring). 2012;20(2):330–42.
40. Greenway FL, Fujioka K, Plodkowski RA, et al. Effect of naltrexone plus bupropion on weight loss in overweight and obese adults (COR-1): a multicenter, randomized, double-blind placebo-controlled, phase 3 trial. Lancet. 2010;376:595–605.
41. Apovian CM, Aronne L, Rubino D, et al. A randomized, phase 3 trial of naltrexone SR/bupropion SR on weight and obesity-related risk factors (COR-II). Obesity (Silver Spring). 2013;21:935–43.
42. Wadden TA, Foreyt JP, Foster GD, et al. Weight loss with naltrexone SR/bupropion SR combination therapy as an adjunct to behavior modification: the COR BMOD trial. Obesity (Silver Spring). 2011;19:110–20.
43. Hollander P, Gupta AK, Plodkowski R, et al. Effects of naltrexone sustained-release/bupropion sustained-release combination therapy on body weight and glycemic parameters in overweight and obese patients with type 2 diabetes. Diabetes Care. 2013;36:4033–9.
44. Slavin J. Fiber and prebiotics: mechanisms and health benefits. Nutrients. 2013;5:1417–35.
45. Adebola OO, Corcoran O, Morgan WA. Synbiotics: the impact of potential prebiotics inulin, lactulose and lactobionic acid on the survival and growth of lactobacilli probiotics. J Funct Foods. 2014;10:75–84.
46. Beserra BT, Fernandes R, doRosario VA, Mocellin MC, Kuntz MG, Trindade EB. A systematic review and meta-analysis of the prebiotics and synbiotics effects on glycaemia, insulin concentrations and lipid parameters in adult patients with overweight and obesity. Clin Nutr. 2014. doi:10.1016/jclnu.2014.10.004.
47. Probiotics. Agency for Healthcare Research and Quality, Rockville, MD. Oct 2014. http://www.ahrq.gov/research/findings/evidence-based-reprots/er200-abstract.html.
48. Srinivas NR. Impact of Roux-en-Y gastric bypass on pharmacokinetics of administered drugs: implications and perspectives. Am J Ther. 2015;PMID:26398718.

Chapter 11
Bariatric Surgery

Key Message

Metabolic and bariatric surgery reverses the pathophysiological effects of obesity and results in significant, sustained weight loss and improvement or remission of obesity-related disease. In other words, surgery essentially reverses the primary defect of adiposopathy or "sick fat" and results in varying degrees of improvement or remission of every disease associated with obesity. Outcomes depend upon the specific surgical procedure utilized, the device utilized, and patient factors. Metabolic and bariatric surgery is so effective against obesity and related disease, particularly type 2 diabetes (T2DM), that it has been called one of the most effective therapies in medicine. The utilization of surgery is limited, however. Patients with obesity must be medically eligible for surgery in the first place, but even then, less than 1 % of eligible patients have access to surgical therapy for a variety of reasons.

Every aspect of bariatric surgery is covered in this chapter, including (1) the indications and contraindications for surgery, (2) the preoperative physical, social and psychological assessments of the patient that should be done prior to surgery, (3) the procedures for obtaining informed consent, and (4) the potential complications of surgery, including the primary 30 day complications for each surgical procedure. This chapter also includes a complete description of the mechanism of action of MBS. It also contains a detailed description of the major surgical procedures approved for use in the United States and the major surgical "devices" approved by the FDA for use in obesity treatment, including the (Laparoscopic (or open) Roux-en Y Gastric Bypass (LRYGB), the Laparoscopic Sleeve Gastrectomy (LSG), the Duodenal Switch/Biliopancreatic Diversion (DS/BPD), the Laparoscopic Adjustable Gastric Band (LAGB), the Gastric Balloon (GB) and the Vagal Blocking Device (VBLOC). Finally, this chapter covers the data on outcomes of MBS on weight loss and obesity-related disease, and the subjects of post-surgical health maintenance and weight regain.

Learning Objectives

1. Identify the mechanism of action of metabolic surgery
2. Distinguish and describe the major surgical procedures currently approved in the United States
3. Describe the surgical devices approved by the FDA for use in obesity treatment
4. Summarize the primary 30 day complications for each procedure
5. Summarize the outcomes of weight loss and obesity-related disease for each approved procedure and understand the recommendations for post-surgical health maintenance, and the incidence and evaluation of weight regain after bariatric devices and procedures
6. Use the knowledge of procedure outcomes to counsel patients about risk-benefit for surgical management of obesity and related disease

Bariatric surgery is that group of surgical procedures that are performed to intervene in the state of obesity. Laparoscopic or minimally invasive techniques (MIS) for doing the procedures are utilized in 98.5 % of primary bariatric cases [1]. Primary cases are defined as the first bariatric intervention a patient undergoes. The intervention can be a medical device or a procedure.

Bariatric surgery includes the use of medical devices approved by the Federal Food and Drug Administration (FDA). Examples of such devices are the adjustable gastric band (AGB) and the more recently approved gastric balloon (GB) and the vagal nerve blocking device (VBLOC). The AGB and VBLOC are placed laparoscopically, whereas the GB is placed endoscopically. All three are usually done as outpatient procedures. The effects of these devices on obesity and related disease are related to the weight loss itself that the devices induce. At one time the adjustable gastric band (AGB) accounted for as much as 37 % of bariatric surgery cases in the United States, but a recent review of case types in an academic center shows the percentage has dropped to 0.8 % [1] (Table 11.1).

In addition to device procedures, bariatric surgery also includes *metabolic procedures* that reverse the pathophysiological effects of obesity as a primary action and, in addition, result in significant sustained weight loss and improvement or remission of obesity-related disease. The improvement or remission of obesity-related disease is often more profound than the weight loss itself and the disease may not reoccur even when weight is partially regained [3, 4].

There is no formal approval process for these procedures on a governmental basis. The American Society for Metabolic and Bariatric Surgery (ASMBS),

Table 11.1 Devices approved by the FDA

Description	Abbreviation	Notes
Laparoscopic adjustable gastric band[a]	AGB	0.8 % of current cases in academic centers Approved for use in BMI of ≥ 30 kg/m^2 [2]
Endoscopic gastric balloon	GB	Recent approval for BMI of ≥ 30 kg/m^2
Vagal blocking device	VBLOC	Recent approval for BMI of ≥ 35 kg/m^2 plus one obesity-related disease

[a]http://www.fda.gov/MedicalDevices/ProductsandMedicalProcedures/ObesityDevices/ucm350134.htm

Table 11.2 Metabolic bariatric surgery procedures approved by ASMBS

Description	Abbreviation	Percentage of current cases[a] (%)
Laparoscopic vertical sleeve gastrectomy	LVSG or LSG	60.7
Laparoscopic (open) gastric bypass Roux-en Y	LRYGB ORYGB	37.0, 1.5
Duodenal switch Biliopancreatic diversion	DS BPD	<3

[a]From Varela and Nguyen [2]

however, has put in place a process to evaluate the data from these procedures and to determine if the data supports safety and efficacy. ASMBS-approved metabolic and bariatric surgery procedures make up the majority of the procedures currently utilized in the United States [2] (Table 11.2).

In some cases new and experimental procedures may be performed in situations where insufficient data exists to support short or long-term safety or effectiveness. Physicians and patients should be cautious about referring patients or going to centers where procedures are being performed without sufficient scientific and experimental support unless the patient is fully informed and the procedure is conducted as part of a clinical trial under the supervision of an Institutional Review Board (IRB) that requires data on safety and efficacy to be reported.

Metabolic surgical *procedures*, as opposed to *devices*, are more effective both at achieving and maintaining weight reduction, as well as for having a more beneficial effect on obesity-related disease. This is because metabolic surgical procedures have multiple primary effects on physiology. On the other hand, devices may be safer to place and may be able to be placed in series, i.e., placement followed by removal followed by replacement. The gastric balloon, only approved for six-month intervals, is designed to function in series.

National Accreditation in Metabolic and Bariatric Surgery

The American Society of Metabolic and Bariatric Surgery (ASMBS) initially implemented national accreditation in bariatric surgery for adults in 2005 in response to the growth in demand for procedures. This was followed almost immediately by a similar effort at the American College of Surgeons (ACS). The goal was to improve safety and provide a mechanism for new programs to be developed. In 2012, the ASMBS and ACS merged the two accreditation programs into one national accreditation program: the *Metabolic and Bariatric Surgery Accreditation and Quality Improvement Program* (MBSAQIP). The MBSAQIP offers accreditation for surgeons for both adult and adolescent patients.

National accreditation requires an accredited surgeon with the training and expertise to meet MBSAQIP standards. In an MBSAQIP center, every patient's data and outcomes must be submitted to a national registry by certified clinical abstractors using standardized definitions and methodology. The purpose of collecting this very high quality data is to provide the center a valid platform for quality improvement at the local level. In addition, each program must establish a Metabolic and Bariatric Surgery Committee to review risk-adjusted data and determine steps to improve care. Finally, each program must establish clinical pathways and protocols with a multidisciplinary team, establish and maintain appropriate equipment, and establish surgeon call schedules and ongoing continuing medical education for all program staff to safeguard patients with obesity undergoing surgical treatment. A surgeon site visitor audits all of these elements every 3 years. Currently the MBSAQIP collaborative has over 785 programs in the U.S. [5].

The effect of national accreditation has resulted in achieving a unique level of safety for these elective, highly complex operations in complex patients. Patients and providers are encouraged to seek out these centers to ensure the best opportunity for success [6].

Indications/Contraindications for Surgery

Indications and contraindications for any medical therapy are based on an analysis of the risk of the proposed treatment versus the risk of continuing to have the disease. In the case of bariatric surgery, the risk of nonsurgical traditional therapy is that patients may remain obese and their level of obesity has a natural tendency to increase over time. This often results over time in patients developing obesity-related diseases including cardiovascular disease, type 2 diabetes, and increased risk for cancer.

In 1991, The National Institutes of Health (NIH) established traditional indications for bariatric surgery [7]. The indications established were:

- BMI of 40 kg/m^2 without obesity-related diseases or
- BMI of 35 kg/m^2 with at least one obesity-related disease
- Previous attempts at weight loss.

The NIH guideline was updated in 1998, but remained relatively unchanged [8]. The most recent guideline was published by the American Heart Association in association with other societies in March of 2011. They are also relatively unchanged from the NIH guidelines but include the recommendation to refer patients with a BMI over 35 to a bariatric surgeon for evaluation [9]. Multiple other societies have supported the use of bariatric surgery, including the American Diabetes Association [10], the American Association of Clinical Endocrinologists (July 2011) [11] the International Diabetes Federation (June 2011) [12]; the U.S. Internal Revenue Service (IRS) [13]; and the Centers for Medicare and Medicaid Services (CMS) (2006) [14].

There is controversy about the guidelines being BMI-based instead of disease-based. There is also controversy about discounting the significant improvement in the safety of bariatric surgery. In 2004, mortality of 0.5 % (1 in 200) was documented using data that primarily reflected the use of an open abdominal technique [15]. Currently, mortality for a gastric bypass performed laparoscopically is 0.06 (1 in 1750) in a nationally accredited bariatric center. This mortality is lower than laparoscopic cholecystectomy mortality [16]. Likewise, morbidity has also improved (21 % vs. 5.5 %) [17]. Clearly the "risk" aspect of the risk-benefit equation has changed.

Despite the fact that our knowledge of obesity has profoundly evolved, our indications for the use of metabolic/bariatric surgery have not. We are still using a gross measure of BMI as a surgical threshold, even though obesity has been shown to cause obesity-related disease at much lower BMI. In addition, strong data now indicates that the sooner a return-to-normal weight is achieved by a patient, the less long-term impact obesity will have, not only on the future health of the patient, but through the passage of epigenetic material during conception and pregnancy to the patient's children. It is this fundamental change in our understanding that argues for moving away from a BMI approach to a more fundamental analysis to identify and select patients most at risk for future obesity-related disease and prescribe for them intensive traditional medical treatment which may eventually progress to surgical treatment if they do not respond to traditional treatment. Early evaluation and recommendations will likely result in better outcomes of traditional weight loss treatment, as well.

Considerations for obesity-related therapy should take into account the following individual patient factors:

- Specific early signs of adiposopathy

    - Endothelial insulin resistance as indicated by

      Fasting insulin level

    - Hyperleptinemia as indicated by

      Serum leptin levels

    - Fatty liver as indicated by

      Elevated liver functions
      Ultrasound evidence

- Biochemical signs of cardiovascular risk

    - Total cholesterol (TC), low-density lipoprotein cholesterol, high-density lipoprotein cholesterol, (TC/HDL ratio)
    - Triglycerides (TG), TG/HDL ratio
    - HbA1c
    - Homocysteine
    - Lipoprotein A
    - CRP

- Physical factors
    - Immobility (frailty)
    - Joint Pain in lower extremities indicating early sign of inflammation
    - Disability
- End stage disease
    - Type 2 Diabetes
    - Metabolic Syndrome/Poly Cystic Ovarian Syndrome [18]
    - Obstructive Sleep Apnea
    - Steatohepatitis
    - Gastroesophageal Reflux
    - Pulmonary Hypertension
    - Cardiac Disease

A growing body of evidence suggests that the earlier bariatric surgery is utilized, the less risk there is and the better the outcome. Bariatric surgery in the metabolically healthy morbidly obese (MHMO) population achieves remission of early cardiovascular risk factors and improves quality of life [19–21].

True contraindications for metabolic and bariatric surgery are rare, but include active drug or alcohol use, uncontrolled psychiatric disease, binging/bulimia, noncompliance, or inability to give consent or assent. Moreover, a patient with obesity and significant related disease may be challenging and may present an increased risk for surgery. Most significant medical problems previously considered as contraindications, however, like pulmonary hypertension, cirrhosis, uncontrolled diabetes, chronic kidney disease, advanced age, or new cancer diagnosis, can be managed with rehabilitative strategies that allow patients in these categories to achieve safe and effective bariatric surgical outcomes.

It is time to align the recommendation and use of bariatric surgery around the effects it has on the obesity-related diseases it is designed to treat, rather than basing the decision upon a relatively arbitrary gross measure of weight like BMI.

Mechanism of Action of MBS

Disease driven indications should be used to make therapeutic decisions about obesity treatment because metabolic surgery has been shown to work in ways that were completely unexpected. When a patient loses a certain amount of weight with diet and exercise they get hyperphagia rebound, oftentimes resulting in a rapid regain of the weight. *Hyperphagia rebound is missing* in patients who lose weight with bariatric surgery, which is exactly the opposite from what we would expect in the human being adapting to fasting [22]. In addition, the profound decrease in hyperglycemia that a bariatric patient with type 2 diabetes experiences after surgery prompts the question: how do these procedures work?

The traditional hypothesis of mechanism of action for bariatric surgical procedures was based on the assumption that the weight loss resulted from a mechanical food restriction versus the voluntary food restriction of a diet. *This theory of mechanism of action has been largely disproved* [23–26]. In fact, mechanical restriction when it occurs is an undesirable outcome and contributes to less weight loss in an individual patient because it keeps the flow of nutrients from reaching the part of the intestine where the nutrient's effects are maximized [27]. Weight loss itself also has an impact on obesity-related disease. The beneficial effect of surgery that results from weight loss itself is a secondary effect of surgery. One example of this is the decrease in leptin that results from a decrease in body fat percentage [28, 29].

Metabolic bariatric surgical procedures, sleeve gastrectomy, gastric bypass, and duodenal switch/biliopancreatic diversion have been shown to affect a variety of body systems. These procedures impact obesity and related disease in profound ways. The weight loss itself will reverse the defects of sick fat; however these procedures also have mechanisms of therapeutic value that are "weight independent." For example, changes in body systems brought on by bariatric surgical procedures can have a profound effect on cardiovascular risk: reducing lipids, reducing type 2 diabetes, and reducing hypertension [30]. Long term, these reductions are shown to decrease mortality, stroke, and myocardial infarction. An additional benefit is a decrease in cancer occurrence and reoccurrence [31].

Epigenetic Changes

Earlier in this textbook we studied the way epigenetic changes, also called genetic resetting^{TM}, affect the predisposition of an individual to obesity. We are quick to think of these acquired epigenetic changes as a type of long term, static change; however, *epigenetic changes are dynamic*. In fact, it appears that acquired epigenetic changes may be reversible. Epigenetic reversibility has been studied in cancer, including hepatocellular cancer, but researchers are just beginning to understand the role of epigenetic changes in chronic disease and how they can be reversed [32]. New data show that epigenetic changes that lead to non-alcoholic fatty liver disease are reversible with bariatric surgery [33]. Studies are ongoing, but the profound and sustained effect of weight loss and fat loss after bariatric surgery on obesity-related disease argues in favor of reversibility and "genetic resetting^{TM}."

Enteroplasticity

Metabolic procedures manipulate the body systems (like the gut-brain axis) that provide the major source of input to the brain regarding the environment and state of health of the organism. Surgery restructures the internal gastrointestinal anatomy of the microbiome.

This restructuring causes a physiological reaction that "fixes" many of the problems in the gut caused by obesity. The restructuring of the gastrointestinal system alters the response to stimuli. This ability of the gut to make these changes is referred to as the "plasticity of the gut" or "enteroplasticity" [34]. After a metabolic procedure, the gastrointestinal system changes in at least four major ways: (1) morphology, (2) nervous system, (3) gut hormones, and (4) nutrient sensing [35].

The gastrointestinal system includes the entirety of the gut and its microbes. The epithelial cells that line the intestine turn over every 3–5 days and have a unique ability to respond to the stimuli of food [36, 37]. In general, macronutrients are absorbed in the proximal small intestine and micronutrients are absorbed in the ileum or distal intestine. This morphology changes under the pressure of different stimuli, including dietary changes. This was first demonstrated in patients who underwent small bowel resection [37].

Moreover, high-fat diets create changes that contribute to many of the complications of obesity [38]. The alternation of microbiota is one of the drivers of mechanism in the gastric bypass [39]. Gastric bypass in rats has been shown to result in significant morphological changes [40].

Some of these changes involve the enteric nervous system that is independent of the autonomic nervous system and controls motor function of the intestine, blood flow, mucosal transport and secretions, and modulates immune and endocrine function. The enteric nervous system spans the entire gastrointestinal tract [41]. Mice that underwent a gastric bypass where the vagus nerve was spared showed greater weight loss, possibly modulated by the celiac branch of the vagus nerve [42, 43]. Thus, sparing the vagus nerve during the gastric bypass may result in a better outcome.

In addition to the changes caused by bariatric surgery in the nervous system, there is also a major change in the enteroendocrine system. Similar foods result in markedly different increases in GI peptides [44]. The change in the signal produced in response to food may be due to the chronically high gastric emptying rate as a direct result of the changes made in anatomy [45]. Anatomical surgical changes alter the amount and composition of bile acids and nutrient flow in both the laparoscopic vertical sleeve gastrectomy (LVSG), laparoscopic roux-en-y gastric bypass (LRYGB) and duodenal switch/biliopancreatic diversion (DS/BPD). LVSG in particular results in increased flow of bile acids resulting in changes in pH that promote the growth of some bacteria and the death of other strains. Some recent data suggests that bile acid concentrations increase progressively over the first year [46]. Metabolic procedures alter the type of bacteria in the gut to improve downstream effects like insulin sensitivity [47].

With *all* the metabolic surgical procedures there is a change in the signaling of ghrelin, a hormone produced primarily in the stomach. These changes specifically occur in the the acetylated active form of ghrelin. In the duodenal switch/biliopancreatic diversion, the gastric bypass and sleeve gastrectomy there is a marked improvement in hyperglycemia of diabetes. The change in ghrelin signaling may be important in that effect, as demonstrated in the STAMPEDE prospective trial [48].

Finally, food is broken down into nutrients. Nutrients have a dual role as fuel and as signaling molecules. Sensing cells are found not only in the mouth, but throughout the gastrointestinal track as well. Metabolic bariatric procedures alter the way nutrients are sensed in these cells [49].

In summary, metabolic bariatric procedures produce a number of adaptations in the gastrointestinal system that lead to an improvement in obesity and its downstream complications.

Changes in Reward Pathways

There is a debate about whether food is "addictive" to certain people (ones affected by obesity) similar to the way drugs and alcohol can be addictive. This debate is in part fueled by the way in which the neural pathways for drug addiction and food stimulation overlie each other. The neural pathways are different in people who suffer obesity versus those who are lean. However, mounting evidence suggests that the reward pathways in patients with obesity may be able to be "rewired," thus indicating that while there may be a predisposition to food addiction, some of the "food reward" pathways may be reversible.

Food reward behavior is etched into the fabric of human life by the need to find and eat food as a daily necessity. Food reward provides the motivation to overcome almost all adversity in obtaining food. Food reward is one of the most powerful reinforcements of behaviors. During the three recognized phases of this behavior (procurement, consummatory and postconsummatory), the expectancy of a reward created by the brain's neural regulatory systems is the driver. Even in the postconsummatory phase the neural sensors of the gastrointestinal track provide essential chemical signaling to the reward centers of the brain [50]. The entire brain seems to be engaged in the reward processes. Increased consumption of highly palatable sweet or high-fat foods is due to the brain's increased "liking" of the food [51].

Patients with obesity have a different food reward system than lean people. There is an increased "liking" of food as a function of sweetness and increased BMI in patients with obesity as compared to patients who are lean [52]. Interestingly, a low concentration of fat and sugar shows no increase in liking. Patients who exhibit binge-eating behavior show an increased liking for all food [53].

This effect has been compared in obese rats with a sham gastric bypass versus true gastric bypass. The rats with true gastric bypass exhibited a flat concentration–response curve to sweetness or high fat. This relationship held against rats who were never obese, or who were formerly obese with weight reduction through caloric restriction. In short, rats with a gastric bypass exhibited a marked change in their food reward response to sugar and fat [54].

In humans, obesity confers an increased liking and desire for highly palatable sweet and fatty foods. This is augmented by conditions of high stress [55]. Patients who undergo gastric bypass have a sustained change in their food reward system, contributing to the long-term weight reduction seen in these patients. This may be due to a decrease in dopamine signaling [56].

Changes in Energy Expenditure

The body burns energy based on body composition. Weight loss from traditional approaches leads to an eventual decrease in energy expenditure mediated by the brain, a process called metabolic adaptation. This is the primary mechanism of weight regain after voluntary restriction of food (dieting). One of the most paradoxical findings about bariatric surgery, prompting investigation into the true mechanism of action of bariatric surgery, is that body weight-adjusted resting energy expenditure *increases* in humans after gastric bypass by 17.66 % and correlates with weight loss [57]. Resting energy expenditure was increased from 1329 ± 604 kcal/day (55 % of the Harris Benedict predicted expenditure) to 1882 ± 398 kcal/day (88 % of the Harris Benedict predicted expenditure). At the same time, intake dropped to 1373 ± 620 kcal/day at 24 months [58]. In these two studies, resting energy expenditure was measured using indirect calorimetry. In a study using a metabolic chamber, weight-adjusted energy expenditure increased along with a statistically significant increase in respiratory quotient [59].

Changes based on the long-term loss of fat itself is the key to maintaining weight loss because it reverses the negative effects of high leptin levels, hypoxia induced inflammation and improves energy generation. This is why an emphasis on "leaning out" a patient as their post-surgical weight loss progresses is critical to the long term avoidance of weight regain. A robust program of postoperative follow-up needs to focus on helping patients to lower their body fat percentage.

As shown above, the net result of altering the gastrointestinal track by metabolic surgery procedures results in profound changes in the physiology of weight regulation and metabolism [60]. In summary, the mechanism of the effectiveness of bariatric surgery is demonstrated by the following:

- Epigenetic Remodeling [61]
- Enteroplasty: A change in the morphology and microbiome of the intestine
- Changes in nerve signaling to and from the brain—Vagus and Enteric Nervous System
- Changes in the amount and timing of gastrointestinal hormones that provide signaling—Ghrelin, GLP-1, PYY [62]
- Changes in the reward system that promotes food intake
- An increase in energy expenditure [63]
- Changes based on fat loss
    - Changes in signaling of fat-related hormones

        Leptin and Adiponectin [64].

Metabolic and Bariatric Surgery: Procedures and Devices

Bariatric surgery can be classified as *primary or secondary*. Primary bariatric surgery is the index procedure or device placement that a person undergoes. Secondary bariatric surgery is any subsequent procedure or device application.

Devices are either temporary (balloon) or fixed (adjustable gastric band or vagal blocking device). All devices are reversible but may result in permanent alterations in the soft tissue of the upper abdomen or alternations in the function of the esophagus and stomach as a result of the procedures (damage to vagus nerves). Devices yield more weight loss in an individual patient over placebo (10–15 %). Although the weight loss from devices is less than from MBS procedures, devices generally are believed to be safer to apply. Some devices (balloon) can be used in series if weight regain reoccurs. Devices sometimes do not work if the patient has not adopted sound principles of dietary management and exercise. In addition, we are not certain exactly how some devices accomplish weight loss. In general, they are believed to affect physiology less and have a more mechanically driven mechanism of action. For instance, the balloon works primarily through occupying space within the stomach, thereby restricting food intake.The balloon may possibly work through distension and stretch receptor feedback to the brain but these mechanisms are speculative. Both devices and metabolic procedures used to achieve weight loss may be enhanced by the use of medications, but the data on combination therapy (procedure or device plus pharmaceutical) is sparse.

Bariatric surgery can be performed through either an open or laparoscopic approach. The laparoscopic approach is used in almost 96 % of cases and has changed the safety of bariatric surgery in a profound way. For a gastric bypass, the death rate in open procedures is 2.1 % versus laparoscopic 0.2 % [65]. Given the relative safety of using laparoscopic surgery in operating upon patients who are obese, physicians should refer those patients when possible to centers specializing in laparoscopic surgical access.

All procedures begin in a similar way. The patient is placed on an operating room table engineered to support their weight and girth. The table is covered with gel foam pads to protect pressure points, a footboard is placed at the feet, and a pillow is placed under the knees to take away any pressure on the lower back. Straps are placed across the thighs and lower legs for security. The arms are placed upon arm boards and secured. The patient usually will void prior to surgery so placing a Foley catheter is rarely necessary. Once the patient is asleep under general anesthesia, the table is placed in steep reverse Trendelenburg. The operation takes place primarily in the upper part of the abdomen above the umbilicus, which is often displaced in the obese phenotype. The steep tilt of the operating table allows the bulk of the intestines to fall away from the operative field—a technique called gravity assistance.

In laparoscopic cases it is necessary to create an "operating theater" inside the abdomen. A small paper clip-like device called a veress needle is inserted into the abdomen through the left upper quadrant. CO_2 gas is then injected to achieve and maintain distension inside the abdomen, creating space or an "operating theater." The air pocket protects the intestines and other organs from injury when inserting additional trocars through which to place instruments. After the distension is adequate, a 5 mm trocar is placed usually above the umbilicus and just to the left of the midline, using the camera with a zero degree scope to achieve direct vision of all layers of the rectus sheath. The scope is changed to a 30° or 45° scope to enhance visualization. The newly created "operating theater" now has light and a camera. Additional trocars are placed under "direct" observation to minimize any injury to intraabdominal organs or blood vessels. The introduction of 5 and 12.5 mm trocars allows the surgeon and assistant to place long-handled instruments into the abdominal space in order to perform the operation.

The currently utilized procedures and devices are:

1. LRYGB or the laparoscopic Roux-en Y gastric bypass
2. LSG or the laparoscopic sleeve gastrectomy
3. LAGB or the laparoscopic adjustable gastric band (device)
4. DS/BPD or the duodenal switch/biliopancreatic diversion
5. Balloons and the vagal blocking device.

Each procedure and device is discussed in more detail below.

Laparoscopic Roux-en Y Gastric Bypass (LRYGB)

The LRGBP is the best-studied and the most successful operation in the history of bariatric surgery. It was first performed by Edward Mason, MD in Iowa and adapted over time to improve specific complications and enhance efficacy. This procedure is considered by many to be the gold standard in the field of bariatric surgery (Fig. 11.1a, b).

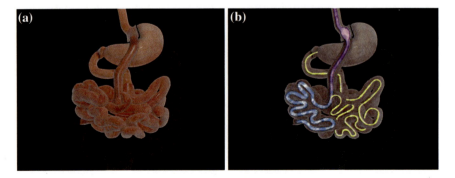

Fig. 11.1 **a** Roux-en-Y gastric bypass. **b** Flow of food and digestive juice (courtesy of Ethicon, Inc.)

Description of LRGBP

Once access to the abdomen is established, as described above, a total of 2–3 5.0 mm trocars and 2–3 12.5 mm trocars are then utilized to perform this operation.

After exploration of the abdomen to identify any unexpected findings, the stomach is divided into two parts, starting from the lesser curve and going up toward the angle of His, which is the junction between the esophagus and stomach. This creates a small gastric pouch connected to the esophagus and completely separates it from the large part of the stomach. Once this is done, food no longer will pass through the stomach. Due to exclusion of the majority of the stomach, patients preparing for gastric bypass often will undergo a screening esophagoduodenoscopy prior to the procedure. The colon is then shifted into the upper abdomen and the Ligament of Treitz, or the beginning of the jejunum, is identified. Counting forward, a length of intestine is measured and then the jejunum is divided. The distal cut end of the jejunum is then brought consistently to the patients' right side and a roux limb length of up to 150 cm is identified. The roux limb is then is reconnected to the proximal end of cut jejunum, creating the jejunal-jejunal anastomosis. All openings between leaves of the intestine (mesentary) are closed with a permanent running suture to prevent herniation. The roux limb is then attached to a drain that allows it to be drawn safely into the upper abdomen behind the colon and stomach and lay on its side against the previously created stomach pouch. Some surgeons perform an antecolic and antegastric roux limb in which case the roux limb and biliopancreatic limbs are usually equal in length. The pouch and jejunal roux limb are then attached to each other and a hand-sewn opening is created between them for the passage of food and liquids. Some surgeons use a stapled anastamosis rather than hand sewn, either with a circular or straight stapler. Food now will pass from the mouth, through the esophagus, and into the small pouch, exiting through the opening between the pouch and jejunal roux limb to the small intestine. Food and fluids take just a few minutes to pass through the small stomach and into the small intestine meaning that food reaches the small intestine very rapidly. Operative time is 126.5 min on average and average length of hospital stay is 2 days [66].

Safety of LRYGB

The current 30-day mortality rate in the National Surgical Quality Improvement Program registry is 0.2 %, morbidity (5.1 %), and reoperations (2.2 %) in a report of 11,617 patients [66]. The readmission rate in this series is is 6.1 % [67].

Complications of LRYGB

The primary concern in the first 24 h is the development of leaks from where the stomach or intestine is divided and reattached, and bleeding. The rate of leak in laparoscopic gastric bypass is currently 0.8 % and 1.5 % in open gastric bypass as reported in a large longitudinal study. Bleeding occurs at an incidence of 1.11 %. The readmission rate is 6.47 % [68]. Laparoscopic RYGB have shorter length of hospital stay, less blood loss and lower mortality as compared with open procedures [65, 69].

Within the first 30 days additional complications may occur. Patients with obesity often have an increased risk for blood clots forming in their legs and sometimes these blood clots break off and float up to block the pulmonary veins or arteries, thereby compromising oxygenation. This is called a pulmonary embolus (PE). These complications are so significant that the patients usually are anticoagulated (the blood made thin by medications) prior to surgery and throughout their hospital stay. In addition, early ambulation is critical. Most patients are up walking every few hours within 6 hours after surgery and must continue ambulating frequently for the first few months after surgery. The incidence of deep venous thrombosis is 0.1 % and PE 0.17 % [68]. The most critical time for a deep venous thrombosis or PE is actually once the patient returns home, making continued ambulation and mobility a key risk factor in preventing complications. There is no indication for vena cava filters; in fact, they tend to increase the rates of complications and bleeding [70].

Additional problems seen in the first 30 days include stricture, usually of the gastrojejunostomy, as well as the nausea/dehydration that arises from the distinct change in eating, and adjustment difficulties.

One of the main differences in complication rates between open and laparoscopic bariatric surgery procedures is in the incidence of surgical site infections (SSI). In open bariatric surgery the rate of infection is as high as 12–16 % versus 4 % in laparoscopic procedures [71, 72, 73]. Longer term complications include marginal ulcer (0.47 %) and bowel obstruction (0.95 %) [68].

Long-term negative effects of surgery can include protein, vitamin, and micronutrient deficiency. The recommendation for daily protein intake after bariatric surgery is 60–120 g daily. This can be difficult for patients to achieve, especially within the first few months after surgery. Patients should be advised to take a daily multivitamin with calcium to supplement their diet and to avoid deficiencies in B vitamins, calcium, and iron. Vitamin D is often deficient prior to surgery and should be replete prior to surgery. Vitamin D should also be included as part of the postoperative regimen. The evaluation and treatment of micronutrient deficiencies is outlined in the manuscript by Bal and associates. [74].

When patients are carrying significant weight their bones are usually healthy. Research indicates that bone mineral density decreases starting as early as the year after surgery, suggesting that attention to fracture prevention may be important especially in the post menopausal woman. [74].

Patients have a risk of developing a new alcohol use disorder (AUD) after bariatric surgery, or of relapsing after previous abstinence. This includes a lifetime risk of alcohol dependence after bariatric surgery of 30.9 % to 33.2 % [75, 76].

Self-harm is an additional concern with a lifetime risk of 3.6 per 1000 patients per year versus 1.2 per 1000 patients per year in the baseline obese population. Self-harm is more prevalent in disadvantaged patients. Ninety three percent of self-harm occurs in patients diagnosed with a mental health disorder during the 5 years prior to surgery.

Benefit of Gastric Bypass Surgery

Total weight loss after gastric bypass is variable. However, all patients lose weight up through 6 months, with only 2.1 % regaining weight for a total weight loss of 10 % at 3 years. The remaining 97.9 % lose from 22 to 45 % total weight loss at 3 years [77] (Fig. 11.2).

Gastric bypass surgery has a profound impact on type 2 diabetes (T2DM). Within the first few days after surgery, the patient's need for glycemic control medication changes drastically, with many patients discharged without any medications to treat hyperglycemia. Many patients seek bariatric surgery due to this specific affect on T2DM. In the prospective STAMPEDE trial with 91 % follow-up

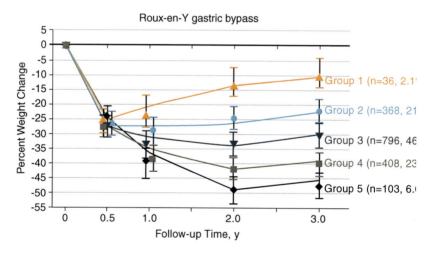

Fig. 11.2 Percent weight change trajectories for Roux-en-Y gastric bypass (from Courcoulas et al. [78]: 310(22), with permission)

at 3 years, and comparing intensive traditional medical treatment to surgical gastric bypass and surgical sleeve gastrectomy, only 5 % of the traditionally treated group achieved a HbA1c of <6.0 % or less versus 38 % in the gastric bypass group and 24 % in the sleeve gastrectomy group [78]. An additional randomized controlled trial compared traditional medical therapy to gastric bypass or biliopancreatic diversion (BPD). At 5 years, 50 % of patients who achieved remission still maintained it (37 % gastric bypass and 63 % BPD) [79]. At 15 years, in the Swedish Obese Subjects perspective trial, the microvascular complications in patients who were diabetic at baseline and treated with traditional medical weight loss therapy was 41.8/1000 versus 20.6/1000 in the surgery group. Macrovascular complications of diabetes in the same group were 44.2/1000 person-years in control patient's versus 31.7/1000 person-years in the surgical group [80]. In addition, studies show that the secondary complications of diabetes like diabetic neuropathy may also improve after gastric bypass surgery [81].

The best way to inform the patient about the probability that he or she will go into *complete remission* from T2DM—defined as HbA1c of <5.7 mg/dl, fasting blood sugar of <100 mg/dl and no medications for 1 year—is to use the DiaRem (Diabetes Remission) Score [82]. The patients are classified as "cured" if complete remission lasts 5 years [83]. Partial remission is defined as HbA1c of <6.5 %, fasting blood glucose <125 mg/dl and no active treatment or ongoing procedures for 1 year. Prolonged partial remission is defined as lasting 5 years. Taking the patients own risk factors into account can help predict the chances of complete remission and set realistic expectations for remission [84].

Gastric bypass has a profound impact on multiple other metabolic diseases in addition to diabetes. A prospective trial of 1156 patients managed with traditional medical treatment versus surgery demonstrates these results [85] (Table 11.3).

LRYGB also has a positive effect on the incidence and mortality of cancer. In the study by Adams et al., the incidence of cancer in the LRYGB group was 3.85 % with 0.62 % mortality versus 5.05 % and 1.13 % mortality in the nonsurgical obese group. This represents a decrease of 24 % in incidence and 46 % in mortality for patients with obesity treated with LRYGB versus traditional medical management [86].

Table 11.3 Health benefits of gastric bypass surgery after 6 years

	Control group 1	Control group 2	RYGB
Follow-up	72.9 % (304/417)[a]	96.9 % (311/321)[a]	92.6 %(387/418)
Mortality (%)	3	1	3
Weight loss	Weight gain 0.2 % from year 2 to year 6	Weight gain 0.0 % year 2 to year 6	Weight loss 34.9 % at year 2 decreasing to 27.7 % at year 6 (7.2 %)
Type 2 diabetes Remission/new onset	8 versus 17 %	6 versus 15 %	62 versus 2 %
Hypertension (%)	18	9	42
Cholesterol (%)	34	18	67

[a]101 participants from control group 1 and 2 underwent bariatric surgery during the 6-year period since the beginning of the trial. These patients are included in the results as intention to treat analysis (results are better because they include surgical patients)
From Cotillard et al. [85], with permission

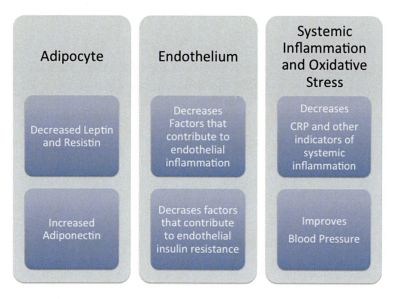

Fig. 11.3 Mechanisms of atherosclerosis and effects of metabolic and bariatric surgery (data from Ashrafian et al. [88]: 2091–203)

Cardiomyopathy from increased leptin levels resolves and results in markedly improved cardiac ejection fraction and function after LRYGB.

In addition, as the table above demonstrates, bariatric surgery impacts cardiovascular disease not only by decreasing fat mass with a corollary decrease in leptin, but through many other mechanisms [87] (Fig. 11.3).

Laparoscopic Sleeve Gastrectomy (LSG)

The LSG has eclipsed the gastric bypass in numbers of procedures performed in the United States in recent years (Fig. 11.4a, b). The sleeve gastrectomy, while currently

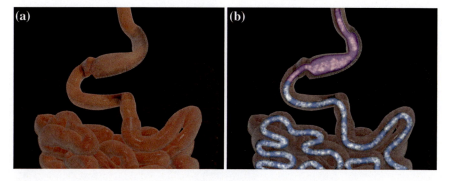

Fig. 11.4 **a** Sleeve gastrectomy. **b** Flow of food and digestive juice (courtesy of Ethicon, Inc.)

performed as a primary procedure meant to be sufficient for remission of obesity and related disease, was initially the first part of a more complex procedure, the duodenal switch/biliopancreatic diversion. It began to be studied as a "stand alone" procedure in approximately 2005. The sleeve gastrectomy is generally perceived as being less difficult to perform than gastric bypass and less subject to frequent complications. These factors, along with the decline in the use of the adjustable gastric band (AGB), have resulted in the sleeve gastrectomy being more commonly performed.

Description of LSG

Once access to the abdomen is established as described above, a total of 2 5.0 mm trocars and 1–2 12.5 mm trocars are utilized to perform the operation.

Once the liver is retracted, a thorough examination of the abdomen is made with notes about the presence or absence of gallbladder inflammation or hiatal hernia. The "starting point" for the division of the stomach is then identified 4–6 cm from the pylorus. Access to the space under the stomach is achieved through the division of the short gastric artery and vein bundles. These vessels are divided using a harmonic scalpel, freeing up the greater curvature of the stomach from the attachments to the spleen and colon. The stomach is then surgically divided into two parts beginning about 4 cm from the pylorus, using a long, articulating stapler. This will divide the stomach into two parts without spilling the contents of the stomach. Approximately 15 % of the stomach is kept in continuity with the esophagus and duodenum. The rest of the stomach, approximately 85 %, is removed from the body in a pastic bag. The specimen is examined for Helicobacter pylori and other pathology. This operation preserves the continuity of the gastrointestinal track but promotes rapid gastric emptying. The operative time averages 93 min on average with 92.8 % of patients staying 1-2 days inpatient [66].

Safety of LSG

The 30-day mortality in a 2014 report from the NSQIP registry is 0.1 %, morbidity is 1.4 % and reoperations rate is 1.6 % in 3069 patients. The preventable readmission rate is 4.3 % [66, 67].

Complications of LSG

In a propensity-matched study from the Michigan Bariatric Surgery Collaborative, serious complications rates of LSG (2.4 %) were similar to Roux-en Y gastric bypass LRYGB (2.5 %) with no significant mortality. Leak/perforation rate was higher in LSG 0.85 % versus LRYGB (0.58 %) as was venous thromboembolic disease (0.47 % LSG vs. 0.34 % LRYGB) [88]. A recently published prospective randomized trial comparing the two procedures showed that LRYGB had a higher rate of major complications (4.5 %) versus LSG (0.9 %) within 30 days after the operation [89].

One important difference in complications between LGBP and LSG is the incidence of gastroesophageal reflux disease (GERD) in the LSG patients. Selecting patients for LSG who have a history of GERD requires an informed consent that specifically addresses this issue as well as a workup that may include barium swallow, upper endoscopy, esophageal manometry, and ambulatory pH monitoring [90]. The incidence of *new onset GERD* in patients who never had it prior to bariatric surgery was 12.5 % and the *remission of GERD* in patients who had GERD prior to bariatric surgery was significantly less in LSG versus LRYGB (50 % vs. 75 %) [89].

Outcomes of LSG

Although some groups have reported that results of sleeve and bypass procedures are equal, the prospective data on sleeve procedures with a high capture of patients with 5-year data is lacking. In an attempt to overcome these deficiencies a recent meta-analysis was done, comparing sixteen studies on 2758 patients. This meta-analysis demonstrated that LRYGB had a stronger effect on type 2 diabetes and weight loss at 1 year as compared with LSG, with similar results in remission of hypertension [91]. Weight loss for LSG at 1 year was about 13 % lower than LRYGB in the Michigan Collaboration study but nearly equal or greater at 3 years in a randomized comparative trial (63.3 % LSG vs. 72.8 % LRYGB). In this most recent report of a prospective trial the remission of type 2 diabetes was 58.7 % LSG versus 67.9 % LRYGB [89].

Laparoscopic Adjustable Gastric Band (LAGB)

The FDA approved the adjustable gastric band (AGB) in 2001 (Fig. 11.5a, b). It enjoyed wide-scale promotion by industry and was utilized by large numbers of patients, with its use peaking in 2009. Although only two companies had approval

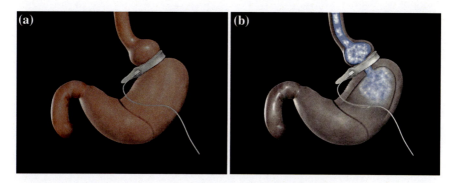

Fig. 11.5 a Adjustable gastric band. b Flow of food and digestive juice (courtesy of Ethicon, Inc.)

for the band in the United States, companies outside the United States produced many more. The band has an excellent safety record and many patients respond initially. Over time, however, weight regain and complications begin to occur in these patients, bringing additional focus to long-term outcomes.

Description of LAGB

Once access to the abdomen is established as described above, one 15 mm trocar and two additional 5 mm trocars are placed under direct vision. The pars flacida is identified and opened with the harmonic scalpel and the crura of the diaphragm is identified. An opening is made at the point where the two crura (right and left) meet, and that opening is then extended across the left crura into the area of the angle of His. Once the opening behind the stomach is made, the band is introduced through the large trocar. The band is grasped and drawn behind the stomach so that it encloses the entire stomach, then the band is closed. A flap of anterior stomach is then secured above the band with suture; thereby creating a flap that helps keep the band in place anteriorly. Posteriorly, the band is locked into place by the soft tissue on either side. The tubing is brought out through one of the 5 mm port sites and then threaded onto the port. A clear area on the anterior abdominal wall fascia is made and the port is sewn securely to the fascia. The port is usually located near the largest incision in the skin of the abdominal wall. This allows the port to be a stable platform for injections of saline that will close the inner tubing in the band and decrease the size of the opening. The operative time is 64 min on average and many patients are sent home on the same day, with 55.5 % staying 1 day as an inpatient [66].

Mechanism of Action of LAGB

When the band was first introduced it seemed apparent that the mechanism of action was restriction created by filling the band with saline. The saline caused the inner lining of the band to swell, allowing only a small opening for food to pass through from the upper part of the stomach to the lower part. Studies demonstrate rapid emptying (3–40 min) of food through the band with no correlation with satiety [92]. An additional study showed gastric emptying to be similar before and after band placement and not correlated with satiety or weight loss [93]. Thus, it now seems that weight loss after gastric banding may not be associated with stomach emptying rate.

Weight regain after gastric banding may result because the banding is mechanically signaling dietary changes to the brain in a way similar to the gut's signaling of dietary changes to the brain after a voluntary restriction of diet. This signaling, whether mechanical or organic, causes the body to try to manipulate obese physiology to regain weight by releasing chronic high levels of ghrelin while decreasing the response of satiety hormones.

At this point in time, the exact mechanism of action of the AGB is not clear.

Safety of LAGB

The band has a very low 30-day mortality (0.1 %). Morbidity (3.7 %) and reoperations (1.0 %) are also low in a study of 5622 patients. The preventable readmission rate is 3.3 % [66, 67].

Complications of LAGB

Some 30-day complications arise in the LAGB procedure, including bleeding (0.1 %) and superficial site infection (0.8 %). Normally, however, there are few serious complications during this period of time. The most important complications are long term and include prolapse of the stomach above the band, erosion of the band into the stomach and esophageal dysmotility with dysphagia and GERD [94].

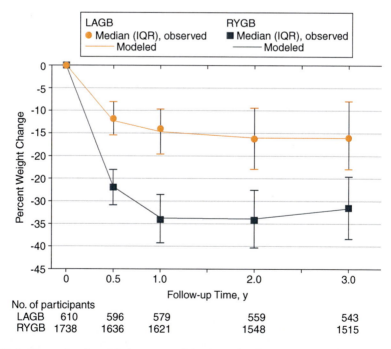

Fig. 11.6 Observed and modeled percent weight change by time point: laparoscopic adjustable gastric band (*LAGB*) and Roux-en Y Gastric Bypass (*RYGB*) (from Courcoulas et al. [78]; 310 (22), with permission)

Outcomes of LAGB

Weight loss with the AGB is highly variable. The Longitudinal Assessment prospective 3-year data shows that 18.9 % of patients lost no weight, 62.4 % lose about 15 % of their weight and only 19 % of patients lose 30 % or more of their weight at 3 years (Fig. 11.6).

At 3 years after LAGB, participants experiencing at least partial remission of type 2 diabetes were 28.6 % versus 67.5 % for LRYGB; remission of dyslipidemia 27.1 % versus 61.9 % for LRYGB, and hypertension 17.4 % versus 38.2 % for LRYGB.

Duodenal Switch/Biliopancreatic Diversion (DS/BPD)

The DS/BPD is the most complex procedure offered in bariatric surgery and is the most frequently performed type of biliopancreatic diversion in the United States after gastric bypass. It can be thought of as a combination of a sleeve and bypass (Fig. 11.7a, b). The DS/BPD is also the most effective procedure for remission of both weight and obesity-related disease. Benefits of this magnitude, however, are tempered by higher risk. For this reason the procedure is usually reserved for people who have the most profound expression of obesity with high BMI and/or burden of obesity-related disease, particularly type 2 diabetes uncontrolled on high-dose insulin. Gastric bypass in this particular subset of patients fails to resolve their burden of obesity and disease in up to 50 % of patients. Obesity in this group of patients is highly resistant to any therapy but can be adequately treated with duodenal switch/procedure. The procedure can be performed through laparoscopic or open access. The DS/BPD is usually performed by surgeons with extensive experience in gastric bypass in a nationally accredited program with substantial clinical support.

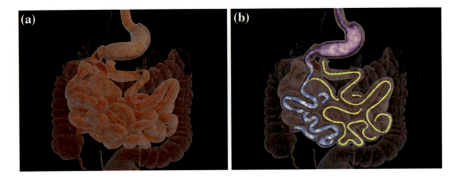

Fig. 11.7 a Duodenal switch. b Flow of food and digestive juice (courtesy of Ethicon, Inc.)

Description of DS/BPD

After access to the abdomen is established as described above, the sleeve gastrectomy is created in a similar fashion as described in the section above on the sleeve. Next, a dissection of the first portion of the duodenum is made and the duodenum is divided. The operation then shifts below the colon and the cecum is identified. Starting at the ileocecal valve a common channel is identified of approximately 150 cm. It is important to note that the shorter the common channel the higher the incidence of malnutrition and gastrointestinal complaints. Once the common channel is marked, an additional 100 cm is measured retrograde from this point and the bowel is divided. The end of the intestine leading to the duodenum (biliopancreatic limb) is connected to the alimentary limb at the previously marked 150 cm mark, creating the jejunoileal anastomosis. The alimentary limb is then connected to the end of the first portion of the duodenum distal to the pylorus, creating a duodenojejunal connection. The duodenal stump staple line is usually over-sewn to prevent leak.

As a result of this procedure, food consumed now traverses the esophagus and the sleeved stomach, crossing the pylorus (which has retained its metering function). The food then proceeds directly into the jejunum as in a bypass. The food then travels to 150 cm proximal to the cecum before being joined by digestive juices coming from the liver and pancreas. The bile and pancreatic enzymes join the food stream at 150 cm from the ileocecal valve. The preservation of the pylorus is believed to be an important part of the procedure.

The procedure, when performed as one stage, has high morbidity and mortality. However, when staged by doing the sleeve procedure first, followed by the bypass portion as a second stage, the risks are reduced and become similar to the risks of the gastric bypass. The mesenteric defects created by the rearrangement of the intestines are closed with a permanent running suture.

The goal of surgery is to complete the procedure in less than 5 hours if done in one stage. The DS/BPD procedure is rarely performed, accounting for 3–4 % of cases in highly specialized tertiary centers.

Safety of DS/BPD

Like every other bariatric procedure the implementation of a laparoscopic approach has improved the safety of this procedure. Mortality at 30 days of 1.4 % and 0.0 % were reported for open versus laparoscopic DS/BPD [95, 96]. Hospital stay was 4.5 days [96].

Complications of DS/BPD

The most feared complication of DS/BPD is a leak at the duodenojejunal anastomosis that occurs in the laparoscopic DS/BPD in 0.7 % of cases. The overall morbidity for major complications was 2.9 % in open DS/BPD and 3.0 % in laparoscopic DS/BPD procedures [94, 95].

Complications include gastrointestinal leaks and deep-vein thrombosis/pulmonary embolism (DVT/PE) that occur around postoperative day 10, after discharge from the hospital. This makes the enhanced recovery protocols critical for identification and communication about a potential leak [97]. Additional complications specific to DS/BPD include a higher incidence of vitamin and protein malnutrition. With the adaptation of longer common channels, the incidence of both of these complications has declined.

Outcomes of DS/BPD

In patients with BMI of ≥ 70 kg/m^2, the staged procedure (sleeve gastrectomy followed by DS/BPD) resulted in average total weight loss of 54.5 %, which was better than either LSG (25.4 %) or LRYGB (43.8 %). A very high percentage of DS/BPD, 98.4 %, were done laparoscopically [98].

The DS/BPD provides more extensive weight loss compared to LRYGB at all statistically significant measured times, including 36 months (68.9 % vs. 54.9 %) [99]. Additional studies corroborate that DS/BPD provides better weight loss than RYGB (excess weight loss 84 % vs. 63.7 %) and less weight regain [100]. In a trial of 60 patients prospectively and randomly assigned to RYGB versus DS/BPD, the resulting reductions in total body weight were 13.6 % versus 22.1 %, respectively. Remission of type 2 diabetes likewise was greater after DS/BPD. Patients undergoing DS/BPD had a higher incidence of postoperative admissions and further surgery as well as more gastrointestinal problems and vitamins deficiencies [101].

The DS/BPD achieves a significant effect in both weight loss and remission of type 2 diabetes in high BMI and insulin dependent patients. The risk is acceptable (as compared to the risk of continuing to be severely obese) but close long-term follow-up is required.

Gastric Balloon (GB) and the Vagal Blocking Device (VBLOC)

In 2015, two additional devices, the vagal blocking device (Fig. 11.8) and the intragastric balloon (Fig. 11.9a, b) were approved.

The vagus nerve is implicated in multiple ways in the communication of signals from the gut to the brain and vice versa. The paired nerves extend from the brainstem to the stomach and have both efferent and afferent signals. The idea to intermittently block the vagus was inspired by reports that patients undergoing bilateral truncal vagotomy for refractory peptic ulcer disease resulted in weight loss. The VBLOC device has two electrodes: one for the anterior and one for the posterior vagus nerves. They are placed on the vagal trunks in order to control all subsequent branches. These are connected to a neuroregulator that is implanted usually against the left lower thorax. The device was studied, as required by the

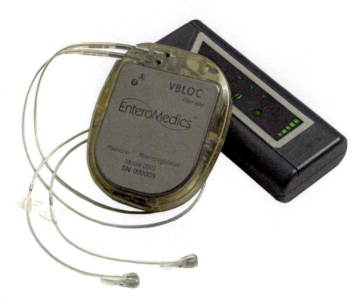

Fig. 11.8 Maestro vagal blocking device (courtesy of EnteroMedics)

FDA, in two trials (Empower and Recharge) the second of which was a randomized, sham controlled trial. Both trials demonstrated the safety of the device with no mortality in either trial. Neither the Empower or Recharge trials met their primary endpoints in that they did not show more than 10 % superiority with respect to excess weight loss over the control group, with the treatment group achieving 24.4 % excess weight loss vs. 15.9 % in the sham group. In the treatment group, 52 % of patients reached 20 % excess weight loss and the primary safety goal was met with 3.7 % adverse events [102].

The gastric balloon (GB) as a device has a long history as an adjunct to weight loss. The FDA recently approved the balloon for use in BMI 30–40 kg/m^2 based on a prospective, sham controlled, double-blinded randomized multicenter trial of 330 patients in 15 sites in the United States. At week 24 the group that did not have a balloon placed (sham) were able to get a balloon implanted. The trial met both primary effectiveness endpoints. Gastric balloon patients had a 25.1 % excess weight loss versus 11.3 % for patients in the sham group.

There were no deaths, intestinal obstructions, gastric perforations or device migrations during the balloon trial. Gastric ulcerations were noted in one-third of patients with unexpected balloon deflation in 6 %. Symptoms of discomfort including nausea, vomiting, and abdominal pain were noted immediately after implantation but abated over time [103]. At this time the cost of GB placement is substantial, requiring endoscopic placement and removal. The VBLOC and GB, however, have the potential to fulfill a treatment gap that provides more weight loss for a lower BMI group of 30–40 kg/m^2. The long-term outcomes in real world settings remain to be determined.

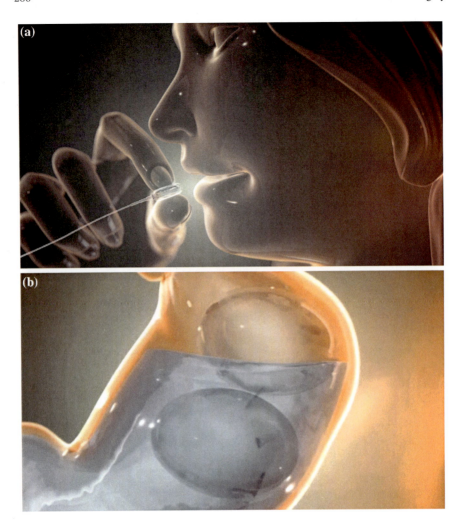

Fig. 11.9 a and **b** Obalon gastric balloon (courtesy of Obalon, Carlsbad, CA)

Variability in Response to Metabolic and Bariatric Surgery: Weight Regain

A fundamental principle that must be observed is that the application of bariatric surgery is very similar patient to patient but the outcomes are different. This variability is not driven by the small or minute changes in the procedures but by the differences in patients in regards to their epigenetic and genetic makeup, their comittment to behavior modification that consolidates the epigenetic change, and perhaps aspects of their individual physiology that we are just now beginning to appreciate. One example of individual physiology that might influence the patient's response to bariatric surgery is the number of specific receptors in the brain for a particular hormonal or bile salt activation pathway. *The Achilles heel of bariatric surgery at this time is that we do not know what procedure to apply to which patient to obtain optimal outcomes with the best safety profile for that individual patient.*

Research into this aspect of bariatric surgery is proceeding quickly at this time. Some early data has identified specific genetic markers that may indicate a less robust response to gastric bypass [104]. These genetic markers are not currently commercially available for patient use.

Although prospective trials document that weight regain at 6 years and 20 years after surgery is about 7 % of body weight, studies of specific genes associated with obesity demonstrate that people with those types of genes may have a variable response with less weight loss or more weight regain in the first 2 years after surgery [105–107]. The melanocortin C4R pathway signaling, described in an earlier chapter, is necessary for weight loss after gastric bypass [108]. Conversely, patients with the I251L allele have better weight loss using traditional methods of weight loss (caloric restriction) and gastric bypass [109]. This appears to be true for monogenic forms of obesity as well [110].

Researchers continue to look for markers that may indicate how weight regain occurs. Ghrelin levels are markedly altered by bariatric procedures but baseline and postoperative measurements of ghrelin and leptin do not appear to be useful as predictors of weight regain [111].

Bariatric surgery even with weight regain, in comparison to nonsurgical treatment of obesity, results in greater body weight loss, more sustainable weight loss and higher remission rates of type 2 diabetes and metabolic syndrome [112, 113].

Cholecystectomy After Metabolic and Bariatric Surgery

Cholecystectomy is required in some patients after bariatric surgery due to gallstone formation. The incidence of gallstones is 34 % in LRYGB patients and 28 % of LSG. In patients who develop gallstones, 12 % become symptomatic and require cholecystectomy [114]. The frequency of cholecystectomy by procedure is about 11 % after LRYGB and 3.5 % after LSG [115]. There is no indication for removal of the gallbladder at the time of surgery as prophylactic removal has been shown to increase complications, length of stay and reoperations if performed during the primary procedure. Concomitant cholecystectomy is reserved for the patient who is symptomatic and has gallstones at the time of the bariatric procedure [116]. The frequency of the development of gallstones is highest within the first few years after surgery, declining to <1 % after 3 years. Ursodiol does not affect post-bariatric surgery cholecystectomy rates and shows no efficacy in the postoperative period as compared to ibuprofen and no therapy [117, 118].

Prehabilitation: Preoperative Assessment and Preparation

Obesity is a foundational disease that affects the entire body and is intimately related to the way the brain and the body functions. The program that surrounds the candidate for bariatric surgery must provide the essential screening and preoperative assessments of the whole person that allow the patient to be as safe and ultimately become as healthy as possible.

In 2009, the Longitudinal Assessment of Bariatric Surgery Consortium identified that a history or diagnosis of deep-vein thrombosis, PE, or obstructive sleep apnea with impaired functional status were each independently associated with increased risk in the laparoscopic era of bariatric surgery [65]. Combining elements of a patient's complex medical history creates a unique program of preoperative interventions that can greatly improve the patient's risk for surgery. Identifying and maximizing the patient's history and health status prior to surgery results in an enhanced patient experience of care and outcomes that are similar to a population of less sick people [119]. *Prehabilitation* is often the term used for this intensive and personalized approach.

The MBS Prehabilitation program takes place in three domains:

- Education: The primary aims of the education program are to establish understanding regarding fundamental principles of weight regulation and nutrition and to promote understanding of the risks and benefits of available procedures (informed consent).
- Physical assessment: The aim of the physical assessment is to: (1) create a shared understanding with the patient of his/her medical complexity through an evaluation of the history and physical exam, and (2) maximize their metabolic acuity and physical function through testing and prehabilitation specifically in regard to mobility.
- Social and Psychological Health assessment: The aim of this assessment is to use psychological screening, testing and the structured interview to determine a patient's psychosocial vulnerabilities and general mental health status, including any historical or current Axis 1 disorders. The assessment can then also be used to identify those patients at risk for alcohol use disorder (AUD) and self-harm. Additional considerations include issues such as postoperative body image, social and sexual relationships, and function after surgery.

A multidisciplinary team that ideally includes a surgeon, a bariatric physician or nurse practitioner, a registered dietician, a physical medicine/rehabilitation physician and a psychologist provides the most comprehensive initial prehabilitation assessment. In programs that also treat adolescents, additional personnel including a pediatric bariatrician and pediatric psychologist may be required. This grouping of practitioners will be in a good position to design a personalized health plan that can decrease risk and achieve long term health by partnering with the patient.

Education and Informed Consent

People with obesity are often affected by the disease for much of their lives, yet they generally have little understanding of how the physiology of obesity works. The onslaught of conflicting and often erroneous information sourced from popular media can be confusing and creates chaos. The lack of understanding of the science behind specific recommendations is one of the key problems the patient faces in achieving good health and long-term weight maintenance.

The education process for the patient with obesity therefore needs to start with fundamental education that includes current science-based primary concepts about obesity itself. This should be followed with options for therapy, including commercially available medically supervised traditional weight loss programs, pharmaceuticals, devices and surgery. Ideally, this generalized education takes place in both group sessions and one-on-one sessions. Data shows that participation in this type of programmed learning can influence the choice of surgical procedure for the patient as well as the decision not to undergo surgery until alternatives are exhausted [120].

The patient's individualized education is usually continued longitudinally through the initial assessment and monthly appointments that focus on the fundamentals of weight management. Education around the specific procedure the patient will undergo should take place both before and after surgery and should continue longitudinally throughout their lifetime [121].

Bariatric surgery is an elective procedure and the burden of obtaining sufficiently informed consent is ongoing and heavy. Documentation of the patient's informed consent begins at the initial public education seminar and continues until the patient and surgeon jointly decide on an optimal procedure. At that point, a frank and detailed discussion about possible adverse events and outcomes, including the limitations of the data available, should take place. The patient's understanding and consent must be sufficiently documented all along the way. This shared decision-making model is an essential part of the process of informed consent for bariatric surgery. Due to the profound effects of surgery, some of which are just beginning to be better understood, as well as the variability in patients' response to different procedures, some element of uncertainty is present and should be included in the consent documentation.

Special risk can be assessed based on the patient's co-morbid disease and this risk should be mitigated as much as possible. These special risks, however, should be clearly discussed with the patient and included in the written consent. A risk calculator can be utilized in order to predict an individual patient's risk [122, 123]. As mentioned previously, outcomes regarding specific motivations for the patient to have surgery, such as the remission of diabetes, should be clearly estimated using the DiaRem score.

Physical Assessment for Surgery

Physical assessment requires that a thorough history and physical exam be conducted as detailed in Chap. 9. The following are additional, more specific assessments that should be done when evaluating a patient for the possibility of bariatric surgery.

An assessment of the patient's micronutrient deficiencies, if any, should be evaluated. It may seem counterintuitive, but anemia and vitamin malnutrition is a common occurrence in patients with obesity. Anemia was found prior to surgery in 14 % of patients undergoing bariatric procedures, of which 98 % were female. These patients had an increased length of stay in the hospital [124]. Vitamin D, thiamine, copper, and zinc also show a marked incidence of deficiency prior to surgery in patients with obesity. Preoperative testing and correction of these deficits is optimal care [125, 126].

Another critical area for assessment is cardiac risk. A recent review of cardiac complications in patients undergoing non-cardiac surgery shows that over 10 million people have a major cardiac-related event in the first 30 days after a surgical procedure. In fact, 1.5 % of patients die within 30 days after a non-cardiac procedure [127]. Reports from large clinical databases show that the incidence of myocardial infarction after bariatric surgery is 0.09 % [66]. Patients with a baseline of cardiac disease and renal insufficiency are at higher risk for cardiac events. This underlying pathology can be exacerbated by perioperative events like bleeding.

Even patients who have not shown any evidence of cardiac disease are also at risk. Cardiac stress testing has been extensively utilized in preparing patients for bariatric surgery, especially in patients who have limited mobility. A meta-analysis, however, shows that up to one-third of patients who have a postoperative myocardial infarction or death had normal preoperative stress test results [128]. Moreover, 65 % of patients with a myocardial infarction do not have symptoms of ischemia, partly due to the use of analgesic medications postoperatively [129].

Measurement of cardiac biomarkers is an alternative to cardiac testing, specifically measuring the B-type natriuretic peptide (BNP) level where a value of >92 ng/l or an N-terminal pro-BNP level of ≥ 300 ng/l indicates an increase in risk. Obtaining a postoperative BNP level also increases the prediction of a postoperative event [130]. Asymptomatic myocardial infarctions are associated with an odds ratio of 4.0 in increased death within 30 days after surgery. Troponin levels, even when not elevated enough to implicate ischemia, are still a good predictor. Obtaining preoperative and postoperative values for comparison in patients with known risk factors may be able to be used to determine who is more at risk for perioperative and postoperative myocardial infarction [131].

The use of aspirin has been extensively evaluated. Current recommendations are that aspirin should be stopped 7 days prior to surgery and resumed 8–10 days after surgery [132].

Perioperative hypotension is a strong independent predictor of stroke and death. A beta blockade could potentially exacerbate hypotension or limit the ability of a patient to respond. In a recent meta-analysis, although the risk of nonfatal myocardial infarction was reduced, the risk of death, nonfatal stroke hypotension and bradycardia were increased [129]. At this time there is no clear recommendation regarding the use of a beta blockade perioperatively. A baseline set of laboratory testing, as set forth in the Table 11.4, is recommended [125–127] (Tables 11.4 and 11.5).

Table 11.4 Suggested baseline preoperative laboratory testing

• CBC	• CMP
• HbA1C	• Ferritin
• Folate	• Vitamin B12
• Calcium, albumin	• Intact parathyroid hormone
• Whole blood thiamine	• Vitamin D
• Serum copper	• Zinc
• Vitamin A	• Bone mineral density
• B-type natriuretic peptide (BNP) ≥ 92 ng/l indicates increased risk for perioperative cardiac events	• N-terminal pro-BNP >300 ng/l indicates increased risk for perioperative cardiac events
• Testosterone (male)	• PSA (male)
• 24-h urinary-free cortisol if >100 µg/24 h then a 1 mg dexamethasone suppression test (young patient with difficult to treat hypertension, diabetes)	• Troponin (baseline)

Data from references [125–127]

Table 11.5 Recommended preoperative testing

• CXR: PA and lateral
• 12 Lead EKG
• Mammogram
– All women age 50 or above must have a current annual mammogram
• Pap test
– Pap smear is required every 3 years for women age 21–65 or every 5 years for women age 30–65 with Pap test and human papillomavirus (HPV) testing
• Colonoscopy required every 10 years at age 50 and above
– More frequent testing is required for high-risk patients
• Endometrial Cancer Screening
– Women who are having post menopausal bleeding are referred for evaluation

Physical Function and Mobility

Limited mobility and poor physical function are among the most significant risk factors for a poor outcome after bariatric surgery. During the initial consultation with the patient, mobility can be assessed and, if compromised, a referral to physical medicine and rehabilitation can be made. A formal assessment and physical therapy preoperatively can improve function, insure that proper appliances (i.e., walker, wheelchair, cane, etc.) are in place, and insure that the patient has ongoing support during and after surgery. In the elderly patient, balance issues contribute to the risk of falling. One machine utilized during physical therapy allows patients to walk on a treadmill "unweighted" by up to 100 lb. The sensation of walking easily, without the burden of excess weight, is motivating for many patients who endure disability from obesity and joint-related inflammation. Patients are usually able to use insurance benefits to access these services, both prior to and following surgery.

Social and Psychological Health Assessment Prior to Surgery

The impact of a patient's social network vis-a-vis their obesity is profound. Culture around food within the family and the social groups to which the patient belongs often dictate much of the learned behavior of eating. These cultural aspects have a profound effect on the level of obesity experienced not only by the patient, but also by their immediate family This was documented in a study utilizing data from the Framingham Heart group. That study showed that when a spouse became obese, the other spouse had a 37 % change of becoming obese. If a sibling became obese, the chance another sibling would be obese increased 40 %. If an individual had a friend who was obese, there was a 57 % chance the individual would also become obese [133]. Social networks promote the spread of obesity and emphasize the impact and importance of "food culture" in many patients who are obese. This begs the question: what would constitute a "network disruption? The culture may be disrupted when one individual in the group, usually prompted by increasing obesity-related problems, decides to address his/her obesity with diet and exercise. However, the network effect may be too strong to overcome without physiological help and "epigenetic resetting" like the genetic resetting^{TM} induced by surgery.

In addition to the cultural and social aspects of obesity, there is a high risk of psychological illness in those who are obese and seek bariatric surgery.

Mental Health Disorders in the Bariatric Population

Generally speaking, there is a high incidence of psychiatric illness and psychological disorders in people with obesity. These disorders should be taken as seriously as any other obesity-related disease in preparing and following patients

Table 11.6 Axis I disorders	Axis I disorders include all clinical psychological disorders
	Disorders diagnosed in infancy, childhood or adolescence (ADHD, learning disorders)
	Delirium, dementia, amnesia and other cognitive disorders
	Mental disorders due to a general medical condition
	Substance-related disorders
	Schizophrenia and other psychotic disorders
	From Christakis and Fowler [134], with permission

treated with surgical therapy. Bariatric surgery, due to the effect of signaling to the brain, has unique effects on psychiatric illness and psychological disorders

The Longitudinal Assessment of Bariatric Surgery studied a representative group of patients undergoing bariatric surgery with the following characteristics: 82.9 % female and Caucasian, median age 46, median body mass index (BMI) 44.8 kg/m^2. In that group, the following incidence of psychological illness was reported:

- 38.7 % lifetime history of depressive disorder
- 33.2 % lifetime diagnosis of alcohol abuse or dependence
- 13.1 % lifetime diagnosis of binge-eating disorder (BED).

In addition, 33.7 % had at least one current Axis I disorder and 68.8 % had experienced at least one Axis I disorder in their lifetime [76, 134] (Table 11.6).

Additional high quality studies support these findings and confirm lifetime rates of psychiatric disorders to be 66.3 % and 72.6 % in bariatric surgery candidates [75, 135].

Psychiatric and psychological disorders impact outcomes of bariatric surgery in the following ways [75, 76]:

- Less weight loss
- Preoperative depression is predictive of postoperative depression
- Depression results in significantly less weight loss at 24 and 36 month follow-ups
- Psychopathology improves immediately postoperatively, but reemerges 2–3 years later
- Lifetime risk of alcohol dependence after bariatric surgery is 30.9 % and 33.2 %
- Risk of self-harm is 3× (3.6 per 1000 patients per year) versus 1.2 per 1000 patients per year in the baseline population—the incidence of self-harm is underestimated by 50 %
- 93 % occur in patients diagnosed with a mental health disorder during the 5 years prior to surgery
- Self-harm is especially prevalent in disadvantaged patients.

It has been a tradition in bariatric surgery to require a psychological interview of all patients prior to any surgical intervention. The interview, however, does not specifically identify a high-risk group for ongoing intervention. The psychological interview may help identify specific social context issues regarding relationships, home or work environments that impact the patient. It can affect the handling of informed consent, and can further clarify risk by assigning a risk group that can be easily identified to all members of the bariatric team [136]. However, few if any studies have demonstrated the value of ongoing intervention in an identified high-risk group.

It may be possible to utilize a screening questionnaire to identify high-risk individuals preoperatively by identifying which questions in the initial history would indicate increased risk. This would include the identification of patients with depressive disorders and BED as well as alcohol and medication misuse. Those high-risk individuals would undergo a structured interview by a licensed psychologist as part of his or her initial evaluation for surgery. Although psychological testing has not been shown to add significantly to the results of the structured interview, many psychologists still add some form of objective testing, usually the Personality Assessment Inventory and Beck Depression Scale to their evaluation [76, 137].

For patients identified as high-risk, longitudinal follow-up with psychology after surgery is indicated. This would include screening questionnaires at every follow-up interval (30 day, 2 month, 6 month, and annual) and reassessment by the psychologist when the screening identifies increased concern. Scheduled meetings with the psychologist would take place at 6 months and annually for patients identified preoperatively to be at higher risk, or more frequently for those who demonstrate increased difficulty on follow up. If a patient is seen in the emergency department for self-harm and has a history of bariatric surgery they should be referred to the program for long-term care. These problems may be more prevalent in patients with less economic resources.

Enhanced Recovery After Metabolic and Bariatric Surgery

Establishing specific enhanced recovery protocols after surgery improves safety and decreases length of stay and cost as compared to groups of patients in whom these specific protocols are not utilized. Studies show no difference, however, in readmission complications or readmission rates [138]. Establishing enhanced protocols for recovery as opposed to implementing standard care has been shown to be effective in bariatric surgery [139, 140].

The areas of perioperative care that are involved in enhanced recovery protocols are: (1) preoperative; (2) morning of surgery; (3) surgery; (4) immediate postoperative period; and (5) discharge.

Specific enhanced recovery protocols include:

Preoperative Prehabilitation

- Confirm the patient's decision for surgery by reviewing specific written informed consent;
- Test the patient's understanding of key principles of the procedure he/she will undergo;
- Review all preoperative tests;
- Review all medications and make adjustments based on recommendations;
- Require chlorhexidine shower protocol [141];
- Ensure that diabetic patients have the capability to check blood glucose at home;
- Communicate between clinic and hospital.

Perioperative

- Triage of scheduling for operation based on acuity
- Prophylaxis
  - Antibiotics
  - Nausea
  - Surgical Team "Time Out"
  - Venous thromboprophylaxis [142]
- Pain management
  - Minimize use of narcotics
- Minimize use of Foley catheters by voiding on call to the OR
- *Medications Note*: The most significant errors in hospitalization occur in regards to medications. Patients with obesity are usually on a high number of significant medications to treat cardiac disease, diabetes and other obesity-related diseases. Particular care and attention to these medications is critical in avoiding perioperative medication errors. Patients often require changes in medications immediately after surgery, a process facilitated by utilizing pharmacy resources during this period of care [143, 144].
- Standardized Procedure.

Postoperative

- Early mobilization (within 6 hours of the procedure end time)
- Stop antibiotic prophylaxis within 24 h
- Per oral liquids/medications when able to control airway

- Rounding 2× per day
- Clear written discharge instructions
- Medication reconciliation and review
- Avoidance of narcotic analgesics
- Post discharge phone call
- Post operative education class at one week to advance diet, answer questions, start vitamins and check on ambulation
- Diabetic patients monitored with daily phone call to manage blood sugar and medications
- Surgeon appointment within 1 month of surgery.

Health Maintenance After Metabolic and Bariatric Surgery

The cornerstone of long-term health is to ask the patient to participate in persistent interaction and follow-up with the team. In each and every encounter the patient should perceive some distinct value in counseling, testing and feedback so that they remain engaged.

Long term testing for protein vitamin and micronutrient deficiency is important. A recent summary suggests the following testing based on current literature [73] (Table 11.7).

It is clear that monitoring the patient's body fat percentage is an important post-surgical goal. The post-surgical patient adopts a lifestyle that includes exercise and food choices that enhance the new physiology. With the corrected signaling, they continue to push their physiology towards leanness and they begin to reverse

Table 11.7 Post operative testing of nutrients after bariatric surgery

• 3 months	– Complete blood count
	– Liver tests
	– Glucose, electrolytes and creatinine
• 6, 12, 18 months	– As for 3 months
	– Folate and Vitamin B12
	– Iron and/or ferritin
	– Albumin and 23-hydroxyvitamin D
	– Serum copper
	– Whole blood thiamine
	– Calcium and intact parathyroid hormone
• 24 months and then yearly	– As for 6 months
	– Zinc
	– Vitamin A
	– Bone mineral density

Data from Bal et al. [74]

the epigenetic changes that have hard-wired their physiology into obesity. They can also improve or reverse many obesity-related diseases.

The effectiveness of surgery comes with a risk of short term and long-term complications. The decision by a patient and surgeon to choose surgical therapy for obesity should be the result of a balanced and careful conversation about risk and benefit. Similar to the variability in response to traditional therapy and medication, response to surgical therapy also varies. The variation in response to surgery resides in the patient. It stems from the patient's baseline genetics and the extent to which the patient's physiology changed as he/she became obese. It also depends on what the patient is willing to do to push the envelope towards better health once the cycle of obesity is broken.

Conclusion

Metabolic and bariatric surgery has a profound effect on obesity and related disease achieving predictable and sustainable control. Among the options for the treatment of obesity, surgery is unequaled in effect. This profound effect is gained at the risk of adverse events, including mortality, either immediately after surgery or in the ensuing years. Although effective in almost all people, bariatric surgery is not a population solution because the application can only be delivered to one patient at a time, the surgical manpower is sufficient to treat only 1 % of affected persons and the cost of delivery of care is substantial. Currently there is no systematic approach to obesity in place that can define what patient is ideal for surgical intervention. Obesity is often still classified as an object of prevention rather than as chronic disease. Patients who adopt diet and exercise habits that augment procedural effects will maximize the genetic resetting™ that occurs with surgery and enhance their lifelong health.

Safety has been and will continue to be a priority for surgeons and interdisciplinary staff who specialize in MBS. The development of safer access (laparoscopic) and systematic care through participation in the national accreditation program, MBSAQIP, has enabled patients to achieve much improved health with very low morbidity and mortality. Scientific study of surgical procedures shows great promise to enhance our understanding of the body systems that control hunger, satiety and metabolism. Delving into new areas of scientific inquiry may yet yield a permanent, nonsurgical solution to the scourge of obesity.

References

1. EstebanVJ, Varela J, Nguyen NT. Laparoscopic sleeve gastrectomy leads the U.S. utilization of bariatric surgery at academic medical centers. Surg Obes Relat Dis. 2015. doi:10.1016/j.soard.2015.02.008.

2. Varela JE, Nguyen NT. Laparoscopic sleeve gastrectomy leads the U.S. utilization of bariatric surgery at academic medical centers. Surg Obes Relat Dis. 2015;11:987–90.
3. Chousleb E, Rodriguez JA, O'Leary JP. History of the development of metabolic/bariatric surgery in the ASMBS textbook of bariatric surgery. New York: Springer Science+Business Media; 2015.
4. Blackstone RP. The history of the American society for metabolic and bariatric surgery in the ASMBS textbook of bariatric surgery. New York: Springer Science+Business Media; 2015.
5. Blackstone RP. Quality in bariatric surgery in the ASMBS textbook of bariatric surgery. In: Nguyen NT, Blackstone RP, Morton JM, Ponce J, Rosenthal RJ, editors. Bariatric surgery, vol. I. New York: Spring Science+Business Media; 2015.
6. Telem DA, Talamini M, Altieri M, Yang J, Zhang Q, Pryor AD. The effect of National hospital accreditation in bariatric surgery on perioperative outcomes and long-term mortality. Surg Obes Rel Dis. 2015;11:749–57.
7. Gastrointestinal Surgery for Severe Obesity. In: Consensus statement NIH consensus development conference. vol. 9(1), 24–27 March 1991.
8. Clinical Guidelines on the Identification, Evaluation, and Treatment of Overweight and Obesity in Adults. The evidence Report. No. 98-4083, September 1998 National Institutes of Health.
9. Poirier P, Cornier MA, Mazzone T, et al. Bariatric surgery and cardiovascular risk factors. Circ J Am Heart Assoc. 2011;123:1–19. Accessed March 2012 from http://circ.ahajournals.org/content/123/15/1683.full.pdf.
10. American Diabetes Association. Standards of medical care in diabetes. Diab Care 2011;32 (S1). Accessed March 2012 from http://care.diabetesjournals.org/content/34/Supplement_1/S11.full.pdf.
11. American Association of Clinical Endocrinologists, The Obesity Society, and the American Society for Metabolic & Bariatric Surgery. Bariatric surgery guidelines; 2008. Accessed March 2012 from http://aace.metapress.com/content/u1w5l4261135n725/fulltext.pdf.
12. Dixon JB, Zimmet P, Alberti KG, Rubino F. International diabetes taskforce on epidemiology and prevention. bariatric surgery: an IDF statement for obese Type 2 diabetes. Diab Med. 2011;28(6):628–42.
13. U.S. Internal Revenue Service. Internal revenue bulletin: rulings and decisions under the internal revenue code of 1986; 2002. Accessed March 2012 from http://www.irs.gov/pub/irs-irbs/irb02-16.pdf.
14. Centers for Medicare & Medicaid Services. Medicare national coverage determinations manual; 2012. Accessed March 2012 from https://www.cms.gov/manuals/downloads/ncd103c1_Part2.pdf.
15. Buchwald H, Avidor Y, Braunwald E, Jensen MD, Pories W, Fahrbach K, Schoelles K. Bariatric surgery: a systematic review and meta-analysis. JAMA. 2004;292(14):1724–37.
16. Morton J. Does hospital accreditation impact bariatric surgery safety? Ann Surg. 2014;260 (3):504–9.
17. Colquitt JL, Pickett K, Loveman E, Frampton GK. Surgery for weight loss in adults. Cochrane Database Syst Rev. 2014; 8(8). doi:10.1002/14651858.DC003641.pub4.
18. Purnell JQ, Selzer F, Smith MD, Berk PD, Courcoulas AP, Inabnet WB, et al. Metabolic syndrome prevalence and associations in a bariatric surgery cohort from the longitudinal assessment of bariatric surgery-2 study. Metab Syndr Relat Disord. 2014;12(2):86–94.
19. Pelascini E, Disse E, Pasquer A, Poncet G, Gouillat C, Robert M. Should we wait for metabolic complications before operating on obese patients? Gastric bypass outcomes in metabolically healthy obese individuals. Surg Obes Relat Dis. 2015; doi:10.1016/j.soard.2015.04.024.
20. Wendling P. Sleeve gastrectomy cut biochemical cardiac risk factors presented by T. Mokhtari at the American College of Surgeons Clinical Congress, October 6; 2015.
21. Dixon JB, Hur KY, Lee WJ, Kim JF, Chong K, Chen SC, et al. Gastric bypass in type 2 diabetes with BMI < 30: weight and weight loss have a major influence on outcomes. Diabet Med. 2013;30(4):e127–34.

22. Ahima RS, Spaer CB, Flier JS, Elmquist JK. Leptin regulation of neuroendocrine systems. Front Neuroendocrinol. 2000;21(3):263–307.
23. Thaler JP, Cummings DE. Minireview: hormonal and metabolic mechanisms of diabetes remission after gastrointestinal surgery. Endocrinology. 2009;150:2518–25.
24. Stefater MA, Wilson-Perez HE, Chambers AP, Sandoval DA, Seeley RJ. Endocr Rev. 2012;33:595–622.
25. Miras AD, LeRoux CS. Mechanisms underlying weight loss after bariatric surgery. Nat Rev Gastroenterol Hepatol. 2013;10:575–84.
26. Odstrcil EA, Martinez JG, Santa Ana CA, Xue B, Schneider RE, Steffer KJ, et al. The contribution of malabsorption to the reduction in net energy absorption after long-limb Roux-en-Y gastric bypass. Am J Clin Nutr. 2010;92:704–13.
27. Akkary E, Sidani S, Boonsiri J, Uy S, Dziura J, Duffy AJ, Bell RL. The paradox of the pouch: prompt emptying predicts improved weight loss after laparoscopic Roux-Y gastric bypass. Surg Endosc. 2009;23(4):790–4.
28. Diabetes Prevention Program Research Group. Reduction in the Incidence of type 2 diabetes with lifestyle intervention or metformin. N Engl J Med. 2002;346:393–403.
29. Look AHEAD Research Group, Wing RR, Bolin P, Brancati FL, Bray GA, Clark JM, Coday M et al. Cardiovascular effects of intensive lifestyle intervention in type 2 diabetes. N Engl J Med. 2013;369(2):145–54.
30. Ricci C, Gaeta M, Rausa E, Maccitella Y, Bonavina L. Early impact of bariatric surgery on type II diabetes, hypertension, and hyperlipidemia: a systematic review, meta-analysis and meta-regression on 6,587 patients. Obes Surg. 2014;24(4):522–8.
31. Sjostrom L. Review of the key results from the Swedish Obese Subjects (SOS) trial-a prospective controlled intervention study of bariatric surgery. J Intern Med. 2013;273:219–34.
32. Ammerpohl O, Pratschke J, Schalmayer C, Haake A, Faber W, Von Kampen O, et al. Distinct DNA methylation patterns in cirrhotic liver and hepatocellular carcinoma. Int J Cancer. 2012;130:1319–28.
33. Ahrens M, Ammerpohl O, von Schonfels W, Kolarova J, Bens S, Itzel T, et al. DNA methylation analysis in nonalcoholic fatty liver disease suggests distinct disease-specific and remodeling signatures after bariatric surgery. Cell Metab. 2013;18:296–302.
34. Drozdowski LA, Clandinin MT, Thomason ABR. Morphological, kinetic, membrane biochemical and genetic aspects of intestinal enteroplasticity. World J Gastroenterol. 2009;15:774–87.
35. Seeley RJ, Chambers AP, Sandoval DA. The role of gut adaptation in the potent effects of multiple bariatric surgeries on obesity and diabetes. Cell Metab. 2015;21:369–78.
36. Groos S, Hunefeld G, Luciano L. Epithelial cell turnover-extracellular matrix relationship in the small intestine of human adults. Ital J Anat Embryol. 2001;106:353–61.
37. Shaw D, Gohil K, Basson MD. Intestinal mucosal atrophy and adaptation. World J Gastroenterol. 2012;18:6357–75.
38. Cani PD, Amar J, Iglesias MA, Poggi M, Knauf C, Bastelica D, et al. Metabolic endotoxemia initiates obesity and insulin resistance. Diabetes. 2007;56:1761–72.
39. Liou AP, Paziuk M, Luevano JM, Machineni S, Turnbaugh PJ, Kaplan LM. Sci Transl Med. 2013;5(78r):a41.
40. Le Roux CW, Borg C, Wallis K, Vincent RP, Bueter M, Goodlad R, et al. Gut hypertrophy after gastric bypass is associated with increased glucagon-like peptide 2 and intestinal crypt cell proliferation. Ann Surg. 2010;252:50–6.
41. Bitar KN, Raghavan S, Azkhem E. Tissue engineering in the gut: developments in neuromuscualture. Gastroenterology. 2014;146:1614–24.
42. Bueter M, Lowenstein C, Ashrafian H, Hillebrand J, Bloom SR, Olbers T, et al. Vagal sparing surgical technique but not stoma size affects body weight loss in rodent model of gastric bypass. Obes Surg. 2010; 20:616–22.

43. Hao Z, Townsend Rl, Mumphrey MB, Patterson LM, Ye J, Berthoud HR. Vagal innervation of intestine contributes to weight loss after Roux-en-Y gastric bypass surgery in rats. Obes Surg. 2014;24:2145–51.
44. Peterli R, Steinert RE, Woelnerhanssen B, Peteres T, Christoffel-Courtin C, Gass M, et al. Metabolic and hormonal changes after laparoscopic Roux-en-Y gastric bypass and sleeve gastrectomy: a randomized, prospective trail. Obes Surg. 2012;22:740–8.
45. Nguyen NQ, Debreceni TL, Bambrick JE, Bellon M, Wishart J, Standfield S, et al. Rapid gastric and intestinal transit is a major determinant of changes in blood glucose, intestinal hormones, glucose absorption and postprandial symptoms after gastric bypass. Obesity (Silver Spring). 2014;22:2003–9.
46. Steinert RE, Peterli R, Keller S, Meyer-Gerspach AC, Drewe J, Peters T, Beglinger C. Bile acids and gut peptide secretion after bariatric surgery: a 1-year prospective randomized pilot trial. Obesity (Silver Spring). 2013;21(12):E660–8.
47. Aron-Wisenewsky J, Clement K. The effects of gastrointestinal surgery on gut microbiota: potential contribution to improved insulin sensitivity. Curr Atheroscler Rep. 2014;16:454.
48. Malin SK, Samat A, Wolski K, Abood B, Pothier CE, Bhatt DL, et al. Improved acylated ghrelin suppression at 2 years in obese patients with type 2 diabetes: effects of bariatric surgery vs. standard medical therapy. Int J Obes (Lond). 2014;38(3):364–70.
49. Li B, Lu Y, Srikant CB, Gao ZH, Liu J. Intestinal adaptation and Reg gene expression induced by antidiabetic duodenal-jejunal bypass surgery in Zucker fatty rats. Am J Physiol Gastrointest Liver Physiol. 2013;304:G635–45.
50. Berridge KC, Robinson TE. Parsing reward. Trends Neurosci. 2003,26.507–13.
51. Pecina S, Berridge KC. Opioid site in nucleus accumbens shell mediates eating and hedonic "liking" for food: map based on microinjection Fos plumes. Brain Res. 2000;863:71–86.
52. Bartoshuk LM, Duffy VB, Hayes JE, Moskowitz HR, Snyder DJ. Psychophysics of sweet and fat perception in obesity: problems, solutions and new perspectives. Philos Trans R Soc Lond B Biol Sci. 2006;361:1137–48.
53. Finlayson G, Arlotti A, Dalton M, King N, Blundell JE. Implicit wanting and explicit liking are markers for trait binge eating. A susceptible phenotype for overeating. Appetite. 2011;57:722–8.
54. Berthoud HR, Zheng H, Shin AC. Food reward in the obese and after weight loss induced by calorie restriction and bariatric surgery. Ann NY Acad Sci. 2012;1264:36–48.
55. Lemmens SG, Rutters F, Born JM, Westerterp-Plantenga MS. Stress augments food "wanting" and energy intake in visceral overweight subjects in the absence of hunger. Physiol Behav. 2011;103:157–63.
56. Dunn JP, Cowan RL, Volkow ND, Feurer ID, Li R, Williams DB, et al. Decreased dopamine type 2 receptors availability after bariatric surgery: preliminary findings. Brain Res. 2010;1350:123–30.
57. Faria SL, Faria OP, Buffington C, deAlmeida Cardeal M, Rodrigues de Gouvea H. Energy expenditure before and after Roux-en-Y gastric bypass. Obes Surg. 2012; 22(9). 1450–5.
58. Fiancbaum L, Choban PS, Bradley LR, Burge JC. Changes in measured resting energy expenditure after Roux-en-Y gastric bypass for clinically severe obesity. Surgery. 1997;122 (5):943–9.
59. Werling M, Fandriks L, Olbers T, Bueter M, Sjostrom L, Lonroth H, et al. Roux-en-Y gastric bypass surgery increases respiratory quotient and energy expenditure during food intake. PLOS ONE. 2015; doi:10.1371/journal.pone.0129784.
60. Seeley RS, Chambers AP, Sandoval DA. The role of gut adaptation in the potent effects of multiple bariatric surgeries on obesity and diabetes. Cell Met 2015; doi:10.1016/j.cmet.2015. 01.001.
61. Ahrens M, Ammerpohl O, von Schonfels W, Kolarova J, Bens S, Itzel T, et al. DNA Methylation analysis in nonalcoholic fatty liver disease suggests distinct disease-specific and remodeling signatures after bariatric surgery. Cell Metab. 2013;18:296–302.

62. Yousseif A, Emmanuel J, Karra E, Millet Q, Elkalaawy M, Jenkinson AD, et al. Differential effects of LSG and LGB on appetite, circulating acyl-ghrelin, peptide YY3-36 and active GLP-1 levels in non-diabetic humans. Obes Surg. 2014;24:241–52.
63. Werling M, Olbers T, Fandriks L, Bueter M, Lonroth H, Stenflo K, LeRoux CW. Increased postprandial energy expenditure may explain superior long term weight loss after Roux-en-Y gastric bypass compared to vertical banded gastroplasty. PLOS ONE. 2013;8(4):e60280.
64. Woelnerhanssen B, Peterli R, Steinert RE, Peters T, Borbely Y, Beglinger C. Effects of Post bariatric surgery weight loss on adipolines and metabolic parameters: comparison of laparoscopic Roux-en-Y gastric bypass and laparoscopic sleeve gastrectomy-a prospective randomized trial. Surg Obes Relat Dis. 2011;7:1561–8.
65. The Longitudinal Assessment of Bariatric Surgery (LABS) Consortium. Perioperative safety in the longitudinal assessment of bariatric surgery. N Engl J Med. 2009;361:445–54.
66. Sanni A, Perez S, Medbery R, Urrego HD, McCready C, Toro JP, Patel AD, Lin E. Postoperative complications in bariatric surgery using age and BMI stratification: a study using ACS-NSQIP data. Surg Endosc. 2014;28(12):3302–9.
67. Sweeney JF, Davis SS. Postoperative complications in bariatric surgery using age and BMI stratification: a study using ACS-NSQIP data. Surg Endosc. 2014;28(12):3302–9.
68. Patterson Wl, Peoples BD, Gesten FC. Predicting potentially preventable hospital readmissions following bariatric surgery. Surg Obes Relat Dis. 2015; 11:866–73.
69. Hutter MM, Schirmer BD, Jones DB, et al. Fist report form the American college of surgeons bariatric surgery center network: laparoscopic sleeve gastrectomy has morbidity and effectiveness positioned between the band and the bypass. Ann Surg 2011;2254(3):410–20 (discussion 420–2).
70. Nguyen NT, Goldman C, Rosenquist CJ, et al. Laparoscopic versus open gastric bypass: a randomized study of outcomes, quality of life, and costs. Ann Surg. 2001;234(3):279–89.
71. Birkmeyer NJ, Finks JF, English WJ, Carlin AM, Hawasili AA, Genaw JA, et al. Risks and benefits of prophylactic inferior vena cava filters in patients undergoing bariatric surgery. J Hosp Med. 2013;8(4):173–7.
72. Christou NV, Jarand J, Sylvestre JL, McLean AP. Analysis of the incidence and risk factors for wound infections in open bariatric surgery. Obes Surg. 2004;14(1):16–22.
73. Schauer PR, Ikramuddin S, Gourash W, Ramanathan R, Luketich J. Outcomes after laparoscopic Roux-en-Y gastric bypass for morbid obesity. Ann Surg. 2000;2324:515–529.
74. Bal BS, Finelli FC, Shope TR, Koch TR. Nutritional deficiences after bariatric surgery. Nat Rev Endocrinol. 2012;8:544–56.
75. Rodriguez-Carmona Y, Lopez-Alavez FJ, Gonzalez-Garay AG, Solis-Galiia C, Melendez G, Serralde-Zuniga AE. Bone mineral density after bariatric surgery. A systematic review. Int J Surg. 2014;12(9):976–82.
76. Kalarchian MA, et al. Psychiatric disorder among bariatric surgery candidates: relationship to obesity and functional health systems. Am J Psychiatry. 2007;164:328–34.
77. Mitchell JE, et al. Psychopathology prior to surgery in the longitudinal assessment of bariatric surgery-3 (LABS-3) psychosocial study. Surg Obes Relat Dis. 2012;8(5):533–41.
78. Courcoulas AP, Christian NJ, Belle SH, Berk PD, Flum DR, Garcia L, et al. Weight change and health outcomes at 3 years after bariatric surgery. JAMA. 2013; doi:10.1001/jama.2013.280928.
79. Schauer PR, Bhatt DL, Kirwan JP, Wolski K, Brethauer SA, Navaneethan SD, et al. Bariatric surgery versus intensive medical therapy for diabetes—3-year outcomes. N Engl J Med. 2014;370(21):2002–13.
80. Mingrone G, Panunzi S, De Gaetano A, Guidone C, Iaconelli A, Nanni G, Castagneto M, Bornstein S, Rubino F. Bariatric-metabolic surgery versus conventional medical treatment in obese patients with type 2 diabetes: 5 year follow-up of an open-label, single-center, randomized controlled trail. Lancet. 2015;386:964–73.
81. Sjostrom L, Peltonen M, Jacobson P, Ahlin S, Adnersson-Assarsson J, Anveden A, et al. Association of bariatric surgery with long-term remission of type 2 diabetes and with microvascular and macrovascular complications. JAMA. 2014;311(22):2297–304.

82. Muleer-Stich BP, Fischer L, Kenngott HG, Gondan M, Senft J, Clemens G, et al. Gastric bypass leads to improvement of diabetic neuropathy independent of glucose normalization-results of a prospective cohort study (DiaSurg 1 study). Ann Surg. 2013;258(5):760–5.
83. Still CD, Wood GC, Benotti P, Petrick AT, Gabrielsen J, Strodel W, Ibele An, Seiler J, Irving BA, Celaya M, Blackstone RP, Gerhard GS, Argyropoulos G. Preoperative prediction of type 2 diabetes remission after Roux-en Y gastric bypass surgery: a retrospective cohort study. Lancet Diab Endocrinol. 2014;2(1):38–45.
84. Buse JB, Caprio S, Cefalu WT, et al. How do we define cure of diabetes? Diabetes Care. 2009;32(11):2133–5.
85. Cotillard A, Poitou C, Duchateaus-Nguyen G, et al. Type 2 diabetes remission after gastric bypass. What is the best prediction tool for clinicians? Obes Surg. 2015;25(7):128–1132.
86. Adams TD, Davidson LE, Litwin SE, Kolotkin RI, LaMonte MJ, Pendleton RC, et al. Health benefits of gastric bypass surgery after 6 years. JAMA. 2012;308(11):1122–31.
87. Ashrafian H, Ahmed K, Rowland SP, Patel VM, Gooderham NG, Holmes E, et al. Metabolic surgery and cancer. Cancer. 2011;117(9):1788–99.
88. Ashrafian H, LeRoux CW, Darzi A, Athanasiou T. Effects of bariatric surgery on cardiovascular function. Circulation. 2008;118:2091–102.
89. Carlin AM, Zeni RM, English WJ, Awasli AA, Genaw JA, Kr Krause, et al. The comparative effectiveness of sleeve gastrectomy, gastric bypass and adjustable gastric banding procedures for the treatment of morbid obesity. Ann Surg. 2013;257(5):791–7.
90. Peterli R, Borbely Y, Ker B, Gass M, Peters T, Thurnheer M, et al. Early results of the swiss multicenter bypass or sleeve study. A prospective randomized trial comparing laparoscopic sleeve gastrectomy and Roux-en-Y gastric bypass. Ann Surg. 2013;258(5):690–5.
91. Patti MG, Allaix ME, Fisichella M. Analysis of the causes of failed antireflux surgery and the principles of treatment a review. JAMA Surg. 2015;150(6):585–90.
92. Li P, Fu P, Chen J, Wang LH, Wang DR. Laparoscopic Roux-en-Y gastric bypass vs. laparoscopic sleeve gastrectomy for morbid obesity and diabetes mellitus: a meta-analysis of sixteen recent studies. Hepatogastroenterology. 2013;60(121):132–7.
93. Pedersen JB, Laresen JF, Drewes Am, Arveschoug A, Kroustrup JP, Gregersen H. Weight loss after gastric banding is associated with pouch pressure and not pouch emptying rate. Obes Surg. 2009;19(7):850–5.
94. De Jong JR, van Ramshorst B, Gooszen HG, Smout AJ, Tiel-Van Buul MM. Weight loss after laparoscopic adjustable gastric banding is not caused by altered gastric emptying. Obes Surg. 2009:19(3):287–92.
95. LePage PA, Kwon S, Lord SJ, Lord RV. Esophageal dysmotility after laparoscopic adjustable gastric band surgery. Obes Surg. 2014;24(4):625–30.
96. Anthone GJ, Lord RVN, DeMeester TR, Crookes PF. The duodenal switch operation for the treatment of morbid obesity. Ann Surg. 2003;238(4):618–28.
97. Biertho L, Simon-Hould F, Marceau S, Lebel S, Lescelleur O, Biron S. Current outcomes of laparoscopic duodenal switch. Ann Surg Innov Res. 2016;10(1): doi:10.1186/s13022-016-0024-7.
98. Spaniolas K, Kasten KR, Sippey ME, Pender JR, Chapman WH, Pories WJ. Pulmonary embolism and gastrointestinal leak following bariatric surgery: when do major complications occur? Surg Obes Rel Dis. 2015. doi:10.1016/j.soard.2015.05.003.
99. Eldar SM, Heneghan HM, Brethauser SA, Khwaja HA, Singh M, Rogula T, et al. Laparoscopic bariatric surgery for those with body mass index of 70–125 kg/m^2. Surg Obes Relat Dis. 2012;8(6):736–40.
100. Prachand VN, DaVee RT, Alverdy JC. Duodenal switch provides superior weight loss in the super-obese (BMI > 50 kg/m^2) compared with gastric bypass. Ann Surg. 2006;244(4):611–9.
101. Topart P, Becouarn G, Ritz P. Weight loss is more sustained after biliopancreatic diversion with duodenal switch than Roux-en-Y gastric bypass in super obese patients. Surg Obes Relat Dis. 2013;9(4):526–30.

102. Risstad H, Sevik TT, Engstrom M, Aasheim ET, Fagerland MW, et al. Five-year outcomes after laparoscopic gastric bypass and laparoscopic duodenal switch in patients with body mass index of 50–60: a randomized clinical trial. JAMA Surg. 2015;150(4):352–61.
103. Ikramuddin S, Blackstone RP, Brancatisano A, et al. Effect of reversible intermittent intra-abdominal vagal nerve blockade on morbid obesity: the recharge randomized clinical trial. JAMA. 2014;312(9):915–22.
104. Ponce J, Woodman G, Swain J, Wilson E, English W, Ikramuddin S, et al. The REDUCE pivotal trial: a prospective, randomized controlled pivotal trail of a dual intragastric balloon for the treatment of obesity. Surg Obes Relat Dis. 2015;11:874–81.
105. Still CD, Wood GC, Chu X, Erdman R, Manney CH, Benotti PN, et al. High allelic burden of four obesity SNP's is associated with poorer weight loss outcomes following gastric bypass surgery. Obesity. 2011. doi:10.1038/oby.2011.3.
106. Adams TD, Davidson LE, Litwin SE, Kolotkin RL, LaMonte MJ, Pendleton RC, et al. Health benefits of gastric bypass surgery after 6 years. JAMA. 2012;308(11):1122–31.
107. Sjostrom L. Review of the key results from the Swedish Obese Subjects (SOS) trial—a prospective controlled intervention study of bariatric surgery. J Intern Med. 2013;273:219–34.
108. Rodrigues GK, Resende CM, Durso DF, Rodrigues LA, Silva JL, Reis RC, et al. A single FTO gene variant rs9939609 is associated with body weight evolution in a multiethnic extremely obese population that underwent bariatric surgery. Nutrition. 2015;31(11–12):1344–50.
109. Hatoum IJ, Stylopoulos N, Vanhoose AM, Boyd KL, Yin DP, Ellacott KL, et al. Melanocortin-4 receptor signaling is required for weight loss after gastric bypass surgery. J Clin Endocrinol Metab. 2012;97(6):E1023–31.
110. Mirshahi UL, Still CK, Mirshahi T. The MC4R (I251L) Allele is associated with better metabolic status and more weight loss after gastric bypass surgery. J Clin Endocinol Metab. 2011;96(12):E2088–96.
111. Elkhenini HF, New JP, Syed AA. Five-year outcome of bariatric surgery in a patient with Melanocortin-4 receptor mutation. Clin Obes. 2014;4(2):121–4.
112. Pellitero S, Perez-Romero N, Martinez E, Granada ML, Moreno P, Balibrea JM, et al. Baseline circulating ghrelin does not predict weight regain neither maintenance of weight loss after gastric bypass at long term. Am J Surg. 2015;210(2):340–4.
113. Gloy VL, Briel M, Bhatt DL, Kashyap SR, Schauer PR, Mingrone G, et al. Bariatric surgery versus non-surgical treatment for obesity: a systematic review and meta-analysis of randomized controlled trials. BMJ. 2013;347:I5934.
114. Colquitt JL, Pickett K, Loveman E, Frampton GK. Surgery for weight loss in adults. Cochrane Database Syst Rev. 2014;8. doi:10.1002/14651858.CD003641.pub4.
115. Coupaye M, Castel B, Sami O, Tuyeras G, Mskia S, Ledoux S. Comparison of the incidence of cholelithiasis after sleeve gastrectomy and Roux-en-Y gastric bypass in obese patients: a prospective study. Surg Obes Relat Dis. 2015;11:779–84.
116. Tsirline VB, Keilani ZM, Djouzi EL, Phillips RC, Kuwada TS, Gersin K, Simms C, Stefanidis D. How frequently and when do patients undergo cholecystectomy after bariatric surgery? Surg Obes Relat Dis. 2014;10(2):313–21.
117. Worni M, Guller U, Shah A, Gandhi M, Shah J, Rajgor D, et al. Cholecystectomy concomitant with laparoscopic gastric bypass: a trend analysis of the nationwide inpatient sample from 2001 to 2008. Obes Surg. 2012;22(2):220–9.
118. Wudel LJ, Wright JK, Debelak JP, Allos TM, Shry Y, Chapman WC. Prevention of gallstone formation in morbidly obese patients undergoing rapid weight loss: results of a randomized controlled pilot study. J Surg Res. 2002;102(1):50–6.
119. Adams LB, Chang C, Pope J, Kim Y, Liu P, Yates A. Randomized, prospective comparison of Ursodeoxycholic acid for the prevention of gallstones after sleeve gastrectomy. Obes Surg. 2015. doi:10.1007/s11695-015-1858-5.
120. Blackstone RP, Cortes MC. Metabolic acuity score: effect of major complications after bariatric surgery. Surg Obes Rel Dis. 2010;8(2):274–81.

121. Giusti V, De Lucia V, Calmer JM, Heralef E, Gaillard RC, Burckhardt P, Suter M. Impact of preoperative teaching on surgical option of patients qualifying for bariatric surgery obesity. Obes Surg. 2004;1(4):1241–6.
122. Wee CC, Pratt JS, et al. Best practice updates for informed consent and patient education in weight loss surgery. Obesity. 2009;17(5):885–8.
123. Finks JF, Kole KL, Yenumula PR, English WJ, Krause KR, Carlin AM et al. Predicting risk for serious complications with bariatric surgery: results from the Michigan bariatric surgery collaborative. Ann Surg. 2011;254(4):633–40.
124. Ramanan B, Gupta PK, Gupta H, Fang X, Forse RA. Development and validation of a bariatric surgery mortality risk calculator. J Am Coll Surg. 2012;214(6):892–900.
125. Khanbhai M, Dubb S, Patel A, Ahmed A, Richards T. The prevalence of iron deficiency anaemia in patients undergoing bariatric surgery. Obes Res Clin Pract. 2015;9:45–9.
126. Bal BS, Finelli FC, Shope TR, Koch TR. Nutritional deficiencies after bariatric surgery. Nat Rev Endocrinol. 2012;8:544–56.
127. Gudzune KA, Huizinga MM, Chang H, Asamoah V, Gadgil M, Clark JM. Screening and diagnosis of micronutrient deficiencies before and after bariatric surgery. Obesity. 2013;23(10):1581–9.
128. Devereaux PJ, Sessler DI. Cardiac complications in patients undergoing major noncardiac surgery. N Engl J Med. 2015;373:2258–69.
129. Beattie WS, Abdelnaem E, Wijeysundera DN, Buckley DN. A meta-analyses comparison of preoperative stress echocardiography and nuclear scintigraphy imaging. Anesth Alalg. 2006;102:8–16.
130. Devereaux PJ, Xavier D, Pogue J, Guyatt G, Sigamani A, Garutti I, et al. Characteristics and short-term prognosis of perioperative myocardial infarction in patients undergoing noncardiac surgery: a cohort study. Ann Intern Med. 2011;154:523–8.
131. Rodseth RN, Biccard BM, Le Manach Y, Sessler DI, Lurati Buse GA, et al. The prognostic value of pre-operative and post-operative B-type natriuretic peptides in patients undergoing noncardiac surgery: B-type natriuretic peptide and N-terminal fragment of pro-B-type natriuretic peptide: a systematic review and individual patients data meta-analysis. J Am Coll Cardiol. 2014;63:170–80.
132. Weber M, Luchner A, Seeberger M, Mueller C, Liebetrau C, Schlitt A, et al. Incremental value of high-sensitive troponin T in addition to the revised cardiac index for peri-operative risk stratification in non-cardiac surgery. Eur Heart J. 2013;34:853–62.
133. Wijeysundera DN, Duncan D, Nkonde-Price C, et al. Perioperative beta blockade in noncardiac surgery: a systematic review for the 2014 ACC/AHA a guideline on peri-operative cardiovascular evaluation and management of patients undergoing non-cardiac surgery: a report of the American College of Cardiology/American Heart Association task force on practice guidelines. Circulation. 2014;130:2246–64.
134. Christakis NA, Fowler JH. The spread of obesity in a large social network over 32 Years. N Engl J Med. 2007;357(4):370–9.
135. The Diagnostic and Statistical manual of Mental Disorders. DSM-5. 5th ed. American Psychiatric Association (APA); 2013.
136. Bhatti JA, et al. Self-harm emergencies after bariatric surgery a population-based cohort study. JAMA. 2015; doi:10.1001/Jamasurg.2015.3414.
137. Blackstone RP, et al. Psychological classification as a communication and management tool in obese patients undergoing bariatric surgery. Surg Obes Relat Dis. 2010;6:274–81.
138. Schlick A, Wagner SA, Muhlhaus B, et al. Agreement between clinical evaluation and structured clinical interviews (SCID for DSM-IV) in morbidly obese pre-bariatric surgery patients. Psychother Psychosom Med Psychol. 2010;60:469–73.
139. Spanjersberg WR, Reurings J, Keus F, van Laarhoven CJ. Fast track surgery versus conventional recovery strategies for colorectal surgery. Cochrane Database Syst Rev. 2011;(2) DC007635.

140. Lemanu DP, Singh PP, Berridge K, Burr M, Birch C, Babor R, et al. Randomized clinical trial of enhanced recovery versus standard care after laparoscopic sleeve gastrectomy. Br J Surg. 2013;100(4):482–9.
141. Awad H, Carter S, Purkayastha S, Hakky S, Moorthy K, Cousins J, Ahmed AR. Enhanced recovery after bariatric surgery (ERABS): clinical outcomes from a tertiary referral bariatric centre. Obes Surg. 2014;24:753–8.
142. Edmiston CE, Lee CJ, Krepel CJ, Spencer M, Leaper D, Brown KR, et al. Evidence for a standardized preadmission showering regimen to achieve maximal antiseptic skin surface concentrations of chlorhexidine gluconate, 4 % in surgical patients. JAMA Surg. 2015;150(11):1027–33.
143. Bartlett MA, Mauck KF, Daniels PR. Prevention of venous thromboembolism in patients undergoing bariatric surgery. Vasc Health Risk Manage. 2015;11:461–77.
144. Quidley AM, Bland CM, Bookstaver PB, Kuper K. Perioperative management of bariatric surgery patients. Am J Health Syst Pharm. 2014;71(15):1253–64.

Chapter 12
Population Health Management of Obesity

Key Message

Obesity is a foundational and systemic disease that underlies most chronic illness in the modern world. The projected cost of American healthcare has been projected to be over $4 trillion by 2017, with 50 % of the costs assigned to "preventable" disease, including heart disease and diabetes [1]. This chapter proposes a whole new paradigm: *patients, health care providers and the public must shift from treating obesity as an individual's choice, to accepting obesity as a chronic disease that is best managed by early recognition, education and treatment.* The three principles of the new paradigm are: Recognition, Education, and Engagement. Implementing a systematic population management strategy for early recognition, education and treatment of overweight and obesity throughout the healthcare system will lower costs, positively effect health outcomes, and improve value in healthcare. Understandably, this is no easy task; a global collaborative effort is required. Patients, health care providers, the public at large, and community leaders in government all must first better understand the science of overweight and obesity, and then be willing to participate in a population management strategy to ensure success of the vision. The paradigm is simple, but its effect would be profound: we can significantly curb, even perhaps cure, obesity and its related diseases if we universally understand, recognize and manage overweight and obesity from its inception in an individual.

Learning Objectives

1. Understand a systematic management system that can be implemented on a local, national, and ultimately global level to identify and treat obesity and obesity-related disease within the population.
2. Discuss the measurement of value and how it applies within the new proposed obesity paradigm.
3. Discuss the public health policies that would likely result in a decrease in obesity in a given population.

The projected cost of American healthcare has been projected to be over $4 trillion by 2017, with 50 % of the costs assigned to "preventable" disease, including heart disease and diabetes [1]. Obesity ranks third, behind smoking and armed violence, in social burdens generated by human beings. It accounts for 2.8 % of the global gross domestic product. The financial cost of obesity to society is obviously very high. An even higher price is being paid when a propensity for obesity is passed onto future generations, sapping their health, their productivity, and their self-esteem. Obesity is associated with related disease including cancer, heart disease, type 2 diabetes, musculoskeletal disease requiring joint replacement, and other chronic illnesses [2]. This association drives the cost of obesity even higher.

Scientific understanding and innovation of disease is continually evolving. Unfortunately, the value of new scientific findings and innovation is ineffective if providers on the front lines continue to deliver care without incorporating the new knowledge into their treatment paradigms [3]. Against the backdrop of busy practices and busy lives, many providers of first line care continue to base therapy on old paradigms. When providers have outdated knowledge or lack knowledge, their treatment paradigms may be impacted by their own bias and strongly held beliefs. This is especially true in managing obesity.

The prevailing belief among healthcare workers, administrators, and the public is that obesity is simply a "calorie in-calorie out" problem exacerbated by a lack of exercise and/or a lack of discipline, compliance or motivation. Simply because a person *ought* to lose weight does not create a moral imperative that they *can* lose weight [4]. The judgment visited on people with obesity is often harsh and unforgiving, and can even provoke anger expressed as verbal or physical abuse. When moral boundaries are crossed, blame is assigned to the person who "could" but "chooses" not to lose weight. Indeed, in some provider's eyes, the only time it is not our moral obligation to do what we ought to do is when it is outside our ability to do so. We have explored this notion in the context of obesity at length within the pages of this textbook. Although some degree of weight control is "chosen" by the patient, the now know that the physiology of obesity, once entrenched, is challenging to reprogram or change. The question is how do we challenge outdated paradigms? How do we communicate the latest science of the disease of obesity and begin to bridge the lack of understanding and prejudice that is too often imposed upon patients with obesity who cannot "self control" their weight?

Multiple stakeholders have launched valiant efforts across the country and around the world to try and bring attention to the deepening crisis of obesity. Public policy is often viewed as the solution. At times the data indicates these efforts are making progress and that risks of obesity are declining [5]. Those positive reports, however, seem to be countermanded by newer reports, such as the 2015 Gallup Well-Being Poll, which indicates that the 2015 U.S. obesity rate set a new record high at 28 % [6].

It is time to take an organized strategic approach to containing and diminishing the disease of obesity [7]. The ideal setting in which to do this is through an integrated healthcare delivery system that will impact large segments of population. Hospitals and health care systems throughout the U.S. and the world must utilize their resources to create powerful partnerships around obesity

Barriers

Accurate Measurement of Obesity Is Essential

Population management of obesity begins with *accurate measurements* of the level of obesity of each individual patient within the population. Currently, all measurement of obesity in the population we are treating *is an estimate* either from self-reported data or from survey data extrapolated to the population. We do not currently have actionable data that arises in our own sphere of influence, such as our clinics, hospitals, and healthcare systems. Without this "actionable data" type of measurement, our clinics, hospitals, and health care systems are reluctant to implement an engaged and systematic care process of management because the cost is unknown. Paradoxically, it is these smaller subunits of influence that can be significantly impacted in a positive way by a comprehensive and systematic process.

Humans have developed a culture of obesity worldwide. This culture is becoming hard wired by the transition of physiology from lean to obese through epigenetic modifications, and these modifications are being passed down to subsequent generations. If the goal is to completely reverse the obesity epidemic and thereby improve the related diseases that accompany it, then we must seek the tipping point where the tide can be turned. This goal first requires a clear understanding of the scientific truth about obesity, not out-dated assumptions about obesity that are rooted in myth or prejudice. A coordinated population management strategy must then be developed and implemented universally by practitioners, payers, healthcare systems, and patients in a strategy that is scalable. The goal must be to bring an end to obesity.

Politicizing Obesity Prevents Action

The issue of obesity is often politicized, with one side placing blame and claiming that obesity is the responsibility of the individual, while the other side wants to implement expensive public policy changes on a large scale to impact the consumer without their awareness. In the context of obesity, this polarization serves only to stymie effective solutions and perpetuate the status quo. Obesity has become urgent not only because of individual health concerns but because obesity and its related diseases affect so many people. Obesity is becoming increasingly expensive for any business, government or patient to manage. According to official estimates Medicare and Medicaid accounted for 20 % and 16 %, respectively, of health care spending in 2014 [8]. Some estimates put the total healthcare expenditure by government at 66 % [9]. Government covers a disproportional share of the aged, disadvantaged, or minorities, which are the groups most affected by obesity. Coverage of obesity by government payers is estimated at $91.6 billion a year and has become an important driver of Medicare and Medicaid spending [10]. Politicians need to understand the truth about obesity. When politics keeps us from reaching effective solutions it penalizes not only the people with obesity but also taxpayers in general.

Prevention Versus Recognition and Treatment of Existing Disease

Obesity is often the target of interventions designed as "prevention". Prevention is always a goal, but focusing only on prevention fails to address the health of the 66 % of people who are already overweight and obese. It also fails to account for the fact that obese parents are passing on epigenetic changes in regulatory DNA that hardwire the physiology of metabolism, giving the offspring a strong predisposition to obesity early in life. In this regard, treating parents who are obese is arguably the most effective prevention of obesity in future generations.

Best practice for population management of obesity requires that all health care providers first recognize obesity as a chronic disease, and then make sure every patient's level of obesity is accurately measured and specifically addressed as part of any health care visit. When obesity is thought of as a "preventable" condition instead of as a chronic disease, physicians often fail to deal with the issue directly. In this way, obesity is treated completely differently than any other disease. Try to imagine a woman getting a mammogram that shows a BIRADS 4 breast mass and the physician not engaging the patient directly in a discussion of the problem or urging a secure plan for treatment! Do we fail to discuss other dangerous medical problems in a patient the way we fail to discuss a patient's obesity? Yet time and again the person with overweight or obesity comes to the office for treatment of obesity-related disease, yet the issue of obesity itself is not discussed. Patients routinely progress from overweight to obesity without recognition of the problem by their primary providers. Moreover, many health care providers fail to recognize that the FOUNDATION of the patient's entire poor health status is built on the pathology of obesity. The patient faces the slippery slope of increasing disability with no warning or help.

In this textbook, there is a demonstration that ineffective and lack of treatment of obesity is too often based on faulty scientific understanding of the disease and the unwillingness of many health care providers to give up their individual bias. Changing the paradigm to an understanding that obesity is a chronic disease is a major shift that brings obesity into view as a medical problem that is treatable. It also opens the door to a systematic approach that begins at the curative stages of overweight (BMI 25–30 kg/m^2) and provides a progressive process of intensifying treatment as patients cross into higher risk categories of disease.

The Epidemic of Obesity Is a Social Disease

Obesity is contagious. Not in the sense that there is a specific bacteria or virus that is passed from person to person, but in the context of a social phenomena. The Framingham Heart Study provides proof of this phenomenon. A comprehensive mapping of the social networks of the participants or "egos" in the Framingham Heart Study was made on the "egos" and their closely associated family and friends over a 32-year period, from 1971 to 2003. This resulted in a densely interconnected network of 12,067 people [11] (Figure 12.1). Each of these people's BMI was assessed repeatedly over this time. The "alters" were people connected with the ego in multiple layers of separation: the first alter knew the ego directly, the second alter was related to the first alter, etc. If the ego became obese during the study interval, the first alter had a 57 % chance of becoming obese, and the second alter had a 20 % chance of becoming obese. If one sibling became obese the other sibling had a 40 % chance of becoming obese. If one spouse became obese there was a 37 % chance the other spouse would become obese. These statistics were not attributed to geographical location, smoking cessation, or other phenomena. In terms of obesity, this study found there were three degrees of separation in terms of an increased likelihood that a person (i.e., an alter) associated with the primary "ego" or participant in the study would become obese if the ego himself became obese over that period of time. Likewise the next person (alter) in the "network" was also affected, but to a lesser degree. The fourth degree of separation showed no affect. The effect was determined to go both ways: if the ego became obese, the alters did, too; but if the ego lost weight, the alters lost weight, too. Thus, the influence among patients with obesity and a few of their close friends and family would seem to extend to three degrees of separation. Earlier in this textbook, we made the case that epigenetics contributes to hardwiring the physiology of obesity in individuals. Now there is evidence that social environments are part of the phenomena [12]. Leveraging the "social network" approach to help tip the obesity epidemic in a curative direction may be very effective in certain groups, especially adolescents and young adults.

A New Paradigm: Management of Obesity, not Acceptance of Obesity

Obesity is nothing short of an epidemic. We need to change acceptance of obesity into effective management of obesity [13]. To do so, we have to restructure the context of managing obesity within the population by implementing a far-reaching strategic plan. Once we accept the concept that managing obesity truly matters, then specific interventions and efforts in the environment can change everything: it can tip the point of obesity. There are tipping points of obesity in the context of both individual patient management as well as general healthcare system management. It

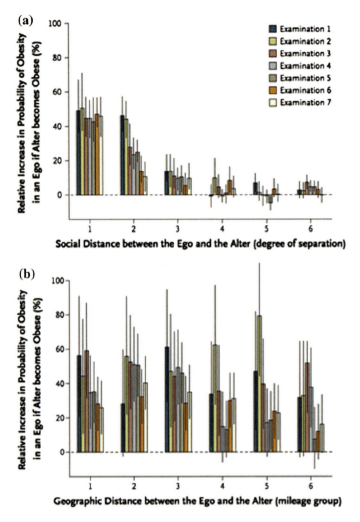

Fig. 12.1 Effect of social and geographic distance from obese alters on the probability of an ego's obesity in the social network of the Framingham heart study (from Christakis and Fowler [11], with permission)

starts with a new paradigm and the use of three principles to tip the population back to better health.

The three principles in the new paradigm are: Recognition, Education, and Engagement. The cornerstone of each principle is outcome measurements. The paradigm is scalable and cost effective. Many leaders in this field support this approach [14].

Recognition

Measure Every Patient, Every Time

The foundation of effective medical treatment is in making the correct diagnosis. The first step in establishing a system of care is to recognize obesity as a foundational problem for the patient and to communicate with the patient about it. Physicians see patients in the office or in the hospital but we often fail to focus on excess weight as a component of the patient's health; therefore the patients fail to do so, too. Thus, the first step of a system of care would be *accurate measurement* of the population.Recognition of obesity as a treatable disease must occur not only in the health care practitioner but also in the patient who may be in denial both about his/her weight and the medical problems that are related to it.

The new paradigm proposes that in *every* portal through which patients flow into the healthcare system *every patient's* weight-related health indicators are *measured* [15]. In some health care settings measurements of weight are currently being done, but height is not routinely being measured. We are taking patients' word for their height and that often results in an inaccurate measurement of BMI. In addition, failing to include the other key components of waist circumference and body fat prevents patients from understanding their level of obesity and the factors that are contributing to their poor health. Recent lay press data report that the BMI in up to 30 % of the population is misleading, leading to miscategorizing people as either normal weight or merely overweight, thus BMI alone is not enough [16]. Medical assistants and other personnel assigned to take specific measurements may lack the knowledge of how to do a proper measurement and the understanding of why it is important to be consistent. They may also not be given enough time to do the necessary measurements properly. These measurements need to become an automatic part of taking a patient's vital signs and the measurements should be incorporated in every patient visit and every hospital admission, every time patients are seen.

The challenge of accomplishing this goal of routinely measuring and recording weight-related health indicators (WRHI) as a normal part of every encounter will require a change in the culture of many clinics/practices. Strategies to help patients feel less defensive even before they come for a visit may be helpful, perhaps by notifying them in advance that this is part of the normal process in the office.

One way to start making this change is to ask every medical student and resident, when they present a patient to their senior mentor, to include BMI in the description of the patient. Inserting BMI, e.g., "This is Cheryl, a 45 year old woman with a BMI of 50 and three days of abdominal pain …" will change the context of the story of that individual patient and allow the whole group of people caring for the patient, as well as the patient herself to "recognize" the patient's medical problems in the context of obesity when warranted. As this becomes the normal way to communicate, attending physicians will also begin to adopt this standard verbal reporting format.

Communicate Level of Risk to Each Patient

The next step in recognition, however, is equally crucial: informing the patient about risk based upon the measurements, so that it fosters a discussion about how weight impacts health. *This step of mutual recognition on behalf of the patient and the provider is essential for change.* Giving the patient a Health Report Card at each and every visit, based on weight-related indicators (WRHI) coded for risk—i.e., red card meaning high risk, orange card meaning moderate risk, yellow card meaning caution, and green card meaning little or no risk—may be just the small nudge the physician and patient need to engage on the topic. Remember, when it comes to epidemics, little changes have big effects. This one change in context immediately transforms the disease of obesity from unseen to seen, from ignored to acknowledged, and from dismissed to discussed—all a major advancement.

There are some providers and groups that may disagree that using objective measured evidence to start the discussion of obesity is best. A more oblique approach to the problem simply preserves the current paradigm of obesity remaining unseen, ignored and dismissed. Indeed, in diagnosing any traditional disease, objectively measured evidence of the disease (i.e., mammograms, blood tests, scans, reflex response, eye pressure, etc.) is usually one of the first things to be accomplished. Similarly, objective measured evidence of a patient's weight is intended to put the conversation about obesity outside of bias, and allow the disease to be medically recognized and discussed. Perhaps most importantly, it puts the patient's weight into the context of the patient's risk to be sick. As with any new recommendation, the requirements of this new paradigm will no doubt be met with some measure of controversy and resistance [17]. Every physician, regardless of discipline, benefits from using objective measurements, especially if measuring conveys a higher risk group that changes treatment approach or compensation for care.

By ensuring that *every* patient is measured and the results communicated you move from an environment where obesity is unseen, ignored and/or stigmatized to one where it is normal to discuss weight as a routine medical issue. It also allows all parts of the system to have real measurements of the population they are treating. This in and of itself is worth the very minimal investment that is made in implementing this simple idea. Recognition and the communication about risk is the first step and can be implemented widely in a short period of time by all healthcare systems and providers.

The approach of using a Weight-Related Health Report Card presented in Chap. 2 (i.e., red, orange, yellow, and green cards) provides a gross measure of risk. It would be effective to use that card as a starting point to also engage patients about their personalized genetic and epigenetic attributes and their physical signs, if any, of early cardiovascular risk. Building a genetic databank linked to a clinical registry may further allow researchers to leverage the knowledge they have gleaned from the databank to benefit all people in finding more effective population-based solutions [18].

Education

Education about what is actually true about obesity and what is myth must be communicated at many levels: to the public at large (both those affected and those not affected by obesity), to patient populations, to individual patients, and to healthcare providers and staff members within the healthcare system. Lack of knowledge drives much of the stigma and discrimination against obesity and is a major barrier to effective care.

Educating *current* students in all health care fields is crucial. Very few medical schools have implemented "obesity" curriculums, and there is often a disjointed approach to teaching about obesity. A systematic approach would require schools to implement a mandatory obesity science didactic curriculum, and experiential training. Obesity curriculum and training should be mandatory in all medical schools, nursing and physician assistants schools, schools that specialize in educating nurse practitioners, registered dieticians and exercise specialists, as well as schools of public health and business administration for the healthcare environment. Mandatory curriculum and training about obesity should be implemented as soon as possible with hard deadlines established by certifying bodies in medicine. Most formal tests in medicine, regardless of discipline, should include questions about patients with obesity both in general, or at a minimum, as it relates to the discipline.

What about currently practicing providers? The immediate educational problem is that most currently practicing front line responders to chronic disease have received little or no education in obesity. Fortunately, we do not have to start from scratch. Education of providers has begun in earnest over the last ten years through the leadership of the Obesity Society, the American Society for Bariatric Physicians, and the American Society for Metabolic and Bariatric Surgery. These groups have organized an effort to provide a board certification in obesity medicine: the American Board of Obesity Medicine for physicians. Similar efforts have been taking place in nursing with the certification of bariatric nurses and registered dieticians. The effort to achieve a baseline fund of knowledge could be accelerated if healthcare systems were to require that each person who works within the system has core training in obesity. Online resources are already available and therefore extremely inexpensive to implement for the population of providers of care [19].

Education of patients takes place in two domains. The first domain is in providing a baseline of education to the public at large. It is essential that we educate the public, both those affected by obesity and, perhaps as importantly, those that are not. Almost every focus group or large-scale survey shows that people are confused about obesity and have little idea where to start in trying to achieve significant change. The inertia of confusion keeps many from taking specific steps. A combination of education around the true science of obesity and what is effective treatment, coupled with consistent personal feedback, has been shown to have impact on the disease. Didactic educational segments could be provided in a series of online education modules or taught to the public within the healthcare system. In addition, patients who consistently use a personal health monitor and provide documentation of calories and exercise could likewise be rewarded. While these ideas all fit into the current paradigm of treatment, leveraging social context and making obesity education "the thing to do" is what will provide a general leaning toward better health. Leveraging education in this manner, if mounted on multiple fronts, could have a major positive effect similar to the efforts and campaign to stop public smoking.

Perhaps the single most important innovation in patient care we can undertake is to clearly communicate risk categories to patients by giving them a visual clue of where they fall in regards to risk by using the Health Report Card. Patients in yellow, orange, and red categories could be encouraged to engage in a series of live or online education sessions that would provide them an accurate basis to understand their obesity. This is roughly the same education as the provider has and so both groups are coming together to engage in the achievement of better health from the same playbook.

The second domain of education for the public relates to a given individual's own risk for disease or disease progression. At this time, we have just the beginning of knowledge of the fundamental genetic and epigenetic science of obesity. We do not know in a given individual how their "obesity" exactly works. We can begin with a survey of information that may give us a better idea of the relative ease or resistance they will have to treatment based on their history. Questions such as whether their mother, father, or siblings are affected by obesity may give us an idea of actual inheritance of core genes. Questions about whether the mother had gestational diabetes or Type 2 diabetes at the time of the patient's gestation can also provide information, but these are crude measures which may or may not be affecting the person before us. The most pertinent information we need is about the patient's current epigenetics, interactome, and microbiome (these are defined and discussed in the Chapter on Biology). The social context of a patient's obesity may also be a driver of continuing obesity or a cause of recurrence or weight regain.

In the context of an epidemic, there are many agents of change. Certain people may be programmed metabolically to make it more likely that they will become big or be diabetic. As they get bigger they also undergo epigenetic changes in the expression of obesity genes that hard wire their physiology into place. The environment then becomes the accelerating factor in this scenario. There is a "stickiness factor" in the resulting set point of obesity in any individual. A major factor in educating the patient is to try and gain some knowledge and educate them about their own genetics. Measuring their genetic and epigenetic risk can be done through currently available technology.

Engagement

Engagement occurs at every level where traditional "treatment" would have occurred. Since the new paradigm for treatment of obesity encompasses a broader definition that includes social context, it applies equally well to individual patient care as well as to community health in general.

The most highly valued currency in healthcare is ongoing engagement of the provider with the patient as a team in addressing the patient's health. It is an allegory for engaging a person's own immune system to fight disease. The capacity for humans to understand and use the power of an emotional connection to change their own health is unlimited. This is the key intervention that should be our focus in solving the problem of obesity.

How to achieve engagement? First, the provider must be willing to engage and have accurate knowledge of the subject. Second, we must leverage the patient's personal stake in the disease of obesity. People who are big know they are big. They live with the inertia of obesity on a daily basis and it saps a good deal of their energy. They make effort after effort to solve the problem, unguided by their health care team. It is an expensive battle in every way expense can be measured. Leveraging the patient's emotion will engage them, because a person who is big takes it very seriously.

What is an individual's tipping point into unacceptably poor health? In other words, at what point does a particular body weight make the patient feel sick, unable to move, have pain? This is akin to asking: what is the "addiction" threshold for an individual patient? When you engage them in a discussion around this they will often be able to tell you.

Busy practices produce busy providers. It is often difficult for the provider of care, who is sitting in the exam room concentrating on putting data into the electronic medical record, to engage on a deep level with anyone, much less a person who is in the office for a cough and cold and who offers the physician a red Weight-Related Health Report Card and says, "What's up, Doc?" The new obesity paradigm proposes that at that moment, the physician needs to lay aside their electronics, engage with the patient and say very clearly, "That red Weight-Related Health Report Card means that although you are here today for your chest congestion, the main health problem you have is that you are carrying too much weight. Let's make an appointment to work on that together.' The more the message is sent, the more it will get through.

Keys to Personal Engagement

The keys to personal engagement are: to engage the patient emotionally in the battle and make sure they know that you are with them in that battle, to see the patient often, to establish a community of social support, and to personalize the approach.

The first step is to construct a system of care that engages the patient often, at least monthly, once an actionable level of obesity is recognized. A structured approach in this context teaches the patient in small bites. The principles of weight management can be delivered by someone other than a physician with less medical training but who is excellent at communicating. It is a given, based on our current knowledge and ability to treat obesity, that the physiology of obesity is likely to cause the patient to regain weight. Once that fact is acknowledged, both provider and patient recognize they are engaged in a battle with a chronic disease. Preparing a person for the specific journey of weight loss and remission avoids frustration for both parties when the inevitable weight regain happens and it helps avoid a negative treatment paradigm. There is evidence that weight loss, even if patients regain part of that weight, is valuable for the legacy effect it has.

The second key to engagement is to help the patient to engage socially and create a community of support that enables them to become comfortable with their process and effort. Education again can form the foundation of this engagement but it might extend to creating group activities that are safe for the patient to engage in. There are many outlets and creative ways this can be accomplished that might utilize social media and the digital community.

The third key to engagement is to utilize technology such as genetic testing, and to correlate that information with clinical data to build specific and personalized approaches, and to test what works for each given person.

Finally, in order to switch from engagement on an individual basis to engagement of the social network of obesity, we need to create groups of influence. Some data shows that a group not larger than about one hundred and fifty people is ideal to impact any given process. Engagement of social networks of disease intersects with biologic networks of disease to influence their course. This could be especially important in achieving obesity recognition and engagement in groups of people who traditionally have strong family cultures and are among the most affected groups of individuals. These groups of influence can create the kind of peer pressure within social networks that will make it impossible for a conciously healthy mother or father to bring cupcakes and soft drinks to school or to games or for teachers or coaches to allow it. Development of networks of groups of influence encourages responsibility and leadership at every level where obesity is managed (Figure 12.2).

Risk Groups in the New Paradigm

Weight-Related Health Indicators (WRHI) will provide four risk groups. Patients in the healthy range of BMI (green card) will require very little to no support on an ongoing basis from the system. They may be the victims of random events, but they rarely have chronic disease.

The focus of the healthcare system and the new paradigm for population management of obesity begins with the BMI Group defined as the "overweight"

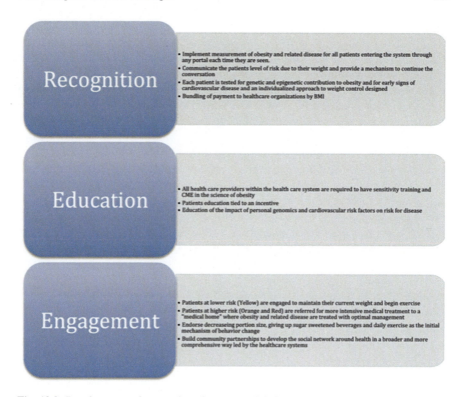

Fig. 12.2 Development of networks of groups of influence encourages responsibility and leadership at every level where obesity is managed

category (BMI 27.0–29.9 kg/m^2) indicating moderate risk (yellow Health Report Card moderated by waist circumference and body fat percentage). It is in this early stage of obesity that fatty liver is established and leptin levels due to high body fat percentage influence cardiac function. In this key group, genetics and cardiovascular disease markers may help to sort out who is actually beginning to get sick based on their level of obesity. It is in this group where the physiology of obesity is not that well established that engagement becomes crucial. Patients in this BMI group usually come in for annual checkups, asthma, cold or flu visits. By leveraging a visit to the clinic to measure obesity and to communicate risk of additional weight gain to the patient allows the provider of care the opportunity to engage and work with the patient to effectuate the immediate loss of the 15–20 lb that will return the patient closer to a BMI of 25–27 (ideal). In this way, *the secondary layering of epigenetic change onto any inherited genetic tendency to obesity may be avoided*. In addition, weight loss has the legacy effect of staving off obesity-related disease, even if the patient regains the weight. These patients should participate in education and ongoing monitoring to convey urgency to the patient that getting that 15–20 lb off is important and needs to happen immediately. This education and monitoring can be inexpensively provided through the online "Fundamentals of

Weight" course, by the patient getting and using a fitness device for monitoring, and by the patient coming in for monthly checkups while they realign their eating and exercise habits to keep their weight in check. Overweight persons are more prone to becoming obese without education and monitoring.

Patients identified in the second orange risk category (orange Health Report Card—which includes patients in the traditional BMI group of 30–39.9 moderated by waist circumference and body fat percentage) need to engage in more intensive obesity management. This could be a part of the primary clinical setting or this could be referred out to a commercial weight loss program or to specialized clinics situated strategically within the healthcare organization to manage all patients with BMI of 30 or greater. The number of clinics needed will depend on the actual burden of the various BMI categories within the system. This is an illustration of how measurement of obesity within the system is important to the successful implementation of a strategic population management plan. Evidence has shown that 8 h of education in a primary care clinic can implement effective weight loss [20].

When patients are already at a high level of risk (red Health Report Card—which includes BMI 40.0 and greater moderated by waist circumference and body fat percentage) at the time of recognition and communication, the healthcare system could invest in and/or provide centralized treatment centers with special expertise that can offer more intensive medical management, including the use and monitoring of pharmaceuticals, devices, and surgery. A recent algorithm for this stepped-up approach to care was published in the 2016 Guideline of the American Board of Obesity Medicine [21]. This paradigm of providing increasing expertise for increasing levels of disease is well understood in medicine.

Measuring Value

The world has focused on healthcare as an increasing part of the gross domestic product of countries. The rising expenditure of health care costs has become even more concerning with the aging of the population. In the United States, health care as a portion of GDP increased between 1950 (4.4 %) and 2011 (17.9 %), but remained relatively flat until 2015, when initial repercussions of the Accountable Care Act (ACA) were realized and costs increased [22]. The increase of healthcare as a percent of GDP has driven serious changes within the health care system, with the most profound change still in the process of evolving: a conversion to a system of care that reflects value. Value in health care is defined as better health outcomes delivered at lower cost [23]. Delivery of value through quality improvement is most successful when physicians are encouraged to modify the intervention to fit their local context [24]. Implementation of any system will require measurement that relates clinical quality and allows for the calculation of cost. Currently, many hospital systems are using either Cerner or Epic electronic health records. Designing and implementing an "obesity module" will allow investigators to align genetic information to disease and treatment outcomes in a big data context. This kind of real world obesity registry data will allow us to understand and track the elements that are necessary to allow more effective engagement.

Our goal is to contain the current level of obesity and begin to reverse the epidemic in a way that conveys value to the patient and the healthcare system and helps prevent the epigenetic transfer of obesity-promoting physiology to children. Policies and programs that are implemented will change the health determinant of interest in this case, decreasing weight and particularly abdominal obesity, in order to achieve optimal health outcomes by reducing obesity-related disease (i.e., lowering blood glucose, blood pressure, and cholesterol). A strong business case can be made for this investment [25].

Michael Porter and Robert Kaplan have proposed moving to a widespread bundled payment system where disease management is the focus and the entire spectrum of care is included [26]. Because obesity is not accounted for in the Chapters of Disease Model of Health Care Financing that is widely used in healthcare, obesity treatment is not included. Unfortunately, the failure to include obesity in the approach to chronic disease treatment dooms all treatment approaches. For example, if a person is being treated for diabetes and achieves better control with medications but goes on to require additional treatment of secondary complications due to obesity, is that of "value" to the individual or to the system? An alternative proposal would be to bundle care of persons by BMI categories and include all their care for the many diseases that they have. BMI are well-established risk categories with known associated disease. So a person with a BMI of 40 and higher risk would have included all their necessary care for diabetes, heart disease or sleep apnea. In order to design an appropriate bundle there are 4 components to be considered: (1) whether the bundle covers care for a medical condition, not for a procedure or treatment episode; (2) whether the bundle is contingent on risk adjusted outcomes; (3) whether payment is based on the cost of efficient and effective care, not what was charged in the past; and (4) whether there are specific limits of responsibility for unrelated care needs and catastrophic events [26].

Bundling by BMI would have numerous effects. First, the "root cause" medical condition for the majority of metabolic disease would be at the heart of treatment. Second, it would provide financial incentive for healthcare systems to embrace the measurement aspects of the strategic plan for the population management of obesity. Third, it would align the incentives of the health care systems, providers, employers, and patients to focus on weight reduction and would provide meaningful effectiveness in every tier of outcomes.

In establishing a systematic approach to obesity within a healthcare system, measurements of cost using a time-driven activity-based costing approach could be charted. [27]. In addition to the actual cost of treatment, the value to patients as measured by improved quality of life assessment and patient experience of care, and tertiary prevention or treatment of related disease, could be improved. A coalition could be assembled to test cost and to implement a pilot program for this simple scalable plan.

Population Health and Public Policy

The focus of medicine has traditionally been on "mopping up the floor" after disease has already occurred. The focus of population health management is squarely on "turning off the tap" or prevention of disease. The United States has fallen behind its peer countries in health improvement despite having the largest per capita health expenditure of all industrialized nations. Leading risk factors for poor health include obesity and many factors related to it, including high blood pressure, high fasting glucose, and physical inactivity. Almost 50 % of the U.S. health burden is for morbidity and chronic disability [28]. Public reactions to health campaigns, specifically around obesity, are burdened by the stigma and public perception of obesity as self-controlled [29]. There are significant barriers to using public policy to implement a population health solution in obesity [30]. In addition, there is pessimism about the ability of intervention to have an impact on obesity [31].

Population health is defined as the health outcomes of a group of individuals, including the distribution of such outcomes within the group. For the purpose of this approach the population is defined as the overweight and obese individuals in a specific sphere of influence. In order to impact population health we have to create interventions that work in individuals on the local level—i.e., in their own health care systems.

Technological innovation, specifically through the use of a personal wearable mobile health platform, is one way to impact obesity. The only disconnect is that it is rarely tied to any type of personal intervention and therefore loses some of its impact. However, as part of a comprehensive strategy and way to create networks of influence, it may be extremely useful [32]. The emergence and popularity of wearable personal mobile health monitors gives an example of how the creation of unique partnerships between industry and individuals may benefit the management of obesity. Another intervention called Health Schools Programs, implemented in California, shows that education and obesity prevention in school-aged kids can be part of a comprehensive solution [33].

"Population Health" is often criticized as being overly broad with no individual person taking responsibility for the achievement of better health. Physicians, administrators of health systems, public policy administrators, and advocacy groups often have too narrow a focus to make a difference in the larger goal. In the context of obesity, all individuals regardless of their level of responsibility, including the patient, should act within their circle of influence to implement a common strategy. Whatever a person's role is—as the leader of their own family, church or social group, the director of a clinic, the CEO of a healthcare system or a public state or national official—they must come together to define and support a common strategy that is simple to implement. Public policy is often a substitute when individual interventions have failed. However, in the treatment of obesity, the medical system has never had a serious, organized strategic intervention, nor do we know the relative cost of such an intervention, the cost of prevention, or the cost of a worsening of the disease.

The Institute of Medicine's vision in the landmark publication, "The Future of the Public's Health in the 21st Century," includes six recommendations that provide an ideal setting for tackling the chronic disease of obesity [34]. It is reasonable to expect that the surgeon general could lead a serious and effective national strategy to stop the epidemic of obesity. An effective strategy around obesity would have major impact on the well-being of our citizens and on the economics of the country. Clinical care is important to the individual but may not be enough. Engagement of a wider and broader coalition of partners, including nontraditional ones in business and government, may be required to address obesity [35].

What will make a difference from a public policy prospective? In the executive summary from the McKinsey Global Institute, an analysis of interventions designed to address obesity being attempted elsewhere in the world found that no single solution was sufficient to reverse the obesity trend. The answer to the crisis would require a systematic and comprehensive program of multiple interventions. Education alone was not sufficient, but almost all interventions were cost effective [25].

We do know that some public policy interventions have been successful. One major public health victory was the decision by the Federal Food and Drug Administration in 2015 to remove artificial trans fats from processed food over a three-year period [36, 37]. What about future public policy interventions? Many believe that the two most well documented strategies that could be implemented on a population basis to address obesity are portion control and decreasing the consumption of sugar-sweetened beverages [38]. From a public policy standpoint efforts to regulate sugar in beverages have been met with stern resistance from companies that make them. Yet now the message of the harm those beverages cause is beginning to be entrenched in public conversations and personal conscience, and companies are responding to the change in preferences.

Public policy interventions also may have ethical implications that should be taken into account, as interventions at this level often require a substantial investment of resources. Ethical implications include singling out individuals based on weight; impinging on autonomy, unintended negative effects, and contributing to harm in some people while benefiting others [39]. Solutions that are market-driven will be more palatable to industry.

The most powerful public policy solution may be through education. If persons affected by obesity understood that when they drink a sugar-sweetened beverage it changes their ability to metabolize carbohydrates, would they make a different choice? Perhaps they would. They would likely share that information with others within their social network. The tipping point of the obesity epidemic will be best reached by changing the public mindset through personal engagement of people seeking advice about their weight and health from those they trust. This scenario can then be further leveraged within the context of a social network or through groups of influence [40].

Hopefully, some people who read this textbook will begin to implement the principles outlined. Early adaptors and innovators in each healthcare system will begin to work toward implementing the strategy adjusted for their local situation. Jumping the chasm will be that early minority of people willing to move forward with this new paradigm. It will require specific people that act as the translators, connectors, mavens, and sales people of the strategy. These early adopters will hopefully start to move the needle in implementing a strategic population management plan to contain and overcome obesity as a disease. The late majority will only be convinced when early measurements of improved outcomes, decreased costs and improved health are demonstrated [13].

Conclusion

Obesity is an epidemic. The current fractured approach to obesity is unacceptable and has not achieved the goal of containing or reversing the epidemic. We must contain the current level of obesity and begin to reverse the epidemic by changing acceptance of obesity into effective management of obesity. To do this, we have to implement a far-reaching strategic population plan that starts with a new paradigm. The new paradigm proposes that, in every portal through which patients flow into the healthcare system, every patient's weight-related health indicators are measured, recorded and communicated to the patient. This new paradigm's emphasis on the use of recognition, education, and engagement in the fight against obesity allows it to be both scalable and cost effective. Implementing an effective population management strategy with all the players' support offers our best hope of significantly reducing, even perhaps curing, obesity and its related disease.

References

1. Gallup. http://www.gallup.com/poll/183155/obeisty-rate-lowest-hawaii-highest-mississippi.aspx.
2. Sturm R, Ruopeng A. Obesity and economic environments. CA: A Cancer Journal for Clinicians. 2014;64(5):337–50.
3. Keown OP, Parston G, Patel H, Rennie F, Saoud F, Kuwari HA, Darzi A. Lessons from eight countries on diffusing innovation in health care. Health Aff. 2014;33(9):1516–22.
4. Stern R. Does, "ought" imply "can"? and did kant think it does? Utilitas. 2004;6(1):42–61.
5. Mehta T, Fontaine KR, Keith SW, Bangalore SS, de los Campos G, Bartolucci A, Pajewski NM, Allison DB. Obesity and mortality: are the risks declining? Evidence from multiple prospective studies in the United States. Obes Rev. 2014;15(8):619–29.
6. Gallup well-being poll: U.S. obesity rate climbs to record high in 2015 at 28.0 %. Washington, DC. 15 Feb 2016.
7. Cecchini M, Sassi F. Preventing obesity in the USA: impact on health service utilization and costs. Pharmacoeconomics. 2015;33(7):765–76.

8. https://www.cms.gov/research-statistics-data-and-systems/statistics-trends-and-reports/nationalhealthexpenddata/downloads/highlights.pdf.
9. Pianin E. How the obesity epidemic drains medicare and medicaid. Fisc Times. 2014. http://www.thefiscaltimes.com/2014/12/15/How-Obesity-Epidemic-Drains-Medicare-and-Medicaid.
10. Trogdon JG, Finkelstein EA, Feagan CW, Cohen JW. State- and payer-specific estimates of annual medical expenditures attributable to obesity. Obesity (Silver Spring). 2012;20(1):214–20.
11. Christakis NA, Fowler JH. The spread of obesity in a large social network over 32 years. N Engl J Med. 2007;357(4):70–379.
12. Warin M, Moore V, Davies M, Ulijaszek S. Epigentics and obesity: the reproduction of habitus through intracellular and social environments. Body Soc. 2015. doi:10.1177/1357034X15590485.
13. Gladwell M. The tipping point: how little things can make a big difference. Boston: Little, Brown; 2000.
14. Dietz WH, Baur LA, Hall K, Puhl RM, Taverns EM, Usury R, Copeland P. Management of obesity: improvement of health-care training and systems for prevention and care. Obesity series: paper #5 published online February 18, 2015. doi:10.1016/S0140-6736(14):61748-7.
15. Jensen MD, Ryan HD. New obesity guidelines promise and potential. JAMA. 2014;311(1):23–4.
16. Brody JE. Weight index doesn't tell the whole truth. NY Times, 30 Aug 2010.
17. Gee KA. School-based body mass index screening and parental notification in late adolescence: evidence from Arkansas's act 1220. J Adolesc Health. 2015;57(3):270–6.
18. Wang C, Gordon ES, Stack CB, Liu C, Korunas T, Wewak L, et al. A randomized trail of the clinical utility of genetic testing for obesity: design and implementation considerations. Clin Trials. 2014;11(1):102–13.
19. Melin I, Alstrom B, Berglund L, Samir M, Rossner S. Education and supervision of health care professionals to initiate, implement and improve management of obesity. Patient Educ Couns. 2005;58:127–36.
20. Ryan DH, Johnson WD, Myers VH, Prather TL, McGlone MM, Rood J, et al. Nonsurgical weight loss for extreme obesity in primary care settings: results of the Louisiana obese subjects study. Arch Intern Med. 2010;170(2):146–54.
21. Guidelines certified diplomat, American board of obesity medicine. http://obesitymedicine.org/obesity-algorithm/.
22. Fuchs VR. The gross domestic product and health care spending. New Engl J Med. 2013;369:107–9.
23. Porter ME, Teisberg E. What is the value in health care? New Engl J Med. 2010;363:2477–81.
24. Dixon M. Developing an ex post theory of a quality improvement program. Milbank. 2011;89:167–205.
25. Dobbs R, Sawers C, Thompson F, Manyika J, Woetzel J, Child P, McKenna S, Spatharou A. Overcoming obesity: an initial economic analysis. Discussion paper, McKinsey Global Institute; 2014.
26. Porter ME, Kaplan RS. How should we pay for health care? Working paper published on line in harvard business school number 15-041. 27 Dec 2014.
27. Kaplan R. Improving value with TDABC. Healthc Financ Manag. 2014. http://www.hgma.org/Content.aspx?id=22957.
28. US Burden of Disease Collaborators. The state of US health, 1990–2010: burden of disease, injuries, and risk factors. JAMA. 2013;310(6):591–608.
29. Puhl R, Luedicke J, Peterson JL. Public reactions to obesity-related health campaigns. Am J Prev Med. 2013;45(1):36–48.
30. Barry CL, Brescoll VL, Brownell KD, Schlesinger M. Obesity metaphors: how beliefs about the causes of obesity affect support for public policy. Milbank Q. 2009;87:7–47.
31. Callahan D. Obesity-chasing an elusive epidemic. Hasting Cent Rep. 2013;43(1):34–40.
32. Hamida ST, Hamida EB, Ahmed B. A new mHealth communication framework for use in wearable WBAN's and mobile technologies. Sensors. 2015;15:3379–408.

33. Madsen KA, Cotterman C, Crawford P, Stevelos J, Archibald A. Effect of the health schools program on prevalence of overweight and obesity in California schools, 2006–2012. Prev Chronic Dis. 2015;12:150020. doi:10.5888/pcd12.150020.
34. http://iom.nationalacademies.org/Reports/2002/The-Future-of-the-Publics-Health-in-the-21st-Century.aspx.
35. Isham GJ, Zimmerman DJ, Kindig DA, Hornseth GW. Healthpartners adopts community business model to deepen focus on nonclinical factors of health outcomes. Health Aff. 2013;32(8):1446–52.
36. http://www.fda.gov/ForConsumers/ConsumerUpdates/ucm372915.htm.
37. Brownell KD, Pomeranz JL. The trans-fat ban-food regulation and long-term health. N Engl J Med. 2014;370(19):1773–5.
38. Niederdeppe J, Robert SA, Kindig DA. Qualitative research about attributions, narratives, and support for obesity policy, 2008. Prev Chronic Dis. 2011;8(2). http://www.cdc.gov/pcd/issues/2011/mar/10_0067.htm.
39. Azevedo SM, Vartanian LR. Ethical issues for public health approaches to obesity. Curr Obes Rep. doi:10.1007/s13679-015-0166-7.
40. Krinsman W. A simple model for BMI change in a social network. NURJ Online 2014–15. http://www.thenurj.com/a-simple-model-for-bmi-change-in-a-social-network/.

Index

Note: Page numbers followed by *f* and *t* indicate figures and tables, respectively

A
Adipocytes, 69, 109, 111
Adipokines, 83
   Adiponectin
      anti-inflammatory adipokines, 79
      pro-inflammatory adipokines, 78
   cancer promotion, 112, 113*t*
   leptin
      discovery of, 77
      levels of, 77
      resistance, 78
Adipose tissue
   Adipokines, *see* Adipokines
   chronic low-grade inflammation of, 90
   development of, 68–69
   energy storage and endocrine signaling, 68
   lipogenesis and lipolysis, 72–73
   structure of
      BAT, 69
      blood flow and innervation, 71–72
      BRITE cells, 70–71
      ECM, 71
      fat cells, types of, 69
      macrophages, 71
      WAT, 69, 70
   tipping point, 73
   WAT, hypoxia and inflammation in
      apoptosis, 76
      Cori cycle activity, 74, 75*f*
      HIF1, 74
      lactate production, 75
Adiposity rebound (AR), 137
AdipQ, 113
Adjustable gastric band (AGB), 161, 261, 275*f*
Adult obesity, 5
Adolescent obesity, 133, 134
   bariatric surgery in, 159
   effects of, 4
   PCOS, 145
Adrenocorticotropic hormone (ACTH), 125
Adult patient
   health history
      allergies, 216*t*, 216
      circadian patterns, 202–204
      dietary history, 199–200
      disordered sleep analysis, 202–203
      lifestyle and family culture, 203–204
      medications, 196
      obesity and related disease, family history of, 195
      obesity-related disease, *see* Obesity-related disease
      occupational factors, 203
      physical activity, 204
      psychosocial and psychiatric history, 216
      ROS, 218
      stress factors, 199–200
      surgical history, 217*t*, 216
      weight gain and loss, historical survey of, 196
   metabolic factors, *see* Metabolic factors
Affordable Care Act, 19
Alcohol
   caloric content of, 177
   causative role, 177, 178

major detoxification of, 176
Alpha-linolenic acid, 178
American Association of Clinical
  Endocrinologists, 264
American Medical Association (AMA), 28
American Diabetes Association, 18
American Heart Association, 264
American Society of Clinical Oncology
  (ASCO), 17
American Society of Metabolic and Bariatric
  Surgery (ASMBS), 261, 263
ANS. *See* Autonomic nervous system (ANS)
Antidepressant drugs, 236, 237*t*
Anti-diabetes drugs, 237, 238*t*
Antipsychotic medication, 236, 236*t*
Antiseizure drugs, 237, 237*t*
Antiviral drugs, 236, 238*t*
Anxiety, 184
Apnea–hypopnea index (AHI), 126
Apoptosis, 76
APLN, 113
ASCO. *See* American Society of Clinical
  Oncology (ASCO)
Asian populations, 14
  BMI of 25 is defined as obes, 14
Asthma, 109, 119
  risk factor, 141
Atrial fibrillation (AF), 101–102
Autonomic nervous system (ANS), 60, 62, 63, 268

B
Baby Boomers, 7
Bariatric population, mental health in
  food addiction
    self-control, lack of, 185
    YFAS, 185, 187–188*t*
  psychiatric disorders, 184
Bariatric surgery, 133, 257, 261
  indications/contraindications for
    indications, 264
    nonsurgical therapy, risk of, 264–265
    patient factors, 265–266
    nutrients, postoperative testing of, 296*t*
    psychiatric and psychological disorders, 293
Basal metabolic rate (BMR), 180
BAT. *See* Brown adipose tissue (BAT)
Beckwith–Weiderman syndrome (BWS), 138
Behavioral Risk Factor Surveillance System
  (BRFSS), 16
Bioelectrical impedance analysis (BIA), 225

Biology of weight, 41
BMR. *See* Basal metabolic rate (BMR)
Body adiposity index (BAI), 11–13
Body composition analysis
  bioelectrical impedance scale, 225
  DEXA, 225
  hydrostatic weighing, 225
  MRI, 225
Body Fat Percent, 10
  impedance scale, 10
  pacemakers, 11
  skinfold thickness, 10
  water displacement, 10
Body mass index (BMI), 2*t*, 5, 9, 11–13
  adolphe quetelet, 12
  ancel keys, 12
  risk of deep venous thrombosis and
    pulmonary embolus with, 120, 120*t*
Brain
  body set point, defense of, 48, 48*f*
  GBA
    chemical sensors, 58
    cognitive function and glucose-related
      signaling, 60
    eating, function of, 57
    ghrelin, 58
    GLP-1, 59
    hormone signals, 57
    insulin, 59–60
    microbiome and microbiota, 55–57
    neuroanatomy, 48–49
    nutrient sensing, 47*f*
BMI for Age/Z Score, 10, 133
  BMI-For-Age chart, 15
Breast cancer, 109
  BMI, 114
  breast cancer stem cell, 109
  IL-6, 115
  leptin, 115
  stem cell signaling, 115
  WHI trial, 114
Brown adipose tissue (BAT), 69
B-type natriuretic peptide (BNP), 290
BWS. *See* Beckwith–Weiderman syndrome
  (BWS)
Bundled payment system, 321

C
Calorie, 41, 46–47
Cancer stem cell, 109, 115
Carbohydrates, 171–174
  digestion and absorption, 173*f*

Cardiovascular disease (CVD), 99, 146–147
Cardiovascular drugs, 238*t*
Cell death, 76
Central nervous system (CNS), 60
　antiobesity drug targets outside, 243*f*
　drugs for, 239
　and metabolic disease, 62*f*
Centers for Medicare and Medicaid Services (CMS), 264
Cephalic phase, 58
Changes in energy expenditure, 270
Changes in reward pathways, 269
Chemotherapy drugs, 238*t*
Child and Adolescent Obesity, 4
　Asian, 4
　black children, 4
　Caucasian children, 4
　Hispanic children, 4
　multiracial, 4
　native american, 4
　pacific islander, 4
Childhood obesity, 1, 133
　biobehavioral susceptibility model of, 152–153
　clinical assessment of
　　fasting glucose tests, 152
　　nutritional assessment, 151
　　physical exam, 150, 150*t*
　clinical consequences of
　　disordered sleep, 141
　　endocrine disorders in, *see* Endocrine disorders
　　gastrointestinal problems in, 142
　　respiratory problems in, 141
　effects of, 4
　evaluation of, 139*t*
　genetic influence
　　BMI, 137
　　epigenetic changes, 135–136
　　LGA and SGA, 136
　　thrifty gene, 135
　inheritable physiology, 5
　prevalence of, 4, 134
　rates of, 134
　treatment recommendations for
　　comprehensive multidisciplinary program, 156–157
　　prevention plus, 154–155
　　structured weight management, 156
　　tertiary care, 157–161
　　weight loss goals, 153, 154
　types of
　　common, 137
　　non-syndromic, 138–139
　　syndromic, 138
Chronic kidney disease (CKD), 99
Circadian rhythm, 109
Cirrhosis, 95
Cleveland clinic, 25
Clinically severe obesity, 2
CNS. *See* Central nervous system (CNS)
Colorectal cancer, 109, 112
30 day complications, 262
Common obesity, 133
Coronary heart disease (CHD), 2, 17, 101
C-reactive protein (CRP), 90, 118
Creutzfeldt-Jakob disease (CJD), 199
Cushing's disease, 145
Cytokines, 112

D

Deep vein thrombosis (DVT), 120
Dehydration, 158
Delos "Toby" Cosgrove, 25
Depression, 184
Developmental origins of health and disease, 56
DEXA. *See* Dual energy X-ray absorptiometry (DEXA)
Diabetes, 83, 103, 207*t*
　gestational diabetes, 91
　T2DM, 209, 210. *See also* Type 2 diabetes mellitus (T2DM)
Diabetic cardiomyopathy (DCM), 103
Diagnostic tests for obesity-related disease, 225
Dietary fat, 72, 175
Dietary fiber, 17
Dietary reference intakes (DRIs), 179
Diet-induced thermogenesis (DIT), 180
Direct costs, 17
　diagnostic tests, 17
　drugs, 17
　inpatient services, 17
　insurance, 17
　outpatient service, 17
Disability-adjusted life years (DALY), 3
　DALY, 3
Discrimination, 23
Distribution of body fat, 11
　Heritable trait, 11
Double helix, 50–51
DS. *See* Duodenal switch (DS)
Drosophila, 52
Dual energy X-ray absorptiometry (DEXA), 147, 225
Duodenal switch (DS)
　complications of, 283
　description of, 283

Duodenal switch (DS) (cont.)
    outcomes of, 284
    safety of, 283
DVT. See Deep vein thrombosis (DVT)
Dysbiosis, 112

E
Early adiposity rebound, 133, 137
Edmonton obesity staging system (EOSS), 14
Education, 315–317
EKG changes in a patient with obesity, 194
Electrocardiograms (EKG), 227–228
ENCODE, 54
End stage renal disease (ESRD), 99
Endocrine disease, 109
    infertility, 118
    PCOS, 117
    thyroid hormones, 116–117
Endocrine disorders
    cardiovascular disease, 146–147
    depression, 147–148
    hypothyroidism, 145
    IIH, 145–146
    insulin resistance and type 2 diabetes, 142–143
    metabolic syndrome in, 143–144
    obesity-related disease, 205–207
    orthopedic disorders, 147
    primary Cushing disease, 145
    stigma and discrimination, 147
Endothelial cell, 88
Endothelial dysfunction, 83, 101
Energy expenditure
    BMR, 180
    components, 180
    TEF, 180–181
    thermogenesis
        NEAT, 181
        physical activity, lack of, 181
        skeletal muscle, 182
Enhanced recovery after metabolic and bariatric surgery, 294
Enteroplasticity, 267
Enteric nervous system (ENS), 63
Epigenetic changes, 267
Epigenetics, 133
ESRD. See End stage renal disease (ESRD)
Explicit attitudes, 26
Extreme obesity, 2

F
Fat, 175
Fat phobia scale, 26

Fatty acids, 178
Federal food and drug administration (FDA), 262
Fenfluramine/phentermine (Fen-phen), 241
Fetal programming, 45
Fetal metabolic programming, 52
Fibrosis, 95
Food
    calories and kilocalories, 170
    digestion, 168–169
    eating, recommended mechanics of, 169–170
    energy expenditure
        BMR, 180
        components, 180
        TEF, 180–181
        thermogenesis, 181–183
    food labels, 179–180
    macronutrients
        alcohol/caffeine and sweetened beverages, 175–178
        carbohydrates, 171–174
        dietary fiber, 17
        DRI, 179
        fat, 175
        fatty acids, 178
        protein, 170–171
        vitamins and minerals, 178–179
        water, 175
    micronutrients, DRI for, 179
    reward system, 269
Food addiction
    self-control, lack of, 185
    YFAS, 185, 187–188t
Food and drug administration (FDA), 179
Food culture, 152
Fruit flies, 52
Fuel, 167

G
Gastric balloon (GB), 261, 284–286
Gastric bypass, 261
Gastric bypass surgery, 275–277
Gastroesophageal reflux disease (GERD), 142, 279
Gastrointestinal (GI) tract, 168
GBA. See Gut brain axis (GBA)
Genetic obesity, 4, 5
Gender, 7
Gene, 41
Genetic obesity, 1
Genetic reset™, 3
Genetic resetting, 2

Index

double helix-human genome, 50–51
epigenetic modification, 51
genetic network, 54–55
imprinting, 51
intergenerational metabolic programming, 51–54
Gestational diabetes, 91
Ghrelin, 41
Gila River Pima Indians, 41
Glucagon-like peptide-1 (GLP-1), 59
Glycemic index (GI), 174
Glycemic load (GL), 174
Gut brain axis (GBA), 55
   chemical sensors, 58
   cognitive function and glucose-related signaling, 60
   eating, function of, 57
   ghrelin, 58
   GLP-1, 59
   hormone signals, 57
   insulin, 59–60
   microbiome and microbiota, 55–57

H

Harassment, 23
HbA1c, 225
Head, eyes, ears, nose and throat (HEENT), 220
Healthcare communication, 23
Health care costs, 1
Healthcare environment, 23
Healthcare systems and obesity, 307
Health indicator, 1
Health maintenance after metabolic and bariatric surgery, 296
Health report card, 320
Heart failure, 83, 102–103
Helicobacter pylori, 27, 278
Historical perspective of weight loss medications, 239
Homologous desensitization, 89
Hormone, 41
Human chorionic gonadotropin (HCG), 198
Human genome, 50
Human genome project (HGP), 54
Human growth hormone (HGH), 198
Human microbiome project (HMP), 55
Hydrostatic weighing, 225
Hyperinsulinemia, 85
Hypertension, 2
Hypnotic drugs, 237*t*
Hypothalamic–pituitary–adrenal (HPA), 125
Hypothyroid, 109, 117

I

Idiopathic intracranial hypertension (IIH), 109, 121, 215
   evaluation for, 145
   presentation and demographics of, 146
IL-6, 118
IL-6. *See* Interleukin 6 (IL-6)
Impaired fasting glucose (IFG), 90
Impaired glucose tolerance (IGT), 90
Imprinting, 41, 51, 133, 136
Implicit association test, 26
Incidence, 3
Index of central obesity (ICO), 94
Indirect costs, 17
   absenteeism, 17
   death, 17
   disability pension costs, 17
   loss of productivity, 17
   premature disability, 17
Infertility, 109, 118, 215
Insulin, 41
Insulin resistance (IR), 83, 84
   basic functions, 85
   cardiovascular disease, highest risk of, 86
   glucose, 84
   HOMA-IR model, 86–87
   hyperinsulinemia, 85
   IFG and IGT, 90–91
   inflammation and, 90
   mechanisms of
      genetic association, 87–88
      molecular association, 88–90
   prediabetes, 91
Insulin, 59–60
Interactome networks in human disease, 54
Intergenerational metabolic programming, 51
Interleukin 6 (IL-6), 112, 115, 124, 125
International obesity task force (IOTF), 15
Intestinal dysbiosis, 112
IR. *See* Insulin resistance (IR)

J

Joint pain, 203

K

Korsakoff's syndrome, 220
Key message, 1

L

Laparoscopic adjustable gastric band (LAGB), 279
   complications of, 281
   description of, 280

Laparoscopic adjustable gastric band (LAGB) (*cont.*)
  mechanism of action of, 280–281
  outcomes of, 282–283
  safety of, 281
Laparoscopic Roux-en Y gastric bypass (LRYGB), 272
  complications of, 274–275
  description of, 273
  gastric bypass surgery, benefit of, 275–276
  safety of, 273
Laparoscopic sleeve gastrectomy (LSG), 277
  complications of, 278–279
  description of, 278
  outcomes, 279
  safety of, 278
Laparoscopic vertical sleeve gastrectomy (LVSG), 268
Laurence–Moon (Bardet–Biedl) syndrome (LMBBS), 138
Learning objectives, 2
Leptin, 109
  breast cancer, 115
  discovery of, 77
  levels of, 77
  resistance, 78
Linoleic acid, 178
Lipid panel, 226
Lipopolysaccharide (LPS), 97
Liraglutide (Saxenda)
  clinical evidence, 247
  contraindications, 240
  description, 249
  metabolism, 250
  safety warnings for, 250, 254
  side effects, 254
Liver function tests, 227
Long chain fatty acids, 72
Lorcaserin (Belviq)
  clinical evidence, 247–248
  description, 246
  dosage, 247
  drug, metabolism of, 246
  safety warnings, 247–248
  side effects, 249
LRYGB. *See* Laparoscopic Roux-en Y gastric bypass (LRYGB)

M
M1 Macrophage, 90, 113
Magnetic resonance imaging (MRI), 225
Mechanism of action metabolic and bariatric surgery, 266
  epigenetic changes, 267

Medical expenditure panel survey MEPS, 32
Medicaid, 19
Medicare, 18
Medical devices, 262
  Adjustable gastric band (AGB), 262
  Gastric balloon (GB), 262
Medications that cause weight gain, 236
  Anti-diabetes drugs, 238
  Antidepressant drugs, 237
  Antipsychotic drugs, 236
  Antiseizure drugs, 237
  Antiviral and chemotherapy drugs, 238
  Cardiovascular drugs, 238
  Hypnotic drugs, 237
  Migraine drugs, 237
  Steroid medications, 238
Melanocortin 4 receptor (MC4R), 42, 134
Mental health disorders, 292
Metabolic and bariatric surgery (MBS)
  cholecystectomy, 287
  enhanced recovery protocols
    perioperative, 290
    postoperative, 290
    preoperative prehabilitation, 295
  health maintenance, 296
  mechanism of action
    energy expenditure, changes in, 270
    enteroplasticity, 266–268
    epigenetic changes, 266
    procedures, 262
    reward pathways, 269
  national accreditation in, 259
  prehabilitation
    domains, 288
    education and informed consent, 289
    social and psychological health assessment, 287–292
    surgery, physical assessment for, 287–290
  procedures and devices, 271
    DS, 282–284
    GB and vagal blocking device, 283–284
    LAGB, 278–281
    LRGBP, 272–277
    LSG, 276–278
  weight regain, 285
Metabolic disease, 69
Metabolic disruptors, 57
Metabolic factors
  body composition analysis
    bioelectrical impedance scale, 223
    DEXA, 225
    hydrostatic weighing, 225

Index

MRI, 225
RMR, 224-225
Metabolic inflexibility, 85
Metabolic surgery, 261
Metabolic syndrome (MetS), 83, 84
   cardinal features of, 94
   IDF definition, 94t
   multiple definitions of, 93
Metabolically healthy morbidly obese (MHMO), 266
Metformin, 133, 158
Microbiome, 41, 55
   Archaea, 55
   second genome, 55
Microbiota, 55
Microenvironment, 109
Migraine drugs, 236, 237t
Mitochondria, 88
Mitochondrial plasticity, 85
Mobility, 292
Monogenic obesity, 133, 138
Morbid obesity, 1, 232
Motivational interviewing (MI), 23, 33
Motivational Interviewing Techinques, 26
   Development of discrepancy, 33
   Expression of empathy, 33
   Expression of empathy Motivational Interview Treatment Integrity Scale, 33
   Intrinsic motivation, 33
   Rolling with resistance, 33
   Support for self-efficacy, 33
Myokine, 182

N

National Accreditation in Metabolic and Bariatric Surgery, 263
   MBSAQIP, 263
Naltrexone SR/Bupropion SR
   clinical evidence, 255
   contraindications, 255-256
   description, 254
   dosage, 255
   metabolism, 256
   safety warnings, 256
   side effects, 256
National health and nutrition examination survey (NHANES), 14, 15
Nervous system
   CNS and ANS, 60
   ENS, 63
   parasympathetic nervous system, 63
   SNS, 62
National Institutes of Health (NIH), 264

NIH guideline, 264
Native Americans, 7
New York Heart Association functional classification, 14
NF-kB, 112
Non-alcoholic fatty liver disease (NAFLD), 83, 142
   dysbiosis, 95
   LPS, 97
   pathophysiology of, 96f
   prevalence of, 95
Non-alcoholic steatohepatitis (NASH), 95, 209
Non-exercise activity thermogenesis (NEAT), 181
Normal weight, 2
Nutraceuticals, 257
Nutrition, 168

O

O'Odham Pima/River People, 42
Obesity, 1, 2, 23, 261
   Adolescent, see Adolescent obesity
   adult patient, see Adult patient
   baby boomers, 8
   cancer
      adipokines, 112
      breast, 114-115
      cytokines, 112
      diagnosing and treating, challenge of, 116
      dysbiosis, 112
      risk of, 110
      sex hormones, 112
      TAMS, 111
   Childhood, see Childhood obesity
   classification of, 2t
   disordered sleep
      breathing disorders, 123
      circadian phenotype, 123
      circadian rhythm, 122
      insomnia and stress, 125-126
      night owl chronotype, 123
      OSA, 126
      REM, 124
      sleep duration, issue of, 124
      sleep, lack of, 124
   endocrine disease
      infertility, 118
      PCOS, 117
      thyroid hormones, 116-117
   epigenetic signature of, 53f
   gender, 8
   genetic component of, 135
   healthcare costs

future cost, 18
personal cost, 18–19
social cost, 17
the foundation of modern disease, 84
implement, 19
incidence and prevalence, 3
IR, *see* Insulin resistance (IR)
measurement of
   U.S. survey, health status, 15–16
   WRH1, 9–15
medications, use of
   bariatric surgery, 257
   cause weight gain, 236
   patients, medical problems in, 228–230
   weight loss medications, *see* Weight loss medications
mitochondrial stress, 89f
modern disease, foundation of, 84
native Americans, 8
objectives, 1–3
patient, *see* Patient, obesity
pediatric, *see* Pediatric obesity
physical activity, lack of, 27
population health management
   accurate measurements, 309
   defined, 316
   education, 308–310
   engagement, 317
   measuring value, 320–321
   new paradigm, 311
   politicizing obesity prevents action, 309
   prevention, 310
   public policy, 322
   recognition, 307, 312–314
   risk groups, 318–319
   social disease, 311
populations
   adult obesity, 5
   child and adolescent obesity, 4–5
   prevalence, 5, 6f, 7f
pseudotumor cerebrii, 121
pulmonary disease
   abnormalities of, 119
   asthma, 119
   OHS, 119–120
   VTE, 120–121
QALY and DALY, 3
socioeconomic status, 8–9
treatment, medications for
   liraglutide (saxenda), 249–252
   lorcaserin (belviq), 246–248
   naltrexone SR/bupropion SR, 254
   nutraceuticals, 257
   orlistat (xenical, alli), 252
   phentermine, 245–247
   phentermine/topiramate (qnexa, qsymia), 252
Obesity classification, 1
Obesity hyper/hypoventilation syndrome (OHS), 109, 119–120
   main symptoms of, 141
Obesity measurement, 1
Obesity metabolic programming, 133
Obesity paradox, 97–98
Obesity population management, 307
Obesity rates within minority groups and subpopulations, 7
Obesity-related cardiovascular disease
   AF and stroke, 101–102
   atherosclerosis, 101
   CHD, 101
   dyslipidemia, 98–99
   hypertension, 99–100
   obesity paradox, 97–98
Obesity-related disease, 2, 18
   Arthritis, 18
   cancer, 17, 212
   Cardiovascular disease, 17
   CHD, 18
   degenerative joint disease, 29
   diabetes, 17
   endocrine disorders, 213
   gastrointestinal disease, 211
   gastroesophageal reflux, 29
   heart disease, 209
   high cholesterol/lipids, 29, 207
   hypertension, 17, 208
   IIH, 215
   infertility and low testosterone, 215
   IR, 209t, 210
   laboratory test recommendations, 225
   musculoskeletal disease, 207
   NAFLD, 209–211
   Obstructive sleep apnea, 29
   Osteoarthritis, 17
   patients, physical assessment of
      abdomen, 219
      anthropometrics, 219
      body fat distribution, pattern of, 219
      chest and breast exam, 221
      extremities, 222, 223
      general observation, 220
      HEENT, 220
      neurologic, 223
      pelvic and anorectal exam, 223
      skin and trunk, 222
      vital signs, 220
   PCOS, 209–211

Index

pregnancy, 215
pulmonary disease, 211
Sleep apnea, 17
T2DM, 210*t*
Type 2 diabetes, 18
UI, 212
Obesogen, 56, 57
   metabolic disruptors, 57
OB Gene, 113
Obstructive sleep apnea (OSA), 109, 126, 203
Orlistat (Xenical, Alli), 133, 158, 252
Orthopedic disorders, 147
Over-the-counter (OTC) medications, 239, 240
Overweight, 2, 134. *See also* Obesity
Oxidative stress, 88

P

Parasympathetic nervous system, 63
Patient, obesity
   bias
      inability/unwillingness, 28
      negatively affects medical outcomes, 29–30
   black hole, 32
   blame, 27–28
   BMI, 30–31
   cancer, relative risk of, 111, 111*t*
   current healthcare environment
      biological basis, 26–27
      explicit and implicit attitudes, 26
      prejudiced, 25–26
   discrimination, 24–25
   implement
      encourage patients, risk, 36–37
      staff and colleagues, 35–36
      workplace, physical environment of, 37
   MI
      development of discrepancy, 34–35
      expression of empathy, 33–34
      tenets, 33
   perspective, 23–24
   safety, culture of, 25
   WRC system, 31
   WRHI, 30
Pattern of body fat distribution, 219
Patient's perspective, 24
PE. *See* Pulmonary embolus (PE)
Pediatricians, 4
Pediatric obesity
   childhood obesity, *see* Childhood obesity
   differential diagnosis in, 140*t*
   epidemic, scope of, 134–135
   risk factors for, 137*t*
Personal cost of obesity, 18

cost of assistance or adaptations, 19
higher insurance premiums, 19
lost or lower wages due to obesity discrimination, 18
obesity-related disabilities, 19
out-of-pocket costs for medical care, 18
procedures not covered by insurance, 18
Phenotype, 41, 54
Phentermine
   contraindications, 245
   description, 245
   dosage, 245
   metabolism, 246
   safety warning for, 245
   side effects, 246
Phentermine/Topiramate (Qnexa, Qsymia)
   clinical evidence, 253–254
   contraindications, 254
   description, 252
   dosage, 253
   safety warnings, 254
   side effects, 254
Physical function, 288
Physician bias, 27
Pima Bajo, 41
Pima story, 42–43
Polycystic ovarian syndrome (PCOS), 109, 117
   adolescent obesity, 145
   obesity-related disease, 208–209
Population health management of obesity, 307
   education, 315
   engagement, 317
   recognition, 313
      communicate level of risk to each patient, 314
      measure every patient, every time, 313
Positron emission tomography (PET), 125
Prader–Willi, 133
Prader–Willi disease, 138
Pramlintide/Metreleptin, 244
Prebiotic, 231, 257
Prediabetes, 83
Pregnancy risk categories, 242
Preoperative prehabilitation, 295
Presenteeism, 19
Prevalence rates, 2
Primary care physician (PCP), 195
Private insurance, 19
Probiotics, 231, 257
Protein
   amino acids, 171
   defining characteristic of, 170
   enzymes, 170–171
   plant sources, 171

Pseudotumor cerebrii, 109. *See also* Idiopathic intracranial hypertension (IIH)
Psychiatric disorders, 184
Psychosocial disorders, 216
Pulmonary disease, 109
   abnormalities of, 119
   asthma, 119
   history of, 211*t*
   OHS, 119–120
   VTE, 120–121
Pulmonary embolus (PE), 120, 274

Q

Quality-adjusted life year (QALY), 3*f*
   QALY, 3
Quartiles of poverty, 9
   High-income quartile, 9
   poor income quartile, 9

R

Randomized controlled trials (RCT), 178
Rapid eye movement (REM), 124
Reactive oxygen species (ROS), 88
Redux. *See* Fenfluramine/phentermine (Fen-phen)
Renal function tests, 227
Resting metabolic rate (RMR), 224–225
RETN, 113
Review of systems (ROS), 218
Roux-en-y gastric bypass (RYBP), 161

S

Satiety hormone. *See* Leptin
Sensitivity training, 26
Short chain fatty acids, 72
Sleep disorders
   breathing disorders, 123
   circadian phenotype, 123
   circadian rhythm, 122
   insomnia and stress, 125–126
   night owl chronotype, 123
   OSA, 126
   REM, 124
   sleep duration, issue of, 124
   sleep, lack of, 124
Sleep-disordered breathing (SDB), 122
Sleeve gastrectomy, vertical (VSG), 161, 261, 276, 277*f*
Social cost, 17
Social disease, 311
   Framingham Heart Study, 311
Socioeconomic status, 9
Social network, 311
Steroid medications, 236, 238*t*
Stigma, 23
Stroke, 83, 101–102
SuVar, 52
Sympathetic nervous system (SNS), 41, 62
Synbiotics, 231, 257
Syndromic obesity, 133, 138

T

Taste cells, 58
T2DM. *See* Type 2 diabetes mellitus (T2DM)
Tertiary care intervention
   bariatric surgery
      adolescents, 159
      procedures, 159–161
   dehydration, 158
   metformin, 158
Thermal effect of food (TEF), 180–181
Thrifty gene, 135
Thrifty phenotype, 133
Thyroid disease, 116
Thyroid hormones, 109
Thyroid-stimulating hormone (TSH) test, 226
Thyroxine (T4), 116
Tipping point, 41
TNFα, 118
Triiodothyronine (T3), 116
Tumor microenvironment, 115
Type 2 diabetes (T2D), 2, 83
   mitochondrial stress, 89*f*
   remission of, 282
Type 2 diabetes mellitus (T2DM), 41, 42
   fetal programming, 45
   history of, 43
   lose weight, 46
   Pima story
      generations of, 42
      Gila River Pima, 43
   research results
      application of, 45–46
      NIH/NIDDK and PIMA, 43–45
   risk factors for, 143
   unique side effects of, 93
   weight loss, 92
Type I pattern of unexpected hospital death, 234
Type II pattern of unexpected hospital death, 235
Type III pattern of unexpected hospital death, 235

U

Underweight, 2
Unexplained hospital deaths (PUHD), 233
   Arousal failure, 234

Index

Hyperventilation compensated by
    respiratory distress, 233
  progressive unidirectional hypoventilation, 233
Uric acid, 227
Urinary (stress) incontinence (UI), 212
U.S. Internal Revenue Service (IRS), 264

V

Vagal blocking device, 284–286
Vagus nerve, 63
Venous thromboembolic (VTE) disease, 109, 120–121
Visceral adiposity, 219
Vitamin D, 213, 227
VTE prophylaxis, 232

W

Waist circumference, 10
  location of fat distribution, 11
Waist-to-hip ratio, 11
WAT. See White adipose tissue (WAT)
Weight loss medications, 231
  action, mechanism of, 242
  Bupropion SR, 231
  goal of, 241
  historical perspective of
    FDA, 239, 241
    hCG, 241
    OTC medications, 239–240, 241
    unintended consequences of, 239t
  hormone leptin, 244
  Liraglutide, 231
  Lorcaserin, 231
  medical practitioner, 242
  Naltrexone SR, 231
  Nutraceuticals, 231
  Orlistat, 231
  Phentermine, 231
  pregnancy risk categories, 242
  Topiramate, 231

Weight loss, 27
Weight regulation, 41
  education, 288
  T2DM, see Type 2 diabetes mellitus (T2DM)
  Weight related health indicators (WRHI), 30, 219t, 313
    Asian Americans, 13–14
    BMI and BAI, 11–13
    body fat, 10
    children and adolescents, measurements in, 14–15
    criteria, 9
    EOSS, 14
    height and weight, 10
    waist circumference, 11
  Weight Related Health Indicators (WRHI), 2, 30, 318
    BMI, 2
    WRHI, 10
  Weight related report card (WRC), 30, 31
  Weight stigma, 24–25
  Wernicke's encephalopathy (WE), 223
  White adipose tissue (WAT), 68
    hypoxia and inflammation in, 74–76
    structure of, 69, 70
  Women's health initiative (WHI), 114
  WRHI. See Weight related health indicators (WRHI)

X

X chromosome, 52

Y

Yale food addiction scale (YFAS), 185, 187–188t

Z

Z codes, 11, 12
Zinc, 290

Made in the USA
Middletown, DE
09 March 2018